Principles of Anesthesia Equipment

Principles of Anesthesia Equipment

Second Edition

Editors

Archana Areti MD
Associate Professor
Department of Anesthesia, Critical Care and Pain Medicine
KMCH Institute of Health Sciences and Research
Coimbatore, Tamil Nadu, India

Bhavani Shankar Kodali MD
Chief
Department of Obstetric Anesthesiology
University of Maryland Medical Center
Assistant Director
Maryland Anesthesia Simulation, Training and Research
Professor
Department of Anesthesiology
University of Maryland School of Medicine
Washington, USA

Forewords

M Ravishankar
James H Philip

JAYPEE

JAYPEE BROTHERS MEDICAL PUBLISHERS
The Health Sciences Publisher
New Delhi | London

Jaypee Brothers Medical Publishers (P) Ltd

Headquarters
Jaypee Brothers Medical Publishers (P) Ltd
EMCA House, 23/23-B
Ansari Road, Daryaganj
New Delhi 110 002, India
Landline: +91-11-23272143, +91-11-23272703
+91-11-23282021, +91-11-23245672
Email: jaypee@jaypeebrothers.com

Corporate Office
Jaypee Brothers Medical Publishers (P) Ltd
4838/24, Ansari Road, Daryaganj
New Delhi 110 002, India
Phone: +91-11-43574357
Fax: +91-11-43574314
Email: jaypee@jaypeebrothers.com

Overseas Office
JP Medical Ltd.
83, Victoria Street, London
SW1H 0HW (UK)
Phone: +44 20 3170 8910
Fax: +44 (0)20 3008 6180
Email: info@jpmedpub.com

Website: www.jaypeebrothers.com
Website: www.jaypeedigital.com

Inquiries for bulk sales may be solicited at: jaypee@jaypeebrothers.com

Principles of Anesthesia Equipment

First Edition: 2016

Second Edition: **2025**

ISBN: 978-93-6616-045-0

Printed at: Samrat Offset Pvt. Ltd.

Dedicated to

The memory of Professor Phaneendra Nath Thota,
a teacher par excellence.
His inspiration helped us to embark on this project.

Yasodananda K Areti
Bhavani Shankar Kodali

Dedicated to

In loving memory of Dr Yasodananda K Areti, whose wisdom, kindness, and dedication to his work and loved ones continue to inspire. His unwavering compassion and pursuit of knowledge left an indelible mark on all who knew him.

May this book stand as a tribute to his legacy, a reminder of his profound impact, and a reflection of the values he held dear.

Forever cherished, never forgotten.

Archana Areti

In Loving Memory of Dr Yasodananda K Areti

It is a great honor, but a sad moment at the same time, to write this note. Dr Yasodananda K Areti, known popularly as "Yasoda," and I have had a long bond of togetherness since 1971. We joined Jawaharlal Institute of Postgraduate Medical Education & Research (JIPMER) in 1971 for MBBS. After our postgraduation and stint of Senior Residency at JIPMER, we spent almost 10 years in Barbados, the land of all-time great cricketers such as Garfield Sobers, Hall, Griffith, Garner, Greenidge, etc. We were associated with landmark papers on capnography in the mid-80s. My initiative to study clinical applications of capnography and Yasoda's comprehensive critical analysis of the subject led to the publication of a series of papers. Our bond with the commitment to anesthesiology development in Barbados for a decade and our earlier stint at JIPMER were memorable moments in our lives. We were called "Anesthesiology Twins". Even now, many remember our combo. Later, Yasoda became a Professor of Anesthesiology at Queen Elizabeth Hospital, University of West Indies, Barbados Campus. I continued to visit Barbados as an Examiner during his tenure in Barbados. It was indeed a sad moment when Yasoda left me prematurely without warning. I felt I lost a part of my body and mind at that moment.

Dr Yasodananda K Areti has an extraordinary interest in and understanding of Anesthesia Equipment; only a few anesthesiologists have this rare gene. It was his brainchild to write the book on Anesthesia Equipment in a language every anesthesia resident can understand. Dr Yasoda and I fulfilled his ambition, and the book instantly succeeded. Now, Dr Archana Areti, MD, continues her father's legacy in bringing about the book's second edition.

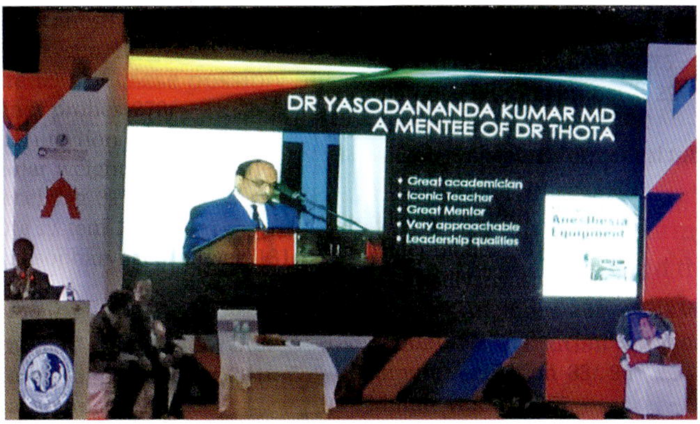
DR YASODANANDA KUMAR MD
A MENTEE OF DR THOTA
• Great academician
• Iconic Teacher
• Great Mentor
• Very approachable
• Leadership qualities

Bhavani Shankar Kodali

A Loving Husband, Father, Teacher, and Friend Dr Yasodananda K Areti

To my dad, whose dream it was to write this book as a comprehensive foundation for the specialty of "Anesthesia." He has always inspired me to strive to be my best and strongest, and I am privileged to continue his legacy of dedication and contribution to our field. He taught me the fundamentals of anesthesia, encouraged me to honor its origins, and instilled in me the highest ethical standards of medical practice. Beyond imparting the knowledge of an anesthesiologist, he served as a role model, demonstrating how to be the best version of oneself.

He also connected me with a legacy of remarkable minds in anesthesia, including Professor Ravishankar, Dr Bhavani Shankar Kodali, Dr Ramkumar Venkateswaran, Professor Hariharan Seetharaman, and Dr N Selvarajan, as well as countless colleagues and friends worldwide who continue to shape my thoughts and help me to grow.

I hope that I will be able to continue his good work in the standards he wished to maintain.

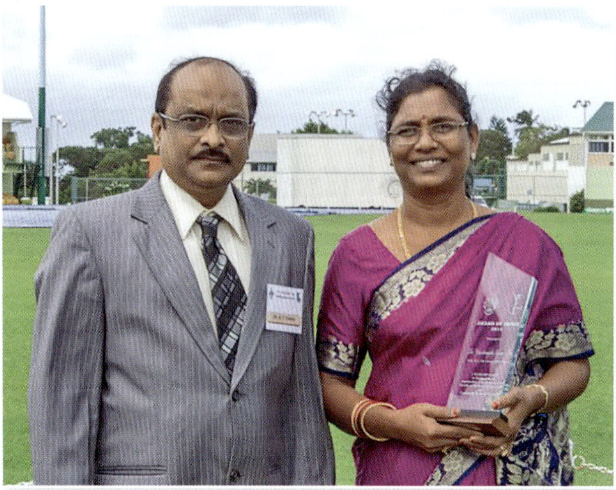

Archana Areti

Contributors

Archana Areti MD
Associate Professor
Department of Anesthesia
Critical Care and Pain Medicine
KMCH Institute of Health Sciences and Research
Coimbatore, Tamil Nadu, India

Yasodananda K Areti MD
Former Professor in Anesthesia
Queen Elizabeth Hospital
University of West Indies
Cave Hill Campus
Barbados, West Indies

TVS Gopal MD
Managing Director
Axon Anaesthesia Associates
Clinical Director
Department of Anaesthesiology
CARE Hospitals
Hyderabad, Telangana, India

Karisha Hinkson-LaCorbinière DM
Associate Lecturer
Faculty of Medical Sciences
The University of the West Indies
Cave Hill Campus
Barbados, West Indies

Ahalya Kodali MD
Instructor of Anesthesia
Washington University School of Medicine
Department of Anesthesiology
St. Louis Children's Hospital
St. Louis, Missouri, USA

Bhavani Shankar Kodali MD
Chief
Department of Obstetric Anesthesiology
University of Maryland Medical Center
Assistant Director
Maryland Anesthesia Simulation, Training and Research
Professor
Department of Anesthesiology
University of Maryland School of Medicine Washington, USA of Maryland School of Medicine
Washington, USA

Akilandeswari Manickam MD
Professor
Department of Anesthesiology
Critical Care and Pain Medicine
Sri Ramachandra University
Chennai, Tamil Nadu, India

Aruna Parameswari MD DNB
Head of Department
Department of Anesthesiology
Critical Care and Pain Medicine
Sri Ramachandra University
Chennai, Tamil Nadu, India

Athma Prasanna MD
Consultant
Anesthesiologist and Pain Specialist
Bengaluru, Karnataka, India

Hariharan Seetharaman MD
Dean of Faculty of Medical Sciences
Professor
Department of Anesthesia and Critical Care
The University of the West Indies
Trinidad and Tobago

Ramkumar Venkateswaran MD
Former Head and Professor
Department of Anesthesiology
Kasturba Medical College
Manipal Academy of Higher Education
Manipal University
Manipal, Karnataka, India

Foreword

For a long time, there was a felt need for a comprehensive book on anesthesia equipment in our continent, written by Indian authors. This is because the standards differ in different countries. Most books on equipment are based on American standards as there are stringent rules prescribed by ASTM (American Society for Testing and Materials, International) to be followed. Moreover, nomenclature differs from one country to another that raises a lot of doubts in the minds of residents. This book has been written predominantly by authors of Indian origin who felt the need for such a book.

The chapters in the book have been logically organized for a better understanding of the subject. Special effort has been taken by the authors to detail the illustrations. The diagram and pictures are laid out to make understanding better. Though it is impossible to cover extensively all the equipment used in anesthesiology, basic principles involved in the design of these equipment are well covered. Most chapters in the book are written by Dr Yasodananda K Areti, whose interest in anesthesia equipment and vision to share the expertise for the benefit of a budding anesthesiologist has resulted in the compilation of this book.

There is a good mix of young as well as experienced anesthesiologists' contribution to the book. It is written in a simple language that makes the reading a pleasure. The chapter on "preuse check of anesthesia equipment" sticks to one practice guideline and clear. The chapter on sterilization is very informative. The chapters on monitoring, neuraxial blocks, and simulation are well illustrated and written.

Overall, the book is a treasure for anesthesiology residents to learn the basics of the equipment used in anesthesia. I hope the book will have acceptance from all quarters.

M Ravishankar DA MD
Director
Department of Center for Digital Resources
Education and Medical Informatics
Emeritus Professor
Department of Anesthesiology
Mahatma Gandhi Medical College
and Research Institute
Sri Balaji Vidyapeeth University
Puducherry, India

Foreword

This book is a treasure trove of facts and detailed information about how things work in anesthesia and the physics, mathematics, and engineering that serve as their basis. Clear and straightforward figures drawn to show basic principles provide great clarity. Simple language effectively teaches both simple and complex concepts. Nomenclature is different in different countries and this book explains their relationships. Adding to Dr Yasodananda K Areti's teaching in developing countries, Dr Bhavani Shankar Kodali's teaching for ventilation monitoring (www.capnography.org; www.capnography.com) based in a well-developed country (USA) for 20 years brings out the latest anesthesia advances.

As I read the book, I found the following to be most striking:

- Chapter 1 on Applied Physics, the relationship of measurement units used in various parts of the world is clearly explained.
- Chapter 3 on Anesthesia Machine or Workstation describes technological progression from the oldest to the newest technical advances and functionalities by major machine manufacturers including EndTidal Control of anesthetic agent on GE Aisys, Draeger Zeus and Maquet FLOW-i in many countries.
- Chapter 5 on Anesthesia Ventilators clearly diagrams and describes modern ventilator capabilities.
- Chapter 7 on Monitoring Technology beautifully describes and diagrams the numerous technologies available.
- Chapter 9 on Electrical Safety, Cautery, and Lasers succinctly and clearly teaches the basic electronics needed by anesthetists in any country.

This book has a great value for anesthetists in all parts of the world. It conveys understanding to those who use the oldest and those who use the newest of the many technologies described.

James H Philip ME (E) MD CCE
Anesthesiologist and Director of Bioengineering
Brigham and Women's Hospital
Professor of Anesthesia
Harvard Medical School
Boston, Massachusetts, USA

Preface to the Second Edition

Anesthesiology is an ever-evolving field, driven by advancements in technology, pharmacology, and clinical practice. A deep understanding of applied physics, equipment, and clinical monitoring is fundamental for safe and effective anesthesia practice. These topics form a significant part of postgraduate education, yet they often pose a challenge due to their complexity.

With this second edition, we continue our effort to present essential principles in a clear and accessible manner. The goal remains to equip anesthesiologists with the knowledge required to use anesthesia equipment safely and interpret monitoring data accurately—both of which are critical for patient safety. We have updated the content to reflect recent developments and improve clarity, ensuring that this resource remains relevant and practical.

We extend our gratitude to all contributors and reviewers who have enriched this edition with their expertise. It is our hope that this book will serve as a valuable guide for postgraduate students and practicing anesthesiologists, fostering confidence in understanding and applying these fundamental concepts.

Archana Areti
Bhavani Shankar Kodali

Preface to the First Edition

"Learning gives creativity, Creativity leads to thinking, Thinking provides knowledge, Knowledge makes you great."

—APJ Abdul Kalam

Applied physics, equipment and clinical monitoring form a major portion of the curriculum for postgraduate students. These topics cover nearly 25% of examination topics. They are quite complicated, and the concepts are difficult to understand for many postgraduate students. We are always challenged with the question as to how much applied physics any anesthesiologist must know. We always opine that if one is armed with knowledge, it will never be regretted. If learning was to be limited, the technological developments in the last five decades would never have been witnessed. Consequently, our specialty and our patients would have been exposed to obsolete technology.

Our aim in producing this postgraduate review is to bring all the essential aspects of applied physics for anesthesiologists into one book and make it simple to understand. One must be able to use equipment safely without placing their patient at risk because of lack of understanding of basic principles. In addition, one must be able to monitor their patients without errors.

We would like to thank all the people who contributed to the preparation of this book. We hope that this venture will be successful in making anesthesiologists acquire the basic knowledge regarding anesthetic equipment.

Yasodananda K Areti MD
Bhavani Shankar Kodali MD

Acknowledgments

We wish to acknowledge the University of the West Indies for facilitating this book. We would like to thank Mr Emmerson Haynes and Mr Muralidhar Areti for their assistance with illustrations.

We would also like to thank Shri Jitendar P Vij (Group Chairman), Mr Ankit Vij (Managing Director), Ms Chetna Malhotra (Senior Director–Professional Publishing, Marketing, and Business Development), and Mr Naman Singh (Development Editor) along with the entire Production team of Jaypee Brothers Medical Publishers (P) Ltd., New Delhi, India for their invaluable support in bringing this project to completion.

Contents

CHAPTER 1

Applied Physics

Archana Areti, Hariharan Seetharaman

INTRODUCTION

Physics is an important component of the curriculum of postgraduate students. A thorough understanding of the physical principles of various pieces of equipment is essential in order to use them safely. This chapter covers the major areas of physics as applicable in anesthesia practice. In each main area, the various details are further explained in alphabetical order, except for some principles that need to be explained together for a better understanding.

- Compressed gases
- Vapors
- Fluids
- Diffusion/osmosis
- Heat
- Humidity
- Electromagnetic (EM) spectrum
- Electricity
- Ultrasound

COMPRESSED GASES

Anesthetists use compressed gases in their day-to-day practice. At room temperature, some agents exist mostly as liquids and some only as gases. A nonliquefied compressed gas is a gas that does not liquefy at ordinary ambient temperatures regardless of the pressure applied. Oxygen and air are examples of such gases. Oxygen, when supplied at very low temperatures, is a cryogenic liquid. A liquefied compressed gas is one that becomes liquid to a large extent in containers at ambient temperature and at pressures from 25 to 1,500 psig (172–10,340 kPa). Examples include nitrous oxide and carbon dioxide. Different principles that require to be understood for safe use of compressed gases are detailed below.

Adiabatic Process

The behavior of gases depends on the constancy of pressure, temperature, or volume. The relationship between these variables is described by ideal gas laws. For a change to occur in the state of a gas, heat energy is either added or taken away from the gas. If the state of a gas is altered without a change in heat energy, it is said to undergo adiabatic change. An adiabatic process describes the change in the state of gas, which occurs without transfer of heat or matter between a system and its surroundings.

Adiabatic Expansion

If compressed gas expands adiabatically, heat energy is taken from the surrounding and cooling occurs. This principle is used in the commercial manufacturing of oxygen and cryoprobe.

Joule-Kelvin or Joule-Thompson effect: The phenomenon was investigated in 1852 by the British physicists James Prescott Joule and William Thomson (Lord Kelvin). When a high-pressure gas is released rapidly through a valve or porous opening, the resulting expansion leads to decrease in temperature. This can result in cooling of the gas, which eventually liquefies. This principle is known as Joule-Kelvin principle and can be used for production of liquid air. By using the fractional distillation of liquid air (due to the different boiling points of nitrogen and oxygen), oxygen can be produced commercially.

The cryoprobe is used for rapid freezing of tissues in the treatment of skin lesions, in gynecology, and in ophthalmic surgery.

Adiabatic Compression

If a gas is rapidly compressed its temperature rises. When a gas cylinder connected to the anesthetic machine is turned on too quickly, the temperature rises in gauges and pipelines, and in the presence of oil or grease may lead to a fire or explosion.

Atmospheric Pressure and Units (Table 1)

The atmospheric pressure is the pressure exerted by the atmosphere at sea level and is the result of the weight of atmospheric gases bearing down on the surface of the earth.

Pressure: Anesthetists make pressure measurements both in patients and in machines, and hence should have a good understanding of pressure and its units of measurement. Pressure is expressed as force per unit area **(Fig. 1)**. The SI unit is Pascal; since this represents a tiny pressure, more commonly, kilopascal (kPa) is used. The other units commonly used are presented in **Table 1**. The relationships between gas volume, pressure, and temperature of compressed gases are shown in **Table 2**.

Critical Temperature and Critical Pressure

Critical temperature is defined as the temperature above which gases cannot be liquefied by applying pressure. Critical pressure is the pressure at which a

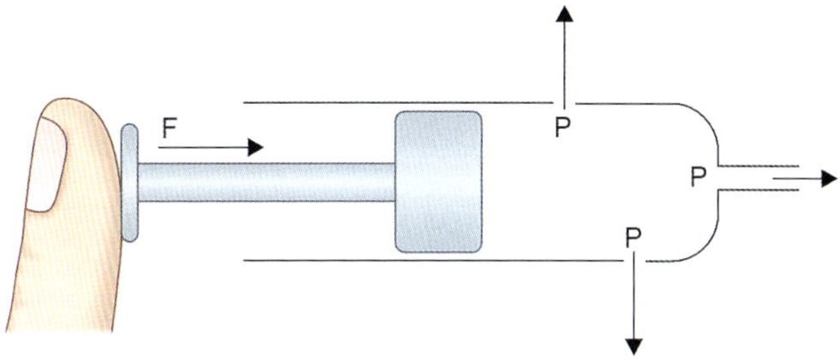

Fig. 1: Force is pressure exerted over an area.

TABLE 1: Units of pressure.

kPa	Kilopascal
cm H_2O	Centimeters of water
psi	Pounds per square inch
mm Hg	Millimeters of mercury
1 kPa = 7.5 mm Hg	
1 mm Hg = 1.35 cm H_2O	
101 kPa = 760 mm Hg = 1,030 cm H_2O = 14.7 psi = 1 atmosphere at sea level	

TABLE 2: Common gas laws.

Gas laws	*Relationship*	*Formula*
Boyle's law	Pressure and volume	P1V1 = P2V2
Charles's law	Volume and temperature	V1/T1 = V2/T2
Gay-Lussac's law	Temperature and pressure	P1/T1 = P2/T2
Ideal gas law	Pressure, volume, temperature	PV = nRT

(n: number of moles; P: absolute pressure; R: universal gas constant; T: absolute temperature; V: volume)

gas can be liquefied at its critical temperature (critical pressure of oxygen—49.7 atm). The critical temperature of nitrous oxide (N_2O) is 36.5°C, and hence N_2O exists as a liquefied gas in the cylinders at room temperature. The critical temperature of oxygen is –118°C and hence at room temperature oxygen exists as compressed gas. Liquid oxygen (LOX) can only be obtained if the oxygen is cooled below its critical temperature and pressurized. In order to maintain this temperature, special insulated and refrigerated containers are required for supply of LOX (Chapter 2).

Poynting Effect

Described by Poynting and also known as pseudocritical temperature, the Poynting effect refers to the phenomenon of physical properties of a mixture of gases, differing from the individual gases. The critical temperature of a gas including its boiling point is altered, when mixed with another gas.

Entonox Cylinder

Oxygen at room temperature exists in gaseous state in compressed gas cylinders because it has a very low critical temperature. Nitrous oxide exists as liquefied gas at room temperature, since its critical temperature is higher. However, when nitrous oxide is mixed with oxygen (Entonox), nitrous oxide remains in a gaseous state even at a pressure of 137 atm. This effect of oxygen, which lowers critical temperature of the mixture (pseudocritical temperature), is attributed to the Poynting effect. This principle allows us to use Entonox cylinder to provide obstetric analgesia and analgesia to transport patients with long bone fractures and in dental practice.

Force (Relation to Pressure)

Force is that which changes or tends to change the state of rest or motion of an object. In SI system force is measured in newtons (N). A newton is that force, which gives a mass of 1 kg an acceleration of 1 meter per second^2 (1 m/sec^2) (kg/ms^{-2}). Force, pressure, and area are interrelated. Force is the pressure acting on unit area **(Fig. 1)**. If force is applied over smaller area (like a smaller syringe) the pressure is higher. Similarly, high pressure acting over small area can be balanced by reduced pressure acting over larger area. This concept is used in the construction of pressure regulators (Chapter 3).

Gas Laws (Table 2)

Avogadro's Hypothesis

Equal volumes of gases at the same temperature and pressure contain equal number of molecules. This number of particles is 6.022×10^{23} and is known as Avogadro's number. One mole of any gas occupies 22.4 L at standard temperature and pressure (STP) and 24 L at room temperature and pressure (RTP) (20°C at sea level). This principle is used to calculate:

- The contents of a cylinder containing liquefied gas
- The amount of vapor that can be generated from a given amount of volatile liquid
- The volume of CO_2 absorbed by soda lime

Boyle's Law

The first perfect gas law; Boyle's law states that at a constant temperature, the volume of a given mass of gas varies inversely with the absolute pressure. Another way to put the Boyle's law is to say that with any increase in the pressure of a gas at a constant temperature, the volume of the gas decreases. Similarly, with any decrease in the pressure, while maintaining a constant temperature, the volume of the gas will increase. Furthermore, any increase or decrease in the volume of the gas at a particular temperature will decrease and increase the pressure of the gas respectively. Two important practical uses of Boyle's law are:

1. Calculation of volume of gas in a cylinder containing compressed gas (Chapter 2)
2. Body plethysmography, where the subject is totally contained in an airtight chamber and attempts to breathe against an occluded airway. Changes in the alveolar pressure are recorded and compared with small changes in lung volume, derived from pressure changes in the plethysmograph. Application of Boyle's law then permits the calculation of lung volume.

Charles's Law

Second perfect gas law states that at a constant pressure, the volume of a given mass of gas varies directly with absolute temperature. This principle is used to calculate the contents of a cylinder containing liquefied gases (Chapter 2).

As per this principle, the volume of a mole of gas at STP is 22.4 L and it becomes approximately 24 L when correction is made for RTP.

Gay-Lussac's Law

Third perfect gas law: At a constant volume, the absolute pressure of a given mass of gas varies directly with temperature. As temperature increases in the cylinders, the pressure increases resulting in the possibility of an explosion. Hence, gas cylinders should not be exposed to extremes of temperatures and stored in cool places and regulations place a limit to filling density of liquefied compressed gas.

The Ideal Gas Law

The ideal gas law relates the four quantities: Pressure, volume, moles, and temperature.

Universal Gas Constant

The three gas laws are combined to give the universal gas constant:

$$P \times V = K1 \qquad V/T = K2 \qquad P/T = K3$$

$$P \times V/T = \text{Universal gas constant "}R\text{"}$$

Using Avogadro's hypothesis at constant T and P, the volume (V) = number of molecules (n).

So, combining all the laws: $PV = nRT$

Measuring the change in the number of moles (n) of a gas in a stream gives a measurement of the number of atoms moving in the flow and is called molar or mass flow. This principle of ideal gas law enables one to understand the principle of partial pressure.

Dalton's Law of Partial Pressures

The Ideal Gas Law for a mixture of two gases can be rewritten as:

$$PV = (n_1 + n_2)\ RT = n_1RT + n_2RT$$

The Dalton's law states that in a mixture of gases, the pressure exerted by each gas is same as the pressure exerted as if it occupied the container alone. The total pressure exerted by the mixture is equal to the sum of pressures exerted by individual gases. The pressure exerted by each gas is proportionate to the percentage of that gas in the mixture.

So partial pressure = Fractional concentration × Total pressure

For example, if air is 20% oxygen and 80% nitrogen, then for an atmospheric pressure of 760 mm Hg, the partial pressure of oxygen will be 152 mm Hg and the partial pressure of nitrogen will be 608 mm Hg. This principle can also be applied to measure partial pressure of different gases in alveoli.

Henry's Law

Henry's law states that at a particular temperature, the amount of a given gas dissolving in a given liquid is directly proportional to the partial pressure of the gas in equilibrium with the liquid (the partial pressure of the gas in gaseous phase is also termed as the tension of the gas in liquid). According to this law, the volume of gas that dissolves in a liquid is equal to its solubility coefficient multiplied by its partial pressure.

$$V = \alpha \times P_{gas}$$

where, V is volume, α is solubility coefficient, and P_{gas} is partial pressure.

Application: This law is used to calculate the amount of oxygen dissolved in plasma at a given partial pressure, where the solubility coefficient for O_2 is 0.003 mL/dL. So, at 100 mm Hg of oxygen tension, the amount of oxygen dissolved would be 0.3 mL.

VAPORS

A gas refers to a substance that has a single defined thermodynamic state at room temperature, whereas a vapor refers to a substance that is a mixture of two phases at room temperature, namely gaseous and liquid phase. A gaseous phase of a volatile liquid below the critical temperature is known as vapor. A vapor can be liquefied using pressure, whereas gas cannot be liquefied unless it is cooled to critical temperature.

Boiling Point

Evaporation occurs at the surface of the liquid when its temperature is below the boiling temperature at a given pressure. The saturated vapor pressure (SVP) of a liquid is independent of the ambient pressure, but increases with increasing temperature. If we continue to heat a liquid, eventually its SVP equals the ambient pressure (usually 101 kPa or 760 mm Hg). The temperature at this point is called as its boiling point of any liquid. Boiling points of some anesthetic agents are listed in **Table 3**.

Latent Heat of Vaporization

Energy is required when a molecule changes from liquid to gas. Latent heat of vaporization is the number of calories required to change 1 g of liquid into vapor without changing temperature. Thus, in the absence of an outside temperature source, volatile liquids will cool significantly and lead to decreasing vaporization. The latent heats of vaporization among the common volatile anesthetic gases are similar.

Since the vaporization process requires heat, it is not surprising that the vaporization process, which draws heat from the liquid anesthetic itself as well as the container, is a cooling process. So, as vaporization proceeds the cooling of the liquid anesthetic would tend to retard the vaporization process. Since vaporization is a temperature-dependent process, if no heat is added, vaporizer output would decline. Accordingly, many vaporizers have temperature compensatory systems to ensure that heat loss due to vaporization is compensated and therefore does not reduce output (Chapter 3).

Saturated Vapor Pressure and Vaporization

In a closed container, molecules from a volatile liquid escape the liquid phase into gaseous phase (vaporization), and vice versa. The pressure exerted by these gaseous molecules on the wall of the container is known as vapor pressure. This process of vaporization will proceed until an equilibrium between the gas and liquid phases is reached. At this point, number of molecules entering gaseous phase equals the number entering liquid phase, and the pressure exerted by the vapor (usually expressed in mm Hg) is called the SVP. The relation between SVP and ATP will enable the manufacturers to

TABLE 3: Boiling points and saturated vapor pressure (SVP) of anesthetic agents.

	Boiling point (°C)	*SVP (mm Hg) at 20°C*
Desflurane	22.8	669
Isoflurane	48.5	238
Halothane	50.2	243
Sevoflurane	58.5	157

determine the splitting ratio of plenum vaporizers (Chapter 3). SVP of some volatile anesthetic agents at 20°C is given in **Table 3**.

FLUIDS

Fluid is a substance that has the ability to flow because its particles are not rigidly attached to one another, and includes both liquids and gases. The behavior of a fluid in flow is predominantly related to two intrinsic properties of the fluid: Density and viscosity.

Density and Viscosity

Density is the pressure exerted by a column of fluid and is defined as the mass of a substance occupying a unit volume. The unit of density is kg/m^3. Density is dependent on temperature and as the temperature of fluid increases the density decreases.

Viscosity is a measure of fluid's resistance to flow and can be thought of as the internal friction of the fluid. It is measured in newtons-seconds per meter^2 (N s/m^2).

Factors Affecting Viscosity

- *Intermolecular forces:* The stronger the intermolecular force, the higher the viscosity.
- *Size of particles:* The smaller the size of the particle, the lower the viscosity.
- *Shape of molecules:* Higher molecular masses have higher viscosities.
- *Temperature:* Viscosity decreases with increasing temperature.

Flow

Flow is the movement of a gas or a liquid through a tube or other system. Flow Q is defined as the volume of fluid passing a point in unit time:

$$Q = V/t$$

Where, V = change in volume

t = the time interval over which the flow is measured

Flow can be described as laminar, turbulent, or a mixture of both.

Laminar Flow/Tubular Flow (Figs. 2A and B)

Orderly movement of a fluid that complies with a model in which parallel layers have different velocities relative to each other. At relatively low flow velocities, the flow can be modeled on layers or cylinders of flow at differing rates, the fastest velocity occurring in the center of the tube and the slowest at the edge where there is friction between the wall of the tube and the fluid. This distinctive velocity profile is maintained as long as laminar flow exists, that is in the absence of eddies or turbulence.

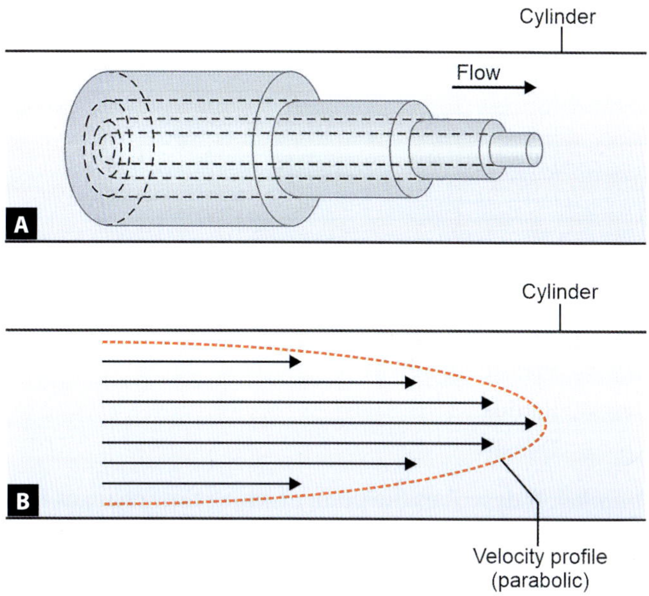

Figs. 2A and B: Laminar flow through a tube with a (A) 3D view or (B) 2D view: Fluid travels in concentric layers of velocity.

Hagen-Poiseuille's law: Hagen (in 1839) and Poiseuille (in 1840) described the laws governing laminar flow through a tube. It applies to laminar flow. It states that flow through the tube is directly proportional to the pressure gradient and the 4th power radius and inversely proportional to the length and viscosity of the gas.

Law follows the formula: Laminar flow $\approx \dfrac{\Delta P.r^4}{\eta L}$

Where,

r = Radius

ΔP = Pressure gradient

L = Length of tube

η = Viscosity

Hagen-Poiseuille's law is applicable at low flows through flow meters.

Turbulent Flow/Orificial Flow (Fig. 3)

Fluid flow which is unpredictable with multiple eddy currents and is not parallel to the sides of the tube through which it is flowing is known as turbulent flow or orificial flow. Turbulent flow is facilitated by corners, irregularities, and sharp angles. Turbulent flow is affected by the density of the gas. The factors that affect turbulent flow and their interrelation are:

$$\text{Turbulent flow} \approx \frac{\sqrt{DP}.\, r^2}{\sqrt{r}}$$

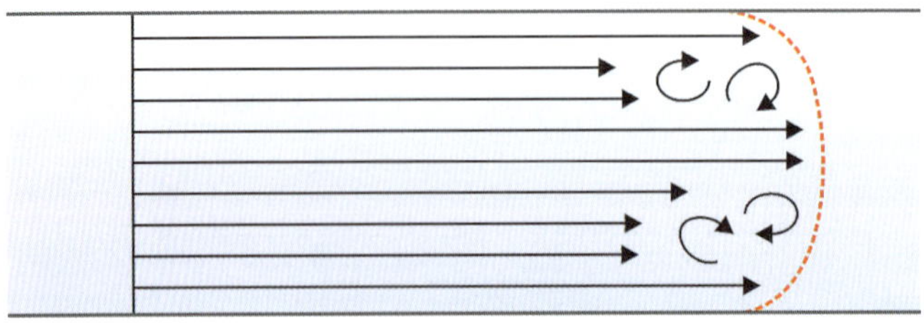

Fig. 3: Turbulent flow.

Where,

ΔP = Pressure gradient

r = Radius

ρ = Density

Reynolds number: It describes the point at which flow changes from laminar to turbulent, and the spectrum in between the two types of flow. The equation for Reynolds number (*Re*) is:

$$Re = \rho\, w\, d_0/\eta$$

Where,

Re = Reynolds number

ρ = Density

w = Flow velocity of the liquid

d_0 = Orifice diameter

η = Viscosity

The Reynolds number is dimensionless, having no units. For numbers <2,000, the flow through a tube tends to be laminar. Between 2,000 and 4,000, the flow pattern is a mix of the two, and above 4,000, the flow is mainly turbulent.

Bernoulli's Principle

Bernoulli's principle is named after the Dutch-Swiss mathematician Daniel Bernoulli who discovered this principle over 300 years ago. In fluid dynamics, Bernoulli's principle states that for an inviscid flow, an increase in the speed of the fluid occurs simultaneously with a decrease in pressure or a decrease in the fluid's potential energy.

Bernoulli's principle is derived from the principle of conservation of energy, which states that in a steady flow, the sum of all forms of mechanical energy in a fluid along a streamline is the same at all points on that streamline. This requires that the sum of kinetic energy and potential energy remains constant. This means that if we alter the energy of one portion of the system, it has an effect on the rest of the system. So, if the kinetic energy rises, the potential energy and pressure must fall.

Bernoulli's equation:

$$P + \frac{1}{2} \times \rho v^2 + \rho gh = \text{Constant}$$

Where,

P = Pressure
g = Acceleration due to gravity (m/s^2)
h = Height of the tube
ρ = Density of liquid
V^2 = Velocity of fluid

Consider a tube with a narrowing as shown in **Figure 4**. There are no leaks, so the volume of fluid at point A is the same at point C. Consequently, the narrowing at point B means that the fluid has to speed up in order to fulfill this continuity. This means that point B has an increase in velocity compared with point A or C, so the pressure falls at this point.

Venturi Effect

The Venturi effect is based on the Bernoulli's principle. The pressure drop induced by the increase in velocity of a fluid passing through a narrow orifice can be used to entrain air or a nebulizer solution.

Venturi tubes are the basis for Venturi injectors which may be used in providing suction or for producing diluted gas mixtures. The venturi tube is shown in **Figure 5**.

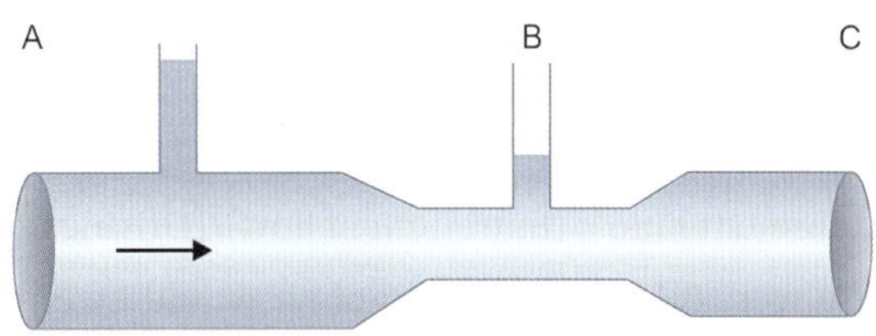

Fig. 4: Bernoulli's principle: When fluid flows from A to C, the pressure at the narrow part B is the lowest.

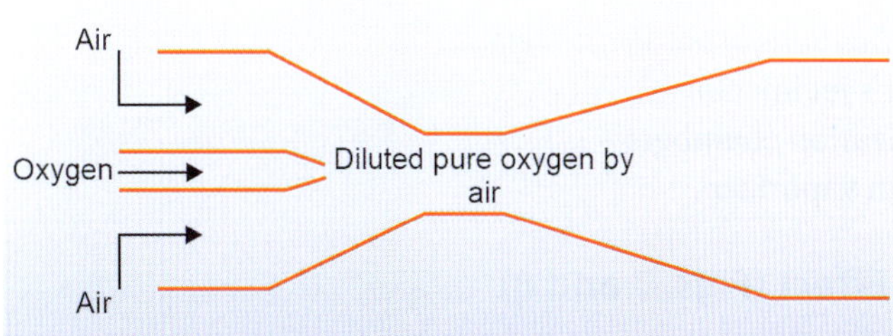

Fig. 5: The Venturi tube.

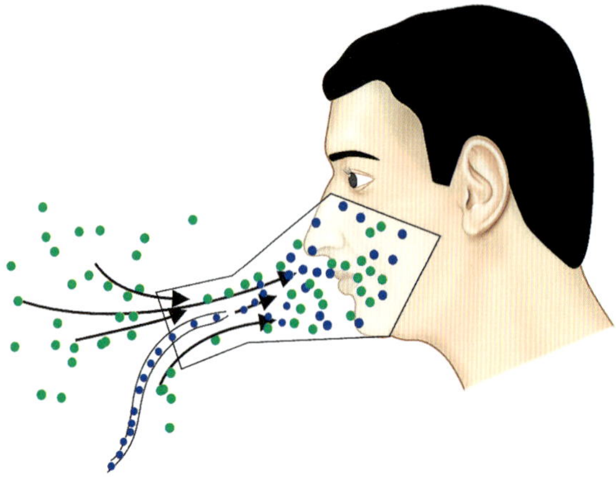

Fig. 6: Venturi mask—an application of the Venturi principle (oxygen molecules—blue, air molecules—green).

The Venturi Mask (Fig. 6)—An Application of the Venturi Tube

The venturi oxygen mask is based on the Venturi principle in that relatively rapidly moving oxygen molecules pull along (entrainment) air molecules by two processes:

1. The first process is based on the Bernoulli effect in which there is a relative reduction in pressure associated with the higher oxygen velocity.
2. The second involves friction between the high-speed oxygen molecules in the lower speed air molecules, which has the effect of pulling air molecules into the higher speed stream. Translational momentum transfer occurs as the air molecules increased their velocity.

   Entrainment ratio can be calculated as a function of the entrainment flow to the driving (oxygen) flow.

   Entrainment ratio = (Entrainment flow)/(Driving flow)

   If the ratio were 8:1, then 8 L/min of air would be entrained by the driving gas (oxygen) of 1 L/min.

Factors that could change the entrainment ratio include transient obstruction, including back pressure, which would ultimately change the oxygen concentration delivered.

Other applications of the Venturi effect:

- Sander's jet injector
- Nebulization chambers
- Modern vaporizers

Coanda Effect (Figs. 7 and 8)

The Coanda effect is an established physical phenomenon of fluid flow. This effect was named after a Romanian aircraft designer Henri Coanda,

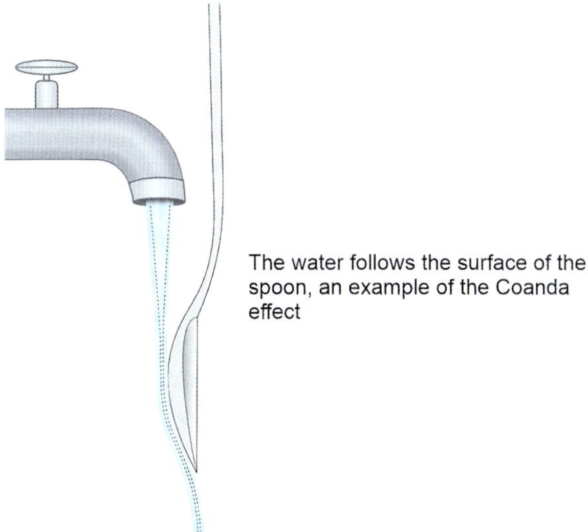

Fig. 7: Coanda effect; spoon and tap.

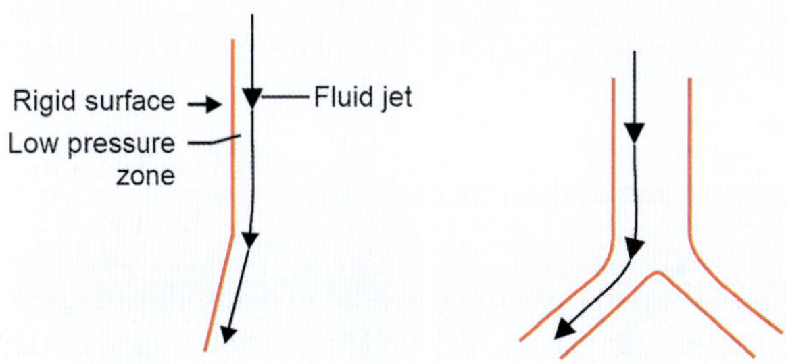

Fig. 8: Diagrammatic depiction of the Coanda effect in branching tube system: By adhering to the nearby surface, the fluid jet is directed into the ipsilateral branch of the bifurcation, depriving the other branch of its share of the fluid flow.

who discovered the effect after an aircraft he designed went up in flames as a consequence of this effect. A jet stream adheres to the boundary wall and therefore produces a lower pressure along the opposite wall. Essentially any fluid coming into contact with a curved surface will cling to this surface and alter its direction of flow. This can be illustrated by running a thin stream of water from a tap and bringing the curved surface of a spoon to touch it. The water follows the surface of the spoon **(Fig. 7)**. It does so because the solid stationary surface of the spoon slows the layer in immediate contact. This has a drag effect on the other layers, in effect pulling them into the line of the curved surface. The Coanda effect is said to explain the maldistribution of air in the pulmonary tree after a constricted portion of bronchiole, as the flow will stream along one fork of the division, leading to unequal distribution of gas flow and V/Q mismatch.

Applications

- Mucus plug at branching of tracheobronchial tree may cause maldistribution of respiratory gases.
- Unequal flow may result because of atherosclerotic plaques in the vascular tree.
- Differential flow produced by Coanda effect is one of the factors responsible for the flow of blood in right atrium of fetal circulation. Because of Coanda effect there is very little mixing of blood flowing from inferior vena cava (IVC) and superior vena cava (SVC).

Surface Tension (Laplace's Law)

Surface tension is the result of attraction between molecules across the surface of a liquid either lining a tube or a sphere. The SI unit for surface tension is newton per meter (N/m).

The Laplace's law describes the relation between transmural pressure, surface tension, and radius. In a tube, the relation between these forces is as follows:

$$\text{Pressure across the wall of a tube} = \frac{\text{Surface Tension}}{\text{Radius}}$$

In a vessel wall drop in pressure can lead to instability of these forces and eventually the vessel collapses, which will be detrimental to perfusion.

In a sphere, like alveoli the forces of the Laplace's law is as follows:

$$\text{Pressure across the wall of a sphere} = \frac{2 \times \text{Surface Tension}}{\text{Radius}}$$

As the radius decreases, there would be unrelenting process proceeding to the collapse of the alveoli. This process is arrested by the presence of surfactant in the alveolar lining, which reduces surface tension. As the radius decreases, the relative concentration of surfactant increases, which prevents collapse. In pathological states where the surfactant is inadequate, respiratory distress occurs as seen in infant respiratory distress syndrome.

DIFFUSION/OSMOSIS

Diffusion

Diffusion is the process by which there is a movement of solute molecules due to their random thermal motion. It is a passive process, and net movement of the solute occurs along a concentration gradient (from high concentration to low concentration).

The rate of diffusion through a membrane is dependent on the concentration gradient, the area of the membrane exposed, the membrane thickness, and the permeability constant k_p.

$$Q = k_p A (C_1 - C_2)/D$$

Where:

Q = Rate of diffusion
k_p = Permeability constant
A = Area of the membrane exposed
$(C_1 - C_2)$ = Concentration gradient
D = Membrane thickness

Osmosis

If two aqueous solutions with different concentrations of particles are separated from each other by a semipermeable membrane, then water will move across the membrane from the solution with the lower concentration to the solution with the higher concentration. The movement of the water will depend on the difference in the concentration of the particles and the nature of permeability of the membrane. This movement of water is termed osmosis and the pressure, which would need to be exerted to halt its movement is called the osmotic pressure. The osmotic pressure is determined by the total number of particles in solution, regardless of molecular nature. The total number of particles will thus depend on the degree of dissociation of solutes **(Fig. 9)**.

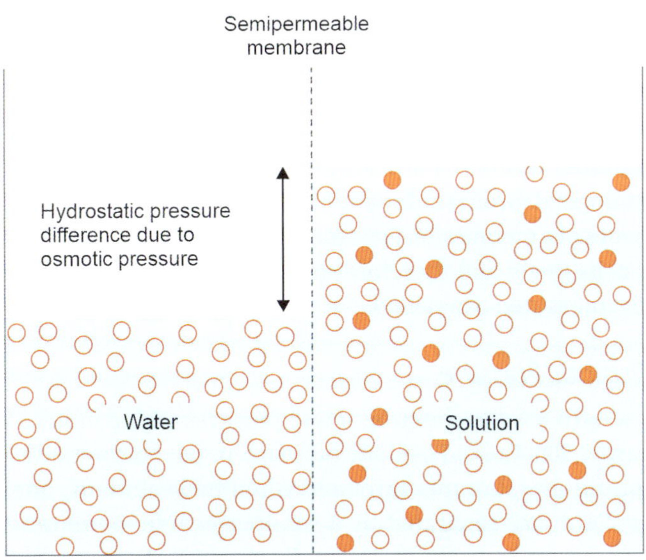

Fig. 9: Osmosis and osmotic pressure.

Osmometry

Osmometry is a technique for measuring the concentration of particles in a solution, i.e., the osmolar concentration. Osmolar concentration can be expressed in two ways:

1. Osmolality expressed as mmol/kg of solvent
2. Osmolarity expressed as mmol/L of solution; osmolality is a thermodynamically more precise expression because solution concentrations expressed on a weight basis are temperature-independent while those based on volume will vary with temperature in a manner dependent on the thermal expansion of the solution.

Based on the total number of solute particles, the plasma osmolarity is 280–300 mOsm/L. 99% of this is contributed by electrolytes such as sodium, chloride, and bicarbonate. Contribution from plasma protein is small (1 mOsm/L).

If a solute is dissolved in a solvent, then the following properties of the solvent change:

- Osmotic pressure increases
- Vapor pressure decreases
- Boiling point increases
- Freezing point decreases

These are known as colligative properties and are all directly related to the total number of solute particles per mass of solvent, i.e., the osmolality. Theoretically, any of the four colligative properties could be used as a basis for the measurement of osmolality. The most commonly used method in the case of physiological fluids is freezing-point depression.

Tonicity

Although the terms tonicity and osmolality are often used interchangeably, there is a clear distinction. Osmolality is a physical property dependent on the total number of solute particles present in a solution, whereas tonicity is a physiological process dependent upon the selectively permeable characteristics of a membrane. For example, solutes such as urea and ethanol permeate cells freely and therefore will have no effect on tonicity but will increase the measured osmolality.

Colloid Osmotic Pressure

Colloid is a term used to describe solute particles with a molecular weight greater than 30,000. Colloid osmotic pressure, or oncotic pressure, describes an equilibrium pressure measurement when two solutions, one of which contains colloid, are separated by a semipermeable membrane. Interest in its measurement has come from studies in critical care medicine in the prediction of intercompartmental body water movements, in particular as a useful prognostic indicator of pulmonary edema, and of mortality in the critically ill.

HEAT

Heat is a form of energy that passes between two samples owing to the difference in their temperatures. Heat energy tends to pass along a temperature gradient from high to low temperatures. Heating a substance gives its constituent molecules increased kinetic energy. This results in a rise in temperature, or changes its state. Loss of heat results in the reverse process.

Units of Heat Energy

Base SI unit for heat energy is joules (J). In terms of other SI units:

$$J = \frac{kg.m^2}{s^2} N.m = Pa.m^3 = W.s = C.V$$

where *kg* is the kilogram, *m* is the meter, *s* is the second, *N* is the newton, *Pa* is the pascal, *W* is the watt, *C* is the coulomb, and *V* is the volt.

Calories or kilocalories are also used as units of heat energy. One calorie is defined as the amount of heat required to raise the temperature of 1 g of water by 1°C (1 calorie = 4.186 kJ).

Temperature

Temperature is the property of matter, which determines whether the heat energy will flow to or from another object of a different temperature. This is expressed according to a comparative scale. It is that property by which we may quantify the heat energy of a substance.

Temperature Scales

The temperature scale most commonly used tends to be the Celsius scale or the centigrade scale (named after 18th century Swedish astronomer Anders Celsius). It uses the boiling and freezing points of water (100°C and 0°C, respectively), at atmospheric pressure.

The Fahrenheit scale (named after 18th century German physicist, Daniel Gabriel Fahrenheit) was set at the lowest freezing point with an ice-water-salt mixture. The freezing point of water is 32°F and the boiling point is 212°F, being 180° apart.

Kelvin temperature scale (named for the British physicist William Thomson, Baron Kelvin) is the base unit of thermodynamic temperature measurement in the International System (SI) of measurement. It is defined as 1/273.16 of the triple point (equilibrium among the solid, liquid and gaseous phases) of pure water. The kelvin (symbol *K* without the degree sign) is also the fundamental unit of the Kelvin scale, an absolute temperature scale.

The Kelvin scale is related to the Celsius scale. The difference between the freezing and boiling points of water is 100° in each, so that the kelvin has the same magnitude as the degree Celsius **(Table 4)**.

Triple Point of Water (Fig. 10)

Water can exist in three phases, as vapor, liquid, and ice. These phases depend on temperature and pressure. The transition between water vapor and water is demarcated by the boiling point of water (*P*), which is 100°C at 1 atm, but which increases with increasing pressure.

Water vapor and water, therefore, coexist along OA **(Fig. 10)**. Similarly, the freezing point of water (0°C at 1 atm) separates water and ice, but decreases

TABLE 4: Different scales for temperature.

	Kelvin (K)	*Celsius (°C)*	*Fahrenheit (°F)*
Water boils	373.15	100	212
Ethanol boils	351.6	78.4	173.1
Human body	310	37	98.6
Room temperature	295	22	72
Water freezes	273.15	0	32
Brine freezes	255	−17.8	0
Mercury freezes	234.3	−38.9	−37.8
Absolute zero	0	−273.15	−459.7

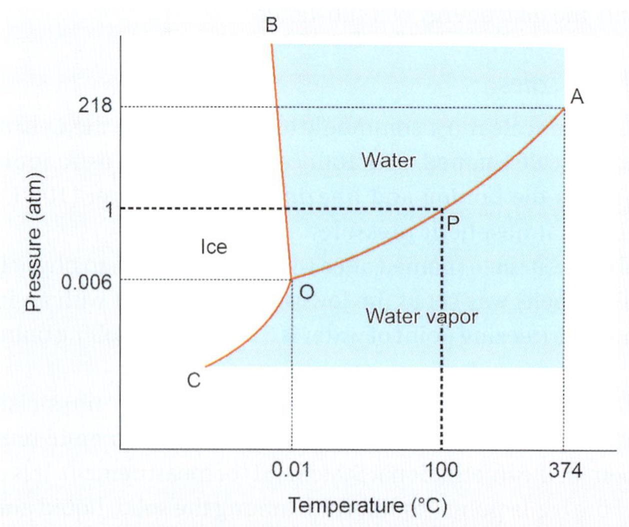

Fig. 10: Triple point.

with increasing pressure (OB). Finally, OC separates ice and water vapor, and these phases coexist along this line. There is only a single point (O) at which the three phases of water coexist, at a pressure of 0.006 atm and 0.01°C. This is the triple point of water.

The internationally agreed temperature "number" of the triple point of water is 2,713.16, because it is the number of units above the recognized absolute zero of temperature, which was deduced from extrapolations of the relationship between pressure, volume, and temperature of gases. Hence, the unit of thermodynamic temperature (Kelvin) is the fraction 1/273.16 of the thermodynamic temperature of the triple point of water. The clinical measurement of temperature is described in Chapter 7.

Specific Heat

The specific heat of a substance is the number of calories required to increase the temperature of 1 g of a substance by 1°C. The concept of specific heat is important to the design, operation, and construction of vaporizers as it is applicable in two ways:

1. The specific heat value for an inhaled anesthetic indicates how much heat must be supplied to the liquid to maintain a constant temperature when heat is being lost during vaporization.
2. The materials used as a body of vaporizers have a high specific heat to minimize temperature changes associated with vaporization (thermostabilization).

Thermal Conductivity

Thermal conductivity is a measure of the speed with which heat flows through a substance. The higher the thermal conductivity, the better the substance conducts heat. Vaporizers are constructed of metals that have relatively high thermal conductivity, thus maintaining a uniform internal temperature.

HUMIDITY

Humidity is an important aspect of delivering gases to patients in theaters and intensive care. The importance of humidity for anesthetists lies in the comfort of the theater environment, safety with regard to static electricity, adverse effects of dry medical gas supplies, and heat loss from the body. Humidity is a measure of the amount of water vapor in a gas. It can be expressed in a number of ways.

Absolute Humidity

Absolute humidity is defined as actual mass of water vapor present in a known volume of gas, and is expressed as mg/mL or g/m^3.

The absolute humidity of air in the upper airway of humans is about 34 g/m^3 and it reaches a peak of 43 g/m^3 as it reaches the alveoli.

Relative Humidity

Relative humidity is defined as the ratio of the mass of water vapor in a given volume of gas to the maximum amount of water vapor that the same gas can hold at the same temperature. Relative humidity is expressed as a percentage.

Measurement of Humidity

Hygrometers are instruments that measure humidity; they can measure absolute humidity, relative humidity, and the dew point—which is the point at which vapor condenses. They range from simple mechanical hygrometers, through psychrometers (wet and dry bulb hygrometer), to more complex electrical and optical instruments.

Some instruments include:

Hair hygrometer: The length of hair increases with increasing humidity.

Wet and dry hygrometer: It involves utilization of two mercury thermometers, one in ambient temperature and one in contact with water through a wick. The difference in temperature readings reflects the rate of evaporation of water, which depends on humidity.

Regnault's hygrometer: Air is blown through a silver tube containing ether. This technique is more accurate than the previous two and gives the relative humidity.

Mass spectrometer: This involves utilizing the principle of reduction in the ultraviolet (UV) light transmitted through the medium containing water vapor.

Humidity transducers: Humidity transducers are used in those places where accurate measurement of humidity is required. They can transform a physical quantity of air humidity into a standard signal, which is transferred to a controller. They are normally used in laboratories, ventilation and air-conditioning systems, and in any other production process where it is necessary to control air humidity. They have an accuracy of ±2% over a range of 0–100% relative humidity. Humidity transducers generate alarms or turn off a ventilation system when the predefined maximum and minimum values are exceeded.

Humidification

While nose-breathing at rest, inspired gases become heated to 36°C and are about 80–90% saturated with water vapor by the time they reach the carina, largely due to heat transfer in the nose. Mouth-breathing reduces this to 60–70% relative humidity. This humidification maintains mucosal integrity, ciliary activity, prevents the drying of secretions, and helps in easy expulsion of respiratory secretions when coughing. Lack of humidification (e.g., ventilating a patient with dry gas through a tracheal or tracheostomy tube) can result in cracking of mucosa, drying of secretions, keratinization of the tracheobronchial tree, reduction in ciliary activity, atelectasis, and infection. Tracheal temperature and humidity fall with increased ventilation, particularly when the inspired gases are cold and dry.

Heat and Water Loss

If totally dry gases were inspired and fully saturated gases exhaled, the total water loss from ventilation at rest would be about 300 mL/day in the average adult. Normally the efficiency of nose and humidity of inspired air minimize this loss by approximately 150 mL/day. Bypassing the nose with an endotracheal tube (ETT) and not humidifying gases cause maximal losses.

Nonrespiratory water losses are typically 300–600 mL/day but are increased if warm moist surfaces are exposed (i.e., burns, open abdomen), particularly if the operating theater is cold and has high-flow air-conditioning.

Advantages of Humidification

- Reduced heat loss
- Reduced water loss
- Prevention of ciliary damage and reduced drying of secretions
- *Microbial filtration:* Some heat and moisture exchanger (HME) filters have viral/bacterial filters.

Disadvantages of Humidification

- Disconnection—some may be bulky and heavy
- Overheating—airway burns
- Overhydration—water intoxication, especially in neonates and infants
- Circuit resistance, dead space, and circuit compliance changes—important consideration for neonates
- Infection
- Water clogging—possible particularly in neonates on continuous flow circuits
- Interference with other devices—possibly affects side stream CO_2 analyzers
- Cost

Methods of Humidification

Humidification can be used with any breathing circuit and may be provided for air, oxygen, and a mixture of anesthetic gases.

Anesthetic Circuits

- Water's to-and-fro type systems generate warm moist gases but are of historical importance.
- Coaxial breathing circuits (Bain's or Lack's) result in both countercurrent heating of the inspired gases and rebreathing of exhaled gas for some humidification, but they probably only are about 10–20% efficient on intermittent positive-pressure ventilation (IPPV) and even less when used for spontaneous breathing (because of the high fresh gas flows required).
- Closed circle circuits warm up after a period of time and do generate water and contribute some moisture.

Heat and Moisture Exchanger and Heat and Moisture Exchanger Filter

Heat and moisture exchanger filters contain materials such as ceramic fiber, paper, cellulose, fine steel, or aluminum fibers in a hygroscopic medium such as calcium chloride or silica gel.

Warm, humidified, expired gas passes through the HME; water vapor condenses within the medium and is then reused for humidification of the inspired gas. The HME is warmed by the latent heat of water condensing on it. This heat is also released during subsequent inspiration. Some filters have bacterial (and/or viral) filtering properties with efficiencies >99.9977.

Microbial filtering property may be due to:

Direct interception: For particle >1 µm, it is physically prevented from passing through the pores.

Inertial impaction: Particles <0.5 µm are held by the filtering medium by Van der Waals electrostatic forces.

Diffusional interception: Particles <0.5 µm move freely and randomly (Brownian movement) and subsequently swell up and get filtered by the pores.

Electrostatic attraction: Charged particles are attracted by oppositely charged fibers.

Advantages of HME filters:

- Easy to use in breathing circuits
- Cheap and disposable
- 60–70% relative humidity achieved
- Temperature achieved ranges from 29°C to 34°C.
- Can be incorporated as a microbial filter.

Disadvantages of HME filters:

- They need replacing every 24 hours (maximum).
- Secretions can block the filter.

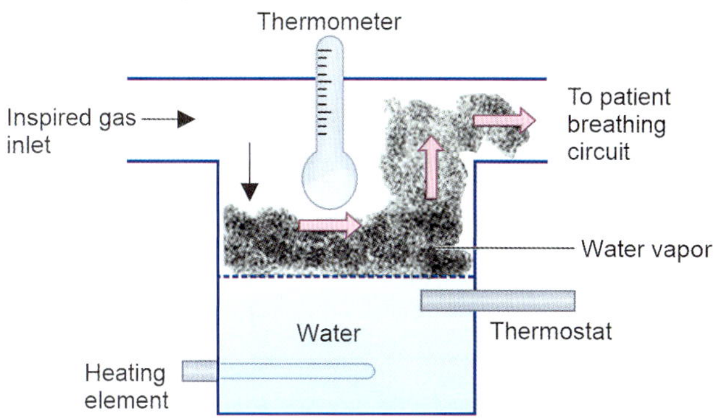

Fig. 11: Heated humidifier.

- Resistance to flow of gas can be up to 2 cm H_2O.
- They can add to the weight of the circuit—may be significant in neonates/ infants.
- They increase circuit dead space.

Water Bath Humidifier

A simple cold-water bath humidifier allows gas to flow through water and carries water vapor as it bubbles out. This type is less efficient as bubbles are large and the loss of heat from the latent heat of vaporization reduces humidity.

The vapor output can be increased by warming the water using electricity (hot-water bath humidifier), but must incorporate a thermostat to maintain an operating temperature at about 40°C **(Fig. 11)**.

At 37°C, near-full saturation can be achieved. A water trap is placed between the humidifier and the patient and is placed below the level of the patient. Vapor output depends on temperature of the water, gas flow, and surface area of contact.

The main problems of hot-water humidifier are:

- Water spillage into the breathing circuit and even into tracheobronchial tree; a water trap will help reduce this problem.
- Airway burns due to thermostat failure and overheating.
- Colonization of water with harmful bacteria can occur. This may be reduced by heating the water to 60°C.

Nebulizers

Nebulizers produce water vapor in the form of microdroplets (1–20 μcm).

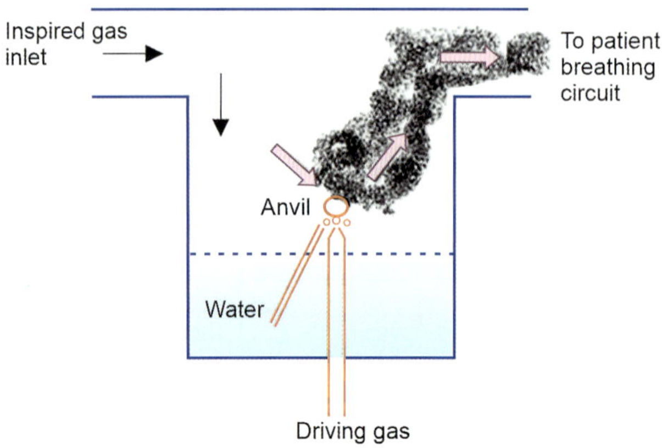

Fig. 12: Nebulizer—based on Venturi principle.

There are three types of nebulizers:

1. *Gas-driven nebulizer* ***(Fig. 12)****:* Gas is passed through a narrow orifice that produces a pressure gradient. This results in water being drawn up through the tube and broken into a fine spray as it comes in contact with the high-speed gas jet. Even smaller droplets can be produced if this spray of gas hits an anvil or a baffle. Most of the droplets are in the range of 2–4 µcm and deposit in the upper airway with a very small amount reaching the smaller bronchioles.
2. *Spinning disk nebulizer:* The rotating disk produces microdroplets when water is drawn onto the disk.
3. *Ultrasonic nebulizer:* Ultrasonic nebulizer has a transducer head immersed in water vibrating at ultrasonic frequency (3 MHz). Ultrasonic nebulizers produce microdroplets <2 µcm, which are capable of reaching alveoli and are therefore a very efficient form of humidification.

   The absolute humidity in different humidifiers is as shown in **Table 5**.

ELECTROMAGNETIC SPECTRUM

The EM spectrum is the range of all types of EM radiations. Radiation is energy that travels and spreads out as it goes—the visible light that comes from a lamp in your house and the radio waves that come from a radio station are two types of EM radiations. The other types of EM radiations that make up the EM spectrum are microwave, infrared (IR) light, UV light, X-rays, and gamma rays **(Fig. 13)**. IR light is used in several clinical monitors (IR analyzers, pulse oximetry, etc.).

Beer–Lambert Law

Beer–Lambert law represents a combination of two laws, which combine to form a mathematical means of expressing how light is absorbed by matter.

TABLE 5: Absolute humidity in different types of humidifiers.

Type of humidifier	*Absolute humidity produced (approx.) (g/m^3)*
• Cold water bath	10
• Heat and moisture exchanger (HME) filter	25
• Hot-water bath	40
• Gas-driven nebulizer	60
• Ultrasonic nebulizer	90

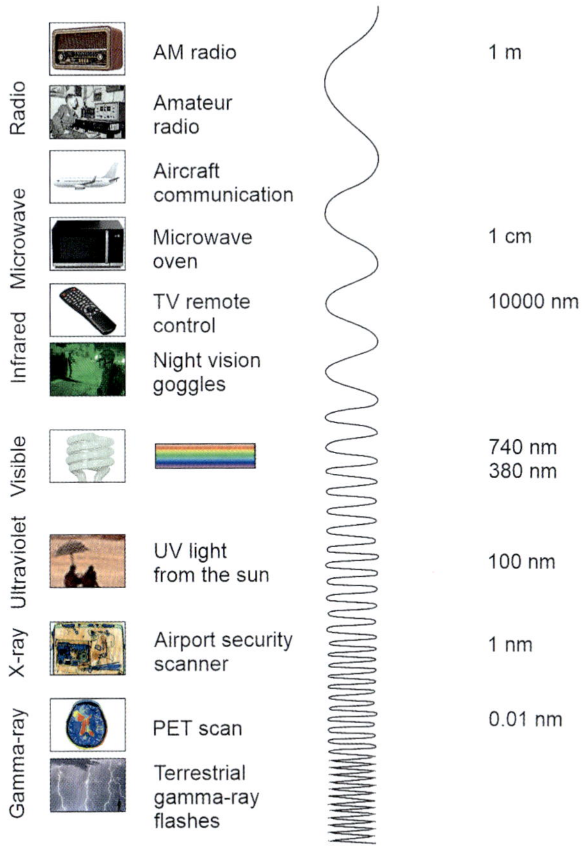

Fig. 13: Electromagnetic spectrum and their wavelengths.

1. Beer's law states that the intensity of transmitted light decreases exponentially as concentration of the substance increases.
2. Lambert's law states that the intensity of transmitted light decreases exponentially as the distance travelled through the substance increases.

Combining the two laws means that the transmission of light through a substance (the inverse of absorbance) is inversely proportional to its molar concentration and thickness.

Beer-Lambert Law: $A = \log_{10} I_i/I_t = \varepsilon LC$

Where

A = Absorbance of light
I_i = Incident light
I_t = Transmitted light
ε = Extinction coefficient
L = Path length
C = Concentration of absorbing media

Clinical Application in Anesthesia

The Beer-Lambert law is relevant to pulse oximetry (Chapter 7), a monitoring technique that works on the basis of spectrophotometry. The pulse oximeter probe, usually placed on a digit, emits light at different wavelengths The blood absorbs a certain proportion of light, which is dependent on the relative concentrations of deoxyhemoglobin and oxyhemoglobin present.

A photodetector placed at a constant path length away on the opposite side of the probe (and thus digit) senses the amount of light that has been absorbed and processes this electronically to give oxygen saturation and pulse waveform, or plethysmograph.

Light

Light is EM radiation within a certain portion of the EM spectrum. The word usually refers to visible light, which is visible to the human eye and is responsible for the sense of sight. Visible light is usually defined as having a wavelength in the range of 400 nanometers (nm), or 400×10^{-9} m, to 700 nm—between the IR (with longer wavelengths) and the UV (with shorter wavelengths). Often, IR and UV are also called light. The wavelength (which is related to frequency and energy) of the light determines the perceived color. The edges of the visible light spectrum blend into the UV and IR levels of radiation.

Most light that we interact with is in the form of white light, which contains many or all of these wavelength ranges within them. Shining white light through a prism causes the wavelengths to bend at slightly different angles due to optical refraction. The resulting light is, therefore, split across the visible color spectrum. This is what causes a rainbow, with airborne water particles acting as the refractive medium. The order of wavelengths is in order of wavelength, which can be remembered by the mnemonic "ROY G BIV" for Red, Orange, Yellow, Green, Blue, Indigo (the blue/violet border), and Violet **(Table 6)**.

Infrared Analyzers

While there is some ambiguity to where the boundaries are for the various "forms" of EM radiation, the IR band is typically taken to begin just beyond

TABLE 6: Visible light spectrum and wavelengths (nm).

Red	*Orange*	*Yellow*	*Green*	*Cyan*	*Blue*	*Violet*
625–740	590–625	565–590	520–565	500–520	435–500	380–435

the red wavelengths of the optical band, around 0.74 μm, and extends up to 300 μm. When IR radiation passes through a sample, some is absorbed by the sample and some of it passes through (transmitted). The resulting spectrum represents the molecular absorption and transmission, creating a molecular fingerprint of the sample. Like a fingerprint, no two unique molecular structures produce the same IR spectrum.

Infrared Spectroscopy

Molecules that contain two or more different atom species absorb IR radiation, because of the nature of the bond between the dissimilar atoms. This property can be used to analyze gases like carbon dioxide, nitrous oxide, and all anesthetic vapors, but not oxygen or nitrogen. Asymmetric, polyatomic molecules absorb the light IR radiation at different wavelengths.

Infrared absorption spectrophotometry devices that detect CO, NO, and inhaled anesthetic agents are used in the operating room; they measure the unique energy absorbed by the gases and vapors, when a sample of the inspired and expired gas is placed into the optical path of an IR beam.

These devices have five components **(Fig. 14)**:

1. IR light source
2. Gas sampler
3. An optical path
4. A detection system
5. A signal processor

Carbon dioxide molecules absorb IR radiation at a wavelength of 4.3 μm. The greater the number of molecules of CO_2 present, the more the radiation at 4.3 μm that is absorbed. All anesthetic vapors absorb IR radiation at 3.6 μm. Because the amount of IR radiation absorbed is a function of the number of molecules present, it is, therefore, also a function of partial pressure. Thus, IR analyzers measure partial pressure. Further details of these monitors are explained in Chapter 7.

LASER (SEE CHAPTER 9)

Ultraviolet Light

Ultraviolet radiation is defined as that portion of the EM spectrum between X-rays and visible light, i.e., between 40 and 400 nm. The UV spectrum is divided into vacuum UV (40–190 nm), far UV (190–220 nm), UVC (220–290 nm),

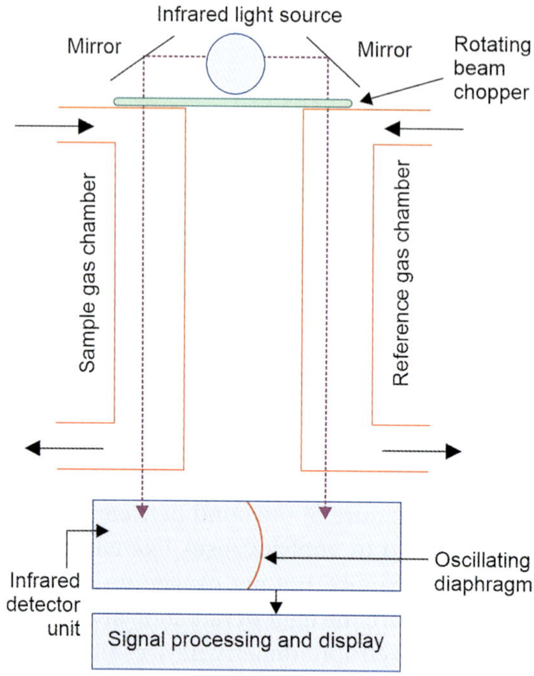

Fig. 14: Diagrammatic depiction of infrared analyzer.

UVB (290–320 nm), and UVA (320–400 nm). The sun is our primary natural source of UV radiation. Artificial sources include tanning booths, black lights, curing lamps, germicidal lamps, mercury vapor lamps, halogen lights, high-intensity discharge lamps, fluorescent and incandescent sources, and some types of lasers [excimer lasers, nitrogen lasers and third harmonic Nd:YAG (neodymium-doped yttrium-aluminum-garnet) lasers]. Unique hazards apply to the different sources depending on the wavelength range of the emitted UV radiation.

ELECTRICITY

Electricity is broad term for the physical phenomena associated with the "flow" of electrons within imbalanced electrodes, usually from a positive to a negative electrode. Electricity may also be described just as the existence of a "charge" between the subatomic particles—electrons and protons, without necessarily having a "flow". In the context of anesthesia and intensive care, it is important to understand the concepts of both electrical "charge" as well as "flow" of the electrically charged particles.

Electromagnetism

The EM force existing within the electrons and protons (and the imbalance existing between them) gives rise to the "electrical charge" of a system.

When this charge is transferred to another point or a system, there is a "flow" of electricity resulting in an electrical "current".

Magnetism is a property of a matter determined by its electronic configuration. When there is zero net orbital motion, the magnetic properties of electrons are nullified mutually, but when the configuration of electrons does not cancel the magnetic properties, the material exhibits "magnetism" and the interaction of these electrically charged subatomic particles gives rise to EM force.

Electrical Charge and Potential

Electrical charge is a physical property exhibited by the subatomic particles of any matter, causing a "force" created by their EM interaction. Thus, conventionally, the charge of an electron is –1 and that of a proton is +1. Like charges repel and opposite charges attract. When charge is transferred between points, there exists a difference of the "electrical potentials" between the points that facilitates the transfer. Thus, the "electrical potential" of a point in a conductor is the work done to move a positive charge from infinity to that point.

- A "conductor" is a medium that conducts or facilitates the flow of an electrical current, e.g., copper wire.
- An "insulator" is a material that does not allow the flow of current through it, e.g., glass.
- A "semiconductor" is a material that has conductivity midway between a conductor and an insulator, e.g., diodes, transistors. Current flow through these semiconductors such as silicon chip occurs either by movement of free "electrons" or through free "holes". Semiconductors are the backbone of modern-day electronics; however, the properties of semiconductors may be unique and may not be similar to that of other electrical phenomena commonly described.

Units, Laws, and Concepts in Electricity

Electrical charge, flow of current, the difference in the electrical potential between conductors, resistance, and the capacitance of the conductors are all interrelated giving rise to the different definitions of the units of measurements in electricity.

Alternating Current and Direct Current (Figs. 15A and B)

- The electrical current when it flows constantly in one direction, this is known as a "direct current" (DC).
- If the current reverses its polarity and alternates its direction of flow cyclically, this is known as "alternating current" (AC).
- Although, in the initial days, DC was predominantly used for all electrical appliances, with the invention of AC, it was actually found to be

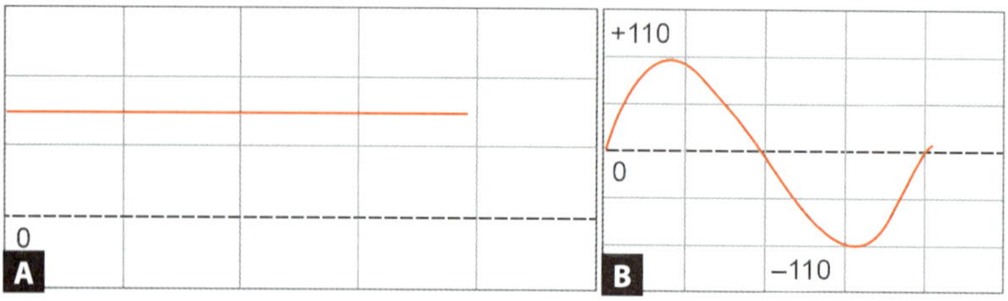

Figs. 15A and B: Direct current (DC) and alternating current (AC).

cost-effective as well as technically advantageous in terms of production and transmission and AC has been adopted throughout the world as the standard current for appliances.

- DC is supplied by batteries including solar cells and flows constantly throughout the cross-section of the conductors such as wires.
- The cycling of AC occurs at the rate of 50 or 60 cycles per second (50 or 60 Hz); the current usually flows toward the periphery of the conductor away from its center.
- AC can be converted to DC by "rectifiers" or adapters, while DC can be converted to AC by "inverters".

Ampere: The SI unit of measurement of current is "ampere", which is one of the basic seven units of the "Système International". One ampere (A) is the amount of transfer of the electric charges (current) passing a point of a conducting system per second. The other units of measurements in electricity are "derived units" and not basic units.

Capacitance

Capacitance in simple terms is the storage of "electrical charge" or energy in a conductor or a set of conductors. When electrical charge is transferred between two conductors, which were not charged earlier, these conductors can then become charged, one positively and another negatively. This results in the establishment of a difference of "electrical potential" between them. Capacitance is calculated as the ratio of the product of the charges of the conductors (numerator) and the potential difference (denominator).

Coulomb: One coulomb (C) of electrical charge is defined as the quantity of charge when a current of one ampere (see below) passes through a conductor within 1 second (A s).

Coulomb's law states that charges repel or attract with a force, which is directly proportional to the product of the charges, and inversely proportional to the square of the distance between them.

Capacitor is an electrical device, which stores the electrical energy in an electrical field and comprises of two conductors separated by one insulator.

Conductance: Electrical conductance is measured in terms of siemens (S).

Farad: One farad (F) is defined as the capacity of system; when charged with 1 coulomb of electricity, has a potential difference of 1 volt.

Impedance and Resistance

Electrical impedance is a concept that extends the property of resistance to ACs.

As illustrated in **Figure 16**, current flows from point A to point B. The difference in the electrical potential between the two points facilitates the current (I) to flow. Herein, there is introduction of another material (R) that opposes or restricts the flow of current between the two points. This is known as the resistance, which reduces the strength of current reaching point B. These three parameters are interrelated as defined by Ohm's law.

Resistance is simply applied to DC, since the flow of current is unidirectional. However, since AC changes the polarity in phases, impedance is a property of the conductor, which takes the phase of the current also into account along with the magnitude of its resistance. In other words, impedance is a complex calculation of resistance that includes the potential difference, the current flow as well as the current phase. Hence, impedance will be the ratio of potential difference to the current incorporating the frequency domain, which is the characteristic feature of AC.

Ohm: One ohm (Ω) is defined as the resistance between two points of a conductor with a potential difference of 1 volt, when 1 ampere of current flows between the points.

Ohm's law: Ohm's law states that the current flow is directly proportional to the potential difference (V) and inversely proportional to the resistance (R). Thus, the relationship between "current" (I), "potential difference" (V), and "resistance" (R) can be expressed as follows:

$$I \propto V \text{ and } I \propto 1/R$$

$$V = I \times R \text{ and } R = V/I$$

The exception to Ohm's law is flow in diodes and batteries where the current flow may not necessarily be linearly proportional to the potential difference. The resistance is determined by factors such as the material with which the conductor is made, shape, and also other factors such as the

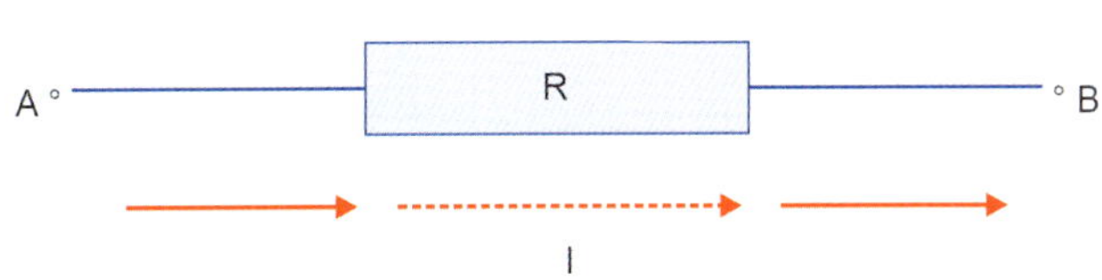

Fig. 16: Concept of resistance.

cross-sectional area. The inverse of resistance is known as conductance, which is the property of a conductor to facilitate the flow of current.

Resistor is an electrical device that imposes a resistance to the flow of current in a circuit, thereby reducing both the potential difference as well as the strength of the current flow. A resistor is different from capacitor in that it does not store electrical energy and may in fact dissipate energy.

Volt: One volt (V) is the difference in the electrical potential energy between two points of a system, when unit charge is transferred from one point to another.

Watt: Watt is a SI unit for measurement of "power", which is the energy converted or transferred per unit time (Joule/second). In electricity, 1 watt (W) is the amount of electrical energy transferred when 1 ampere of current flows between points with a potential difference of 1 volt.

Wavelength and Amplitude

When a current (AC) progresses in a sinusoidal waveform as shown in **Figure 17**, the distance between two consecutive corresponding points in the wave (red arrows) denotes the wavelength (λ). Amplitude is the distance of the highest point of the wave from a zero point (green arrow). Amplitude may also be measured as peak to peak (purple arrow), which is the distance between the highest and the lowest points of the wave.

Static Electricity

Static electricity is the property of a system, caused by the discharge of the "electrical charges" of one system to another, when they are not in

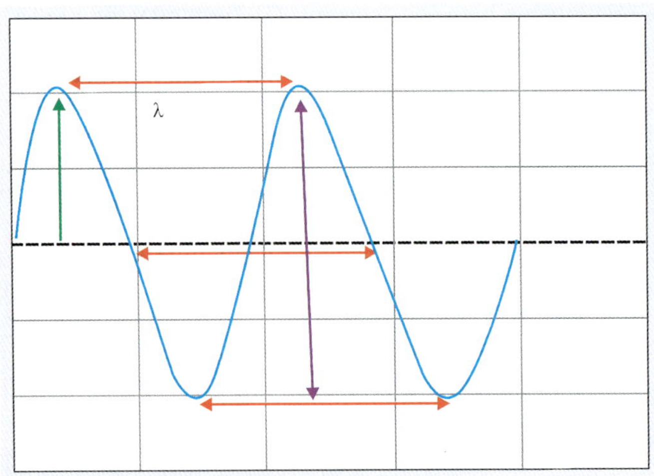

Fig. 17: Wavelength and amplitude.

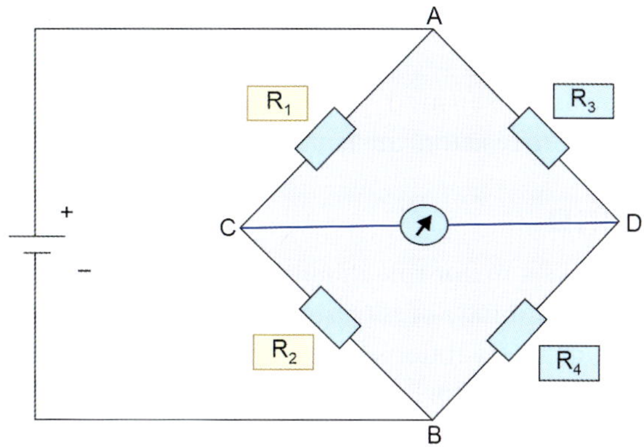

Fig. 18: Wheatstone bridge.

equilibrium. However, when a current flows from one system to another, there is no net gain or loss to any system.

Wheatstone Bridge (Fig. 18)

The principle of Wheatstone bridge is used in many clinical measurements and monitoring like invasive pressure, cardiac output, temperature, etc.

- In modern medical equipment, transducers form an important component. Transducer is by definition a device, which modifies the signal of one form of energy to another. An arterial pulse is sensed by a diaphragm as a mechanical energy signal, which is converted by a transducer to electrical energy and then by a cathode ray oscilloscope to visual signals for this to be displayed in a monitor as a waveform.
- Mechanical energy is usually sensed as "pressure" change by devices known as "strain gauges", or the "diaphragms". This pressure change leads to change in the electrical resistance of the system, which is measured by a device such as a Wheatstone bridge.
- Basically, a Wheatstone bridge is a device to measure unknown resistance in a system. It was originally developed to measure and calibrate resistance in equipment such as ammeters and voltmeters. Modern digital equipment may or may not use Wheatstone bridges; however, these are still helpful to measure very small amount of resistance.
- The bridge consists of two series-parallel arrangements of four resistors in a diamond shape **(Fig. 18)**. When the resistance of three resistors is known along with the voltage, the resistance of the fourth resistor can be calculated using the following formula:

  $$R_1/R_3 = R_2/R_4 = 1$$

  Hence, if R_4 is the unknown resistance

  $$R_4 = R_2 \times R_3/R_1$$

Wheatstone bridges are typically applied in transducers that may include strain gauges also known as "piezo-resistive sensors", light-dependent resistors (photoresistive sensors), potentiometers or positional sensors and thermistors, which are resistors measuring temperature.

ULTRASOUND

The ultrasound plays a major role in anesthesia, pain, and critical care. The rapidly evolving technology of ultrasound in anesthesia, leads away from the typically "blind" interventions based on anatomical landmarks, done at the risk of their very many variations to the normal. Ultrasound guidance is becoming standard practice, and the future generations of anesthetists need to develop a thorough understanding of this technology and practical skills. It should be part of the core training of every anesthetist.

Basic Physics of Ultrasound (see Chapter 10)

The discovery of piezoelectric effect and its utility in construction of high-frequency mechanical vibrating sources coupled with high-frequency electronic drives provided the basis of ultrasound.

Sound is produced when mechanical energy travels through matter as a wave, producing alternate compression and rarefaction. Ultrasound imaging is based on the scattering of sound energy by interfaces formed of materials of different properties. The amplitude of reflected energy is used to generate ultrasound images. Frequencies used for ultrasound are higher than those in the audible range, and typically vary from 2 to 15 MHz for diagnostic procedures.

Propagation of Sound

Ultrasound transducers work on the principle of piezoelectricity. Within the transducer are arrays of piezoelectric crystals, which have the property of changing shape when an electrical voltage is applied. Application of a voltage enables electrical energy to be converted into sound energy.

Modern systems have arrays that are structured to allow the sound waves generated by one crystal to interact with those from other crystals; consequently, the sound waves can be amplified or diminished.

The sound wave is propagated through the body tissues and interactions occur between the wave and the tissues. If the sound is transmitted through a homogeneous structure, the principal interaction is absorption of the sound. The rate of absorption is least in fluids and greatest in solid structures.

The majority of body tissues are not homogeneous and the sound wave strikes a series of interfaces. At each interface, the wave can be reflected or refracted.

Refraction is usually insignificant. The waves that are reflected back to the transducer strike the piezoelectric crystal. The crystal converts sound into electrical energy. The distance of the reflector can be calculated by calculating the time taken for the sound to travel from and to the transducer. The amplitude of the reflected sound can be used to calculate the reflectivity of the object.

The proportion of sound reflected or transmitted at an interface depends upon the difference in acoustic impedance between the tissues forming the interface. The acoustic impedance is measured in Rayls and is the product of the density of the tissue and the velocity with which it propagates sound. Air and bone have different impedances compared to other tissues; therefore, at such interfaces, the majority of sound is reflected **(Table 7)**. Hence, ultrasound cannot be used to image deep to bone or air.

High-frequency transducers produce higher resolution images but the sound waves are absorbed more as they pass through the body. Low-frequency transducers have greater penetration, but poor resolution.

Resolution refers to the ability of the device to differentiate two closely situated objects as distinct structures. Axial resolution is measured along the axis of the ultrasound beam in its direction of propagation. It is directly proportional to the ultrasound frequency. Transverse resolution is measured at 90° to axial resolution. It depends on the width of the pulse beam. Axial resolution is always superior to transverse resolution.

Features of an Ultrasound Image

Recognizing structures on ultrasound takes practice and a good knowledge of the anatomy is a big help. What follows is a brief description of some of the features that make up the image.

Presentation: In almost all applications, the top of the screen represents the probe and as you look further down the screen you are seeing progressively deeper tissues.

Depth: The depth to which you can see is normally shown on a scale running alongside the image. This can be adjusted using the depth adjustor, which will

TABLE 7: Acoustic impedance of different materials.

Material	*Acoustic impedance (Rayls)*	*Typical appearance*
Air	400	Readily reflects echoes (hyperechoic)
Fat	1,380,000	Bright or dark (hypoechoic) subcutaneous fat typically dark
Fluid	1,430,000	Generally dark (anechoic) pus can be bright or dark
Muscle	1,630,000	Moderately reflective (hypoechoic)
Bone	7,800,000	Highly reflective (hyperechoic)

be a prominent control on any scanner. The maximum depth is dependent on the frequency, with lower frequencies penetrating much further, but at the cost of reduced resolution. Hence, lower frequency (2.5 MHz) used in transthoracic echo for visualization of deeper structures. High-frequency probes using frequencies of around 10 MHz are used in transesophageal echocardiography (TEE).

Typical Appearance of Normal Tissue (Table 7)

- Skin appears smooth and bright (echogenic, hyperechoic, highly reflective).
- Fat can be bright or dark (hypoechoic), but subcutaneous fat is typically dark.
- Muscle is also dark, when viewed in cross-section. In long section, sound is reflected back by the muscle fibers and the internal structure of the muscle can be easily seen.
- Fluid, be it blood, effusion, or cyst is generally black (anechoic), though thicker fluids such as pus can be bright or dark.
- Tendons are typically bright, but this varies with their orientation relative to the probe.
- Nerves' appearance is similar to that of tendons. They are typically identified in relation to the relevant anatomy and vasculature.
- Bone appears as a particularly bright line due to the dramatic difference in acoustic impedance between bone and soft tissue. High-frequency ultrasound does not penetrate bone effectively and therefore the screen is generally black deep to the bone.

Components of Ultrasound Imaging

Transducer

- It converts electrical to mechanical energy and vice versa.
- *It serves two functions:*
  1. It converts electrical energy provided by the transmitter into acoustic pulses directed into the patient.
  2. It receives the reflected echoes.

Receiver and Processor

Receiver and processor detect and amplify the backscattered energy and manipulate the reflected signals for display.

Image Display—Modes

- Earliest A-mode devices displayed the voltage produced across the transducer as a vertical deflection on the face of the oscilloscope. Only the position and strength of a reflecting structure could be recorded.

- M-mode ultrasound displays echo amplitude and shows the position of moving reflectors. It represents movement of structures over time. It is used in the evaluation of cardiac chambers, valves, and vessel walls.
- The 2D mode or two-dimensional mode gives a 2D cross-sectional view of the underlying structure and is made up of numerous B mode (brightness mode) scan lines. It is commonly used for ultrasonography (USG) abdomen and Echo.
- Color flow Doppler imaging mode, the velocity, and direction of blood flow are depicted in a color map superimposed on a 2D image.
- Pulse wave Doppler where the Doppler signal arising from a specific position in the scanned tissue is analyzed to depict velocity and direction of flow.
- Continuous wave Doppler mode where a part of the transducer is continuously transmitting, and a part is continuously receiving the Doppler signal along a single line that is placed on the 2D image.

Doppler Ultrasound

The Doppler principle is the phenomenon in which sound transmitted from a moving object is perceived by a stationary observer to be of a different frequency depending upon the velocity and direction of travel. Thus, changes in frequency (frequency shift) can be used to calculate velocity of movement of blood.

Uses of Ultrasound in Anesthesia

Regional Anesthesia (see Chapter 10)

Procedures include:

1. Peripheral nerve blocks
2. Central neuraxial blockade in children and difficult anatomical situations in adults
3. *Chronic pain procedures:* Caudal space injections for low backaches, facet joint injections, lumbar sympathetic blocks, and celiac plexus and stellate ganglion blocks are a few procedures utilizing USG guidance. The advantages of using USG guidance are as follows:
   - Direct visualization of the neural structures
   - Visualization of related structures like blood vessels and tendons
   - Guidance of needle under real-time visualization
   - Avoidance of complications such as intravascular or intraneuronal injection
   - Monitors the spread of the local anesthetic.
   - Allows repositioning of the needle after an initial injection to allow better delivery of local anesthetics to areas, which may not be blocked by a single dose.
   - Can be used in patients with poor twitch response to nerve stimulation.

Transesophageal Echocardiography

Transesophageal echocardiography is used in anesthesia for the following procedures:

1. Assess adequacy of prosthetic valve replacement.
2. Diagnose ongoing ischemia by detecting fresh regional wall abnormalities.
3. Assess volume status in patients with hemodynamic instability.
4. Sensitive tool for early detection of pulmonary embolism
5. Transesophageal stress echocardiography to detect coronary artery disease and viability

Vascular Access

- Central venous cannulation
- Peripheral venous cannulation (obese patients)
- Arterial cannulation.

Advantage of using ultrasound imaging for gaining vascular access:

- Decrease number of "blind" attempts
- Easy identification of variable anatomy
- Avoidance of inadvertent punctures
- Improve overall success rates

Other Applications of Ultrasound

- Assessment of subglottic diameter to calculate appropriate ETT size
- Laryngeal ultrasound to detect patients at risk for postextubation stridor
- Applied to visualize cerebrospinal fluid (CSF) leak in case of postdural puncture headache, and for application of epidural blood patch under real-time depiction
- *Focused assessment with sonography in trauma (FAST):* This is useful in blunt abdominal trauma, stable penetrating trauma, and assessment of the degree of intraperitoneal free fluid.
- *RUSH Examination—Rapid Ultrasound for Shock and Hypotension:* This bedside protocol will enable the clinician to assess and effectively treat patients in shock and who are critically ill. This protocol consists of:
- *To determine the cardiac status:*
  - Detecting cardiac tamponade
  - Left ventricular contractility
  - Right ventricular size
- *Effective intravascular volume status:*
  - Fullness of IVC and internal jugular veins
  - Internal bleeding
  - Decrease in venous return

- *Assess the major vessels:*
    - Aortic aneurysm and dissection
    - Thromboembolic occlusion

SUGGESTED READING

1. Davis PD, Kenny NCG. Basic Physics and Measurements in Anaesthesia, 5th edition. London: Elsevier; 1995.
2. Gilbert-Kawai ET, Wiitenberg MD. Essential Equations for Anaesthesia, 1st edition. Cambridge: Cambridge University Press; 2014.
3. Hill DW. Physics Applied to Anaesthesia, 2nd edition. London: Elsevier; 2013.
4. Jain PN, Ranganthan P. Ultrasound in anaesthesia. Indian J Anaesth. 2007;51(3): 176-83.
5. Magee P, Tooley M. The Physics, Clinical Measurement and Equipment of Anaesthesia Practice for the FRCA, 2nd edition. Oxford: Oxford University Press; 2011.
6. Middleton B, Phillips J, Thomas R, Stacey S. Physics in Anaesthesia, 1st edition. Banbury, UK; Scion Publishing; 2012.
7. Qudaisat Y. Coanda effect as an explanation for unequal ventilation of the lungs in an intubated patient? Br J Anaesth. 2008;100(6):859-60.
8. Seif D, Perera P, Mailhot T, Riley D, Mandavia D. Bedside ultrasound in resuscitation and the rapid ultrasound in shock protocol. Crit Care Res Pract. 2012;2012:1-4.
9. Smith T, Pinnock C, Lin T. Fundamentals of Anaesthesia, 3rd edition. Cambridge: Cambridge University Press; 2009.

CHAPTER 2

Medical Gas Supply, Vacuum, and Scavenging

Yasodananda K Areti

"If anything can go wrong, it will"

INTRODUCTION

Though infrequent several accidents and mishaps have been reported during the use of medical gases. Every precaution possible must be taken to ensure that such accidents do not occur, and adequate backup measures must be drilled into the system in the event of such mishaps.

In the United States, Department of Transportation (DOT) published requirements for manufacturing, marking, labeling, filling, transportation, storage, handling, and maintenance of medical gas cylinders and containers. The Department of Labor (DOL) and the Occupational Safety and Health Administration (OSHA) regulate matters affecting safety and health of employees in all industries. The National Fire Protection Association (NFPA), the Compressed Gas Association (CGA), Canadian Standards Association (CSA), and the International Standards Organization (ISO) have published a number of standards, and many regulatory agencies have made adherence to these standards mandatory. The handling of compressed gases in India is governed by Gas Cylinder Rules (amended in 2010), and Bureau of Indian Standards.

Medical grade gas is supplied to the operating room via two delivery mechanisms, *central supply,* and *portable cylinders.* Most anesthetizing locations will have access to a central supply of the three most commonly used medical gases: oxygen, nitrous oxide, and air. These and all other gases may also be supplied via gas cylinders, most commonly the "E" type cylinder, mounted on the anesthesia machine. A waste anesthetic gas (WAG) scavenging system and a medical suction system for surgical and anesthetic use are also provided centrally.

MEDICAL GASES AND SUPPLY

Oxygen

Medical grade oxygen (99% pure or greater) is a necessity in any operating room. Oxygen is synthesized commercially by first liquefying compressed air (Joule-Kelvin Effect). The boiling points of oxygen (90.2°K) and nitrogen

(77.4°K) are different. Hence, oxygen is separated from liquid air by using fractional distillation. Nitrogen evaporates first leaving liquid oxygen (LOX), which is then evaporated. Oxygen is dried and purified and is supplied as compressed gas in cylinders at ambient temperature. As compressed gases are released to flow meters through cylinder valves, the temperature of gas falls due to adiabatic expansion. This phenomenon can potentially lead to formation of ice crystals if any moisture is left in the gases, leading to interruption of gas flow. Hence, drying the gases before filling cylinders is important.

Medical oxygen is stored as compressed gas in banks of large cylinders (H-type), or LOX bank. A hospital should have at least a 2-day supply of oxygen on-hand, and a backup of at least 1-day supply. Consequently, the system chosen and its capacity will depend on the oxygen demands of the hospital. Even at peak use, the pressure across the network should not result in a larger drop in pressure of >5 psig from the source to the outlet.

Liquid Oxygen

Oxygen can be supplied in cryogenic containers containing LOX **(Fig. 1)**. LOX, though stored as liquid, is used primarily as a gas. It is less bulky and less costly than the equivalent capacity of high-pressure gaseous storage. 1 L of LOX expands to 860 L of gas at 20°C. The physical properties of oxygen, which govern the storage and delivery of LOX, are shown in **Box 1**.

Because the temperature difference between the product and the surrounding environment is substantial (the temperature of LOX has to be

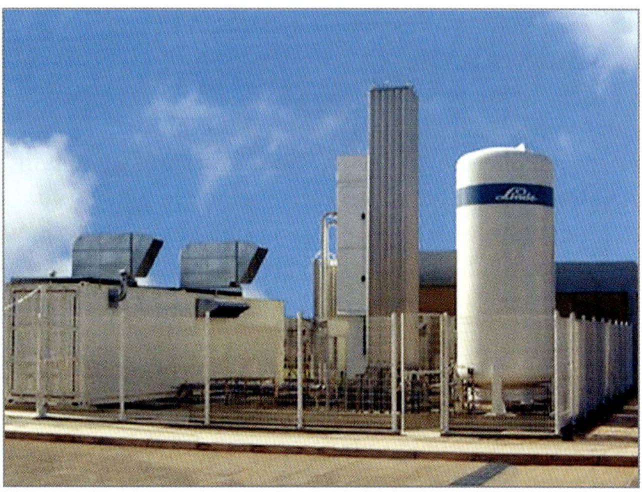

Fig. 1: Liquid oxygen plant (Linde CryoPlants Ltd.).
Source: https://en.wikipedia.org/wiki/Cryogenic_oxygen_plant.

BOX 1: Physical properties of oxygen.

- Boiling point @ 1 atmosphere: 183.0°C (90°K)
- Critical temperature: –118.4°C
- Critical pressure: 729.1 psia (49.6 atm)
- Expansion ratio, liquid to gas, boiling point to 20°C: 1–860.

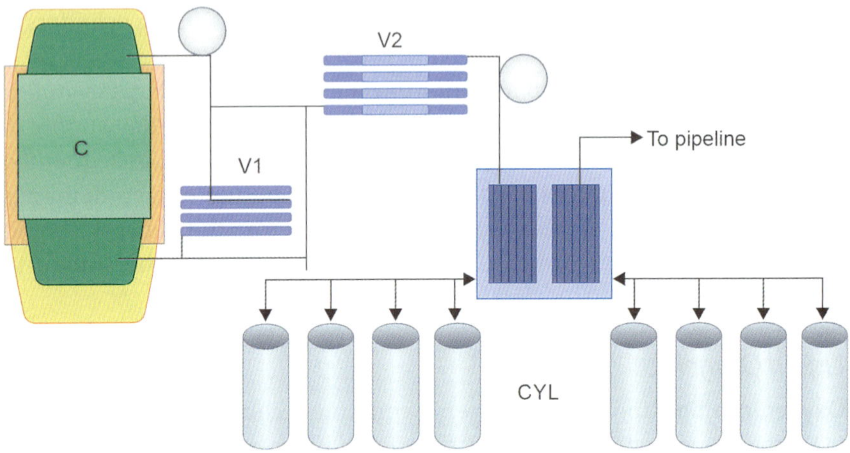

Fig. 2: Medical gas supply to pipeline.
(C: cryogenic container; CYL: cylinder bank; V1 and V2: vaporizer)

maintained below its critical temperature of –118°C), even in the winter, keeping LOX insulated from the surrounding heat is essential. The product also requires special equipment for handling and storage to prevent cold burns for the workers. A typical storage system consists of:

- A cryogenic storage tank
- One or more vaporizers
- A pressure control and pressure relief system, and
- Piping necessary for the fill, vaporization, and supply functions **(Fig. 2)**.

The cryogenic tank is constructed, in principle, like a thermos bottle. There is an inner vessel surrounded by an outer vessel. Between the vessels is an annular space that contains an insulating medium, from which all the air has been removed. This space keeps heat away from the LOX held in the inner vessel.

The liquid oxygen is converted into a gaseous state in the vaporizers. A pressure control manifold then controls the gas pressure that is fed to the pipelines. A backup system may comprise another smaller-sized LOX container or manifold of oxygen cylinders. The backup system should have a separate feedline to the pipeline network to lessen the risk of interrupted supply.

Oxygen Concentrator

Oxygen concentrators are devices, which can be used as a primary source of oxygen in remote locations to feed pipelines. Oxygen is generated onsite using pressure swing adsorber technology. Oxygen in the atmospheric air is concentrated by adsorption of nitrogen by a molecular sieve (zeolite). Oxygen produced by this method has a concentration of only 93% ± 3%. Pressurized air passes through a bed of zeolite contained usually in two containers. As one container adsorbs nitrogen, the other is purged of adsorbed nitrogen and the zeolite is regenerated. The adsorbent has a high affinity for water. Hence, design should include adequate purges, low dead space and heat exchangers. The beds should be sealed so that atmospheric moisture cannot seep into the zeolite. The output concentration of oxygen should be monitored carefully to ensure delivery of adequate oxygen to the pipelines. The size of the adsorption beds determines the output. They must always have a pressurized reservoir that is large enough to cope with peak flows. Portable oxygen concentrators are also available and are quite popular for home oxygen therapy.

Nitrous Oxide

Nitrous oxide is often provided for use as an anesthetic gas. Nitrous oxide is synthesized commercially by heating ammonium nitrate and stored as a liquid at room temperature because the critical temperature of this gas is 36.5°C. Nitrous oxide is usually stored in two banks of large H-cylinders, which are cross-connected via an autoswitching manifold using two-stage pressure regulator (similar to that of oxygen banks). The banks usually have a smaller number of cylinders compared with oxygen supply because of the higher content of liquefied gas and lower consumption of nitrous oxide. As nitrous oxide becomes vaporized from a liquid to a gas, heat will be absorbed from the surrounding. This can lead to the formation of frost on the outside of a gas cylinder.

Medical Air

Air is the natural atmosphere of the earth, a nonflammable, colorless, odorless gas that consists of a mixture of gaseous elements (nitrogen, oxygen, water vapor, a small amount of carbon dioxide and traces of many other constituents). Medical air can be provided from a manifold of cylinders or from a central compressor plant. Usually, two compressors are used, which can run alternately or concurrently depending on the demand. This also ensures that during servicing or repairing, the supply is not interrupted. Air from the intake to the compressors is drawn through a filter and silencer. There usually is an air cooler to cool the compressed air. The air then passes through a nonreturn valve into a large reservoir to maintain a constant air pressure. After leaving the reservoir, the air is cleaned by passing it through baffled separators and filters to remove particulate impurities like oil droplets. The air is then passed through two driers containing a desiccant to remove any excess humidity. Finally, the air is passed through a bacterial filter to ensure removal of any contaminants.

MEDICAL GAS CYLINDERS

Medical gases are stored in metal-alloy cylinders of varying sizes. **Tables 1 and 2** indicate the color codes, state in cylinders, and service pressure for different medical gases. Cylinders are made of aluminum or steel alloys.

TABLE 1: Medical gas cylinders.

Gas	*Formula*	*Color (US)*	*Color (international)*	*PSI at 21°C*	*State in cylinder*	*E-cylinder capacity (L)*
Oxygen	O_2	Green	White shoulder and black body	1,900–2,200	Gas	660
Carbon dioxide	CO_2	Gray	Gray	838	Gas and liquid <31°C	1,590
Nitrous oxide	N_2O	Blue	Blue	745	Gas and liquid <37°C	1,600
Helium	He	Brown	Brown	1,600–2,000	Gas	500
Nitrogen	N_2	Black	Black	1,800–2,200	Gas	660
Air		Yellow	White and black shoulder	1,800	Gas	600

TABLE 2: Size and capacities of various gases in commonly used cylinders.

		Oxygen		*Nitrous oxide*		*Carbon dioxide*	
Type	*Dimensions (mm)*	*Water capacity*	*Gas content*†	*Tare weight*	*Gas content*†	*Tare weight*	*Gas content*†
C	430 × 89	1.2 L	170 L	2.0 kg	450 L	2.0 kg	450 L
D	535 × 102	2.32 L	340 L	3.4 kg	900 L		
E	865 × 102	4.7 L	680 L	5.4 kg	1,800 L	5.4 kg	1,800 L
F	930 × 140	9.43 L	1,360 L	14.5 kg	3,600 L		
G/M*	1,320 × 178	23.6 L	3,400 L	34.5 kg	9,000 L		
J/H*	1,520 × 229	47.2 L	6,800 L	68.9 kg	18,000 L		

(*: alternate nomenclature. The valves may be different, and the contents are slightly different; †: gas content when full).

The parts of cylinder are body, shoulder, neck, and head (valve). Each cylinder is tested by visual inspection and with hydraulic stretch test to assess its integrity when subjected to test pressures 1.66 times the service pressure. Each cylinder should be permanently stamped on the shoulder to indicate the contents, the service pressure, serial number, manufacturer's symbol, owner's symbol, and the test date (original test date and retest date) and the mark of the testing facility.

Filling the Cylinder

The pressure inside a cylinder may vary with ambient temperature. In order to prevent build-up of excessive pressure, a cylinder should not be filled above the service pressure stamped on the cylinder for compressed gases. The filling limit on the cylinders containing liquefied gases is based on the filling ratio or filling density, which is the percent ratio of weight of a gas in cylinder to the weight of water the cylinder would hold at 60°F. The filling density of nitrous oxide and carbon dioxide is 68%.

Safety Pressure Release

Every cylinder is fitted with a safety pressure release device to vent the contents into atmosphere if inside pressure increases to a dangerous level. There are several relief valve models used for this purpose:

- The venting orifice is closed with a disk that ruptures at a given pressure.
- A fusible plug (woods metal), which melts at high temperatures
- A spring-loaded pressure relief valve

In "pin-indexed" valves, this device is present just below the conical depression for the screw clamp and hence care should be taken to prevent any inadvertent damage while mounting the cylinder on the anesthesia machine.

Devices to Open or Close a Cylinder

Large cylinders are fitted with "hand-wheel" to open or close the valves. Small cylinders come with a spindle valve and the spindle can be opened or closed with a wrench or a handle. This wrench is usually fixed to the anesthesia machine to prevent misplacement. While using these wrenches, one must be careful not to handle the hexagonal gland nut that fixes the spindle valve to the cylinder.

Contents of a Cylinder

The contents of a cylinder containing compressed gases like oxygen can be calculated by using Boyle's law, using the pressure inside the cylinder and the water capacity of the cylinder.

$$P1 \times V1 = P2 \times V2;\ V1 - \frac{P2 \times V2}{P1}$$

(P1: atmospheric pressure; V1: volume of oxygen available at atmospheric pressure; P2: pressure in the cylinder; V2: water capacity of the cylinder or volume of oxygen in compressed state)

In type "E" cylinder with a water capacity of 4.7 L, if the pressure gauge reads 100 atmospheres (1,470 psig) then approximate amount of oxygen available (V1) to be used at 1 atmosphere will be:

$$V1 = \frac{100 \times 4.7}{1} = 470\ \text{L or } V1 = \frac{1{,}470 \times 4.7}{14.7} = 470\ \text{L}$$

For all practical purposes, if one learns to read the pressure in the cylinder in atmospheric pressures (the number labeled as kPa × 100), then multiplying this with 4.7 (or even with 5 for approximate values) will give an estimate of the contents of type "E" cylinder for compressed gases. Similarly, the water capacity of type "H" bulk cylinder is 47.2 L. If cylinder pressure reads 100 atmospheres, then each cylinder would contain 4,720 L.

The contents of a cylinder containing liquefied gases (nitrous oxide and carbon dioxide) cannot be estimated by measuring the pressure inside the cylinder, since the pressure remains nearly constant till all the liquid is evaporated. However, they can be estimated using Avogadro's principle. Molecular weight of nitrous oxide and carbon dioxide is same and is 44. As per Avogadro's hypothesis, 44 g would occupy a volume of 24 L at room temperature and pressure (RTP) (20°C, 1 atm; corrected for temperature as per Charles' law). Hence, a liter of nitrous oxide weighs about 1.8 g. The actual weight of the gas in the cylinder should be estimated by the difference between the actual weight and the tare weight of the cylinder. This weight in grams divided with 1.8 (one may use 2 for approximation and ease of calculation) would give us an estimate of the contents of the cylinder. This aspect is particularly useful for the laparoscopic surgeons and their teams to have an idea of the contents of carbon dioxide cylinders prior to starting the surgery.

Valves

The bulk cylinders supplying the pipelines are fitted with bullnose valves with noninterchangeable screw thread system. In order to prevent use of wrong gas the threads on the cylinder should match the threads on the nut. These threads can be either outside or inside the cylinder outlet **(Figs. 3A and B)**. This is different from diameter index safety system (DISS) discussed below **(Fig. 4)**. The type "E" or other type cylinders that fit as backup on anesthesia machine are fitted with pin indexed, spindle valve **(Figs. 5 and 6)**.

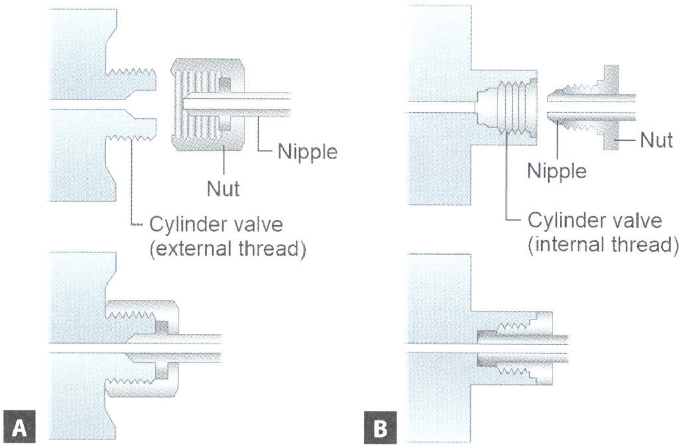

Figs. 3A and B: Valve outlet connections for large cylinders. The threads of the valve outlet must match with the threads on the nut. When the nut is tightened, the nipple seats against the valve outlet. (A) The threads are on the outside of the cylinder valve outlet and the nut screws over the valve outlet; (B) The valve outlet thread is internal so that the nut screws into the outlet.

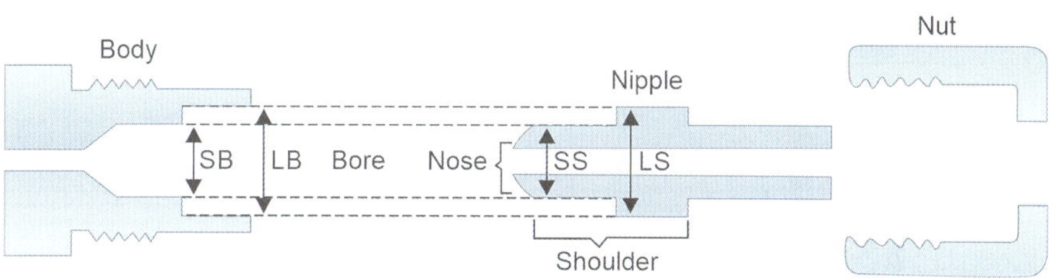

Fig. 4: Diameter index safety system.
(LB: large bore; LS: large shoulder; SB: small bore; SS: small shoulder).
Source: Dorsch JA, Dorsch SE. Understanding Anesthesia Equipment, 5th edition. Philadelphia: Lippincott Williams & Wilkins; 2008.

MANIFOLD AND PIPELINE NETWORK

Normally, the main gas supply to the anesthesia machine is the hospital pipeline system, delivered at approximately 50–55 pounds per square inch gauge. The oxygen supply to the pipeline supply may be from one of the following sources:

- Primary LOX tank with smaller secondary LOX tank as a backup
- Primary LOX tank with a manifold of compressed gas cylinders as backup
- Two banks of compressed gas cylinders with a backup of smaller bank of compressed gas cylinders

The high-pressure source is connected to the pipeline through a two-stage pressure regulator. Where a manifold of cylinders is used, only one

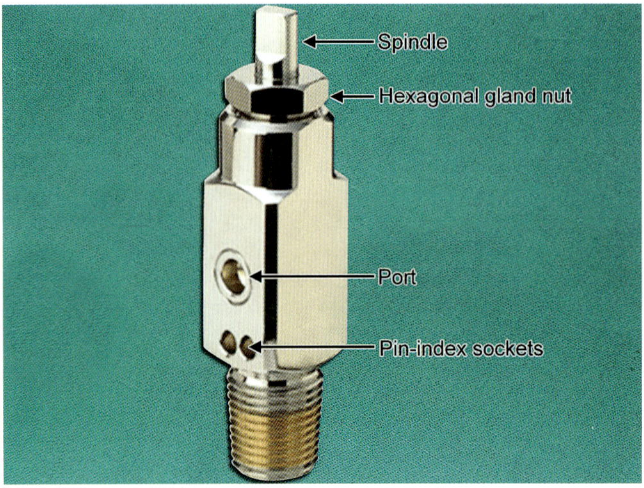

Fig. 5: Parts of spindle valve.

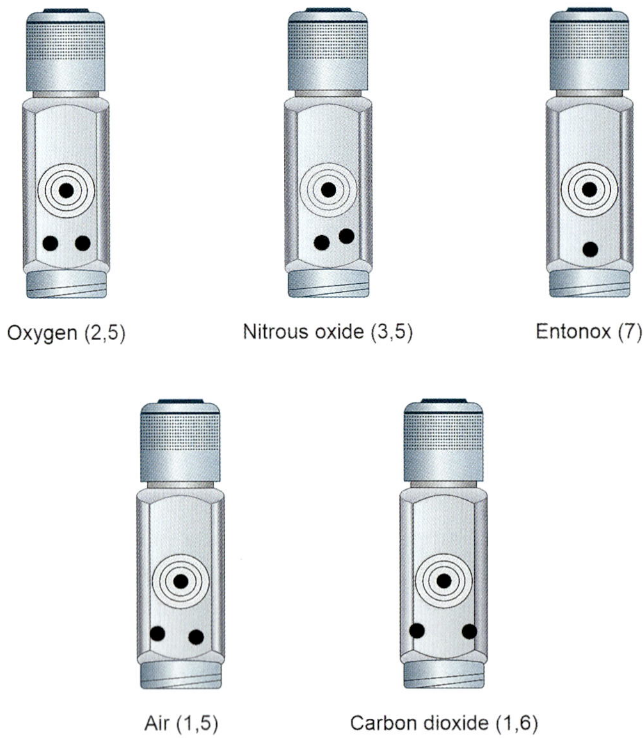

Fig. 6: Pin index safety system for different gases. Two pins in the hanger yoke of anesthesia machine are aligned with two corresponding holes on the cylinder head in order to prevent mounting of a wrong cylinder. Exception being entonox which has one pin on yoke and corresponding hole on cylinder.

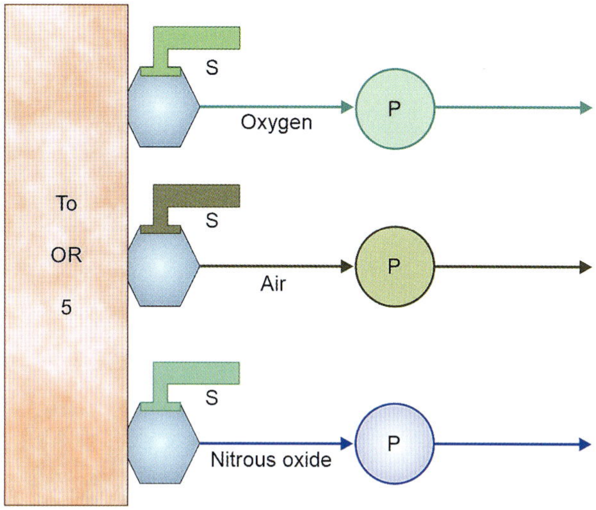

Fig. 7: Pipeline shut off system.

of the two banks supplies the pipeline at any time. When this bank reaches exhaustion, the second bank automatically kicks in. The status of the banks is indicated by visual indicators at the source as well as at a manned control station to enable a prompt change of empty cylinders.

The supply and the manifolds are usually located outside the hospital or free ventilated area. From the manifold, the gases are carried to various points of care through network of pipelines. The pipelines are made of copper. These pipelines should be clearly marked with the label of the gas, color coding, and the direction of gas flow. The pipeline network consists of main pipes, risers (to transport gases from floor to floor) and branches (transport across the floor) to individual areas of the hospital. Each area should have pressure monitors and shut off valves to conduct repairs and maintenance without having to shut down the entire system **(Fig. 7)**.

Outlets

The pipelines end in terminal wall outlets with color-coded plates. These outlets may be either noninterchangeable quick coupling outlets or DISS outlets.

Quick Connectors (Fig. 8)

Quick connectors (automatic quick couplers valves, quick connects, quick-connect fittings, and quick couplers) allow apparatus (hoses, flow meters, etc.) to be connected or disconnected by a single action by using one or both hands without the use of tools or undue force. Quick connectors are more convenient than DISS fittings but tend to leak more. Each quick

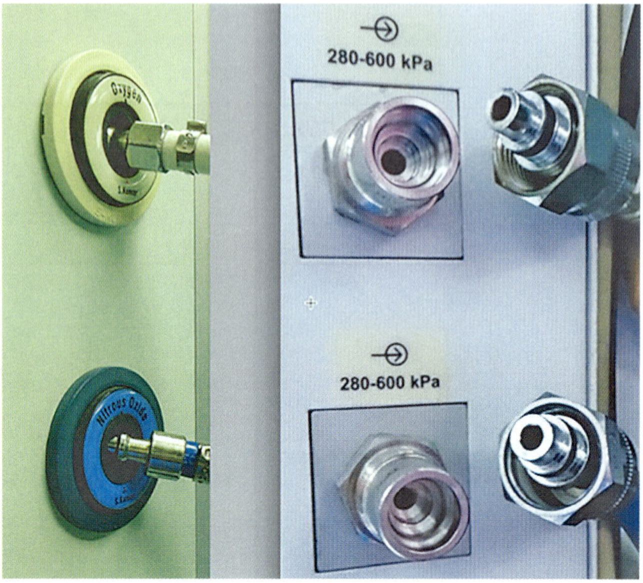

Fig. 8: Quick coupler on the left. Diameter index safety system connectors on right.
Courtesy: Prof M Ravishankar, modified by Mr Muralidhar Areti.

connector consists of a pair of gas-specific male and female components. A releasable spring mechanism locks the components together. Hoses and other equipment are prevented from being inserted into an incorrect outlet by using different shapes and/or different spacing of mating portions.

The Diameter Index Safety System

The DISS was developed to provide noninterchangeable connections for medical gas lines at pressures of 1,380 kPa (200 psi) or less. Each DISS connector consists of a body, nipple, and nut combination **(Figs. 4 and 8)**. There are two concentric and specific bores in the body and two concentric and specific shoulders on the nipple. The small bore (SB) mates with the small shoulder (SS), and the large bore (LB) mates with the large shoulder (LS). To achieve noninterchangeability between different connectors, the two diameters on each part vary in opposite directions so that as one diameter (LS and LB) increases, the other (SS and SB) decreases. These dimensions are unique for each gas and only properly mated parts will fit together and allow the threads to engage.

Safe Use of Cylinders

- The personnel handling the cylinders should be trained adequately.
- In order to prevent injury, gas cylinders must always be properly secured and stored in a cool environment that is protected from fire and open

flame. They should not be subjected to temperatures above 54°C or below -7°C.

- Care should be taken to ensure that cylinders are never dropped or rolled, since damage to a pressurized cylinder can lead to the creation of a fatal projectile.
- They should not be transfilled by the user.
- The cylinders should be kept closed and covered at all times except when they are in use.
- They should never be draped.
- They should be labeled full or empty and stored separately.
- A cylinder should always be opened slowly in order to prevent rapid raise in temperature due to adiabatic expansion.

OTHER MEDICAL GASES OF INTEREST TO ANESTHESIOLOGIST

Entonox

Entonox is a mixture of 50% oxygen and 50% nitrous oxide, stored in cylinders at a pressure around 2,000 psig. Though the critical temperature of nitrous oxide is 36.5°C, in a mixture of gases such as entonox, nitrous oxide remains in gaseous phase. This is sometimes referred to as pseudocritical temperature, or Poynting effect. However, at a temperature below -5.5°C, a liquid phase containing 20% oxygen and 80% nitrous oxide may form below the gas. In order to prevent delivery of hypoxic mixture it is recommended that entonox cylinders should be stored at temperatures above 10°C. Entonox is used mostly for obstetric analgesia and dental analgesia. It is also used for wound dressings and during transport of patients with long bone fractures without any other injuries. It is usually self-administered under supervision of medical or paramedical personnel through a two-stage pressure regulator and a demand valve.

Nitric Oxide

The role of inhaled nitric oxide (iNO) for clinical use has increased remarkably over the last decade. The discovery of iNO's role in pulmonary vascular tone led to a flood of research from basic science to large randomized clinical trials in patients of all ages, resulting in thousands of publications. In 1992, the journal "Science" named nitric oxide the ''Molecule of the Year''. Several researchers received a Nobel Prize in medicine and physiology for their work with nitric oxide in 1998. The only Food and Drug Administration-approved indication for iNO is for the treatment of term neonates with hypoxic respiratory failure associated with pulmonary hypertension as a means to improve oxygenation.

Nitric oxide is supplied as a gaseous blend of nitric oxide (800 ppm) and nitrogen. It is supplied in a nonliquefied form at a cylinder pressure of 2,000 psig at 21°C. Cylinders are constructed of an aluminum or steel alloy. It is administered into the ventilator breathing circuit through a monitoring unit (NOx Box, Nodomo unit, iNO-vent) which operates at 55–60 psig. The most commonly used initial dose is 5–20 ppm by inhalation. Monitoring the levels of inspired nitric oxide, nitrogen dioxide levels, and methemoglobin levels is essential. Weaning should be achieved gradually in decrements of 5 ppm over 6–8 hours.

Heliox

Helium and oxygen mixtures (heliox) have been used for medicinal purposes since 1934. Heliox has been studied and reported to be effective in a variety of respiratory conditions, such as upper airway obstruction, status asthmaticus, decompression sickness, postextubation stridor, bronchiolitis, and acute respiratory distress syndrome. Helium, an inert gas, is odorless and tasteless, and it does not support combustion or react with biologic membranes. Helium is 86% less dense (0.179 g/L) than room air (1.293 g/L). It is seven times lighter than nitrogen, and eight times less dense than oxygen. The lower density of helium reduces the Reynolds number associated with flow through the airways.

Heliox converts areas of extreme turbulence and makes these areas less turbulent. Additionally, heliox converts some areas of turbulence to areas of more efficient laminar flow. Hence, heliox mixtures have the potential to decrease work of breathing in patients with increased airway resistance. However, heliox does not "treat" airway resistance. Heliox also increases the deposition of inhaled particles to the distal airways in patients with severe asthma.

Heliox is commercially available and supplied at the point of care as compressed medical gas cylinders in sizes H, G, and E. Helium and oxygen typically are blended to percentage concentrations of 80/20, 70/30, and 60/40, respectively. Gas regulators manufactured specifically for helium must be used to deliver the gas safely and accurately. The mixture can be administered to the patient via either an endotracheal tube or face mask with reservoir bag.

Xenon

Xenon is a chemical element with symbol Xe and atomic number 54. It is a colorless, dense, odorless noble gas, and inert gas that occurs in the Earth's atmosphere in trace amounts. Xenon has been used as a general anesthetic. Although it is expensive, anesthesia machines that can deliver xenon are about to appear on the European market, because advances in recovery and recycling of xenon have made it economically viable.

Xenon is a high-affinity glycine-site N-methyl D-aspartate (NMDA) receptor antagonist. However, it lacks neurotoxicity of ketamine and nitrous oxide. Xenon inhibits nicotinic acetylcholine α-4 β-2 receptors which contribute to spinally mediated analgesia.

Xenon is a competitive inhibitor of the serotonin 5-HT3 receptor. This action reduces anesthesia-emergent nausea and vomiting.

Xenon gives rapid induction and recovery, due to its low blood/gas partition coefficient (0.15). Xenon has a minimum alveolar concentration of 72%, making it 44% more potent than N_2O as an anesthetic. Xenon is not a greenhouse gas and so it is also viewed as environmentally friendly. Xenon vented into the atmosphere is being returned to its original source, so no environmental impact is likely.

Xenon induces robust cardioprotection and neuroprotection. It was added as an ingredient of the ventilation mix for a newborn baby, whose life chances were otherwise much compromised.

VACUUM

A vacuum is a volume of space that is essentially empty of matter, such that its gaseous pressure is much less than atmospheric pressure (negative pressure). Vacuums are commonly used to produce suction. Suctioning is an important part of anesthesia practice to remove and/or collect solids, gases, and liquids from the patient, airway devices, and the patient's environment.

The most common source of vacuum in healthcare facilities is the pipeline system **(Fig. 9)**. The system must be capable of maintaining a vacuum of approximately 40 kPa (300 mm Hg) at the user end **(Fig. 10)**. The suctioning apparatus is connected to a wall inlet through a noninterchangeable coupler, similar to those used for medical gas pipelines. The pipelines are connected to a central vacuum source. These pipelines are constructed of copper and are slightly larger than the medical gas pipelines. Vacuum is created by two pumps connected in parallel. These pumps are essentially air compressors

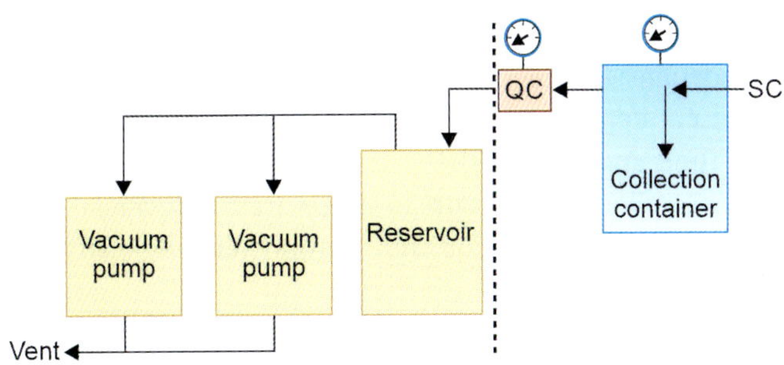

Fig. 9: Complete suction system. Normally, liquids and solids do not move any further than the collection container. (SC: suction catheter; QC: quick coupler in operating room).

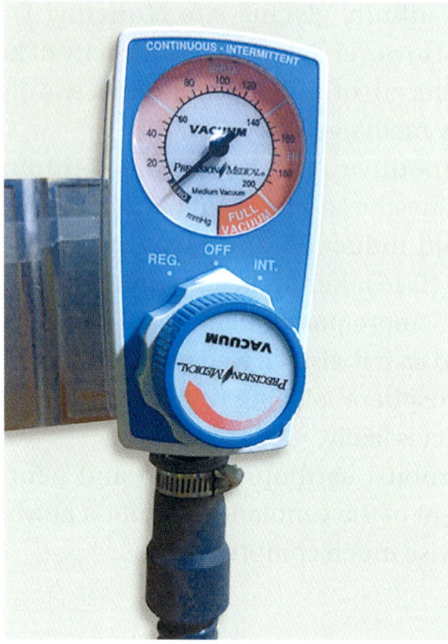

Fig. 10: Testing vacuum in operating room using vacuum gauge.

mounted in reverse to create vacuum. There is a reservoir between the pumps and the pipeline to even out the vacuum and collect any fluids or debris that may enter the system.

SCAVENGING SYSTEMS (FIGS. 11 AND 12)

The anesthetic gases and vapors that leak into the surrounding room during medical procedures are considered waste anesthetic gases (WAGs). It is estimated that >250,000 healthcare professionals in the US, who work in hospitals, operating rooms, dental offices, and veterinary clinics, are potentially exposed to WAGs. The relationship between exposure to trace concentrations of WAGs in the operating room and the possible development of adverse health effects has concerned healthcare professionals for numerous years. Some potential effects of exposure to WAGs are nausea, dizziness, headaches, fatigue, and irritability, as well as sterility, miscarriages, birth defects, cancer, and liver and kidney disease, among operating room staff or their spouses (in the case of miscarriages and birth defects). The reports on the effects of exposure to WAGs are controversial. The evidence that trace anesthetic gases are harmful is at present suggestive rather than conclusive.

However, scavenging of WAGs is recommended for all areas, and work practices to reduce contamination. The maximum recommended trace gas levels are recommended as particles per million (ppm) and vary between different countries **(Table 3)**. In addition, there should be a program for

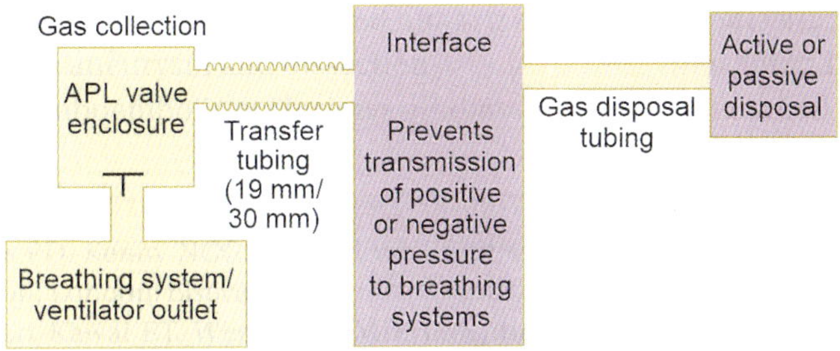

Fig. 11: Schematic representation of the components of scavenging system. (APL valve: adjustable pressure-limiting valve)

Typical active AGSS transfer hose assembly incorporating pressure relief valve

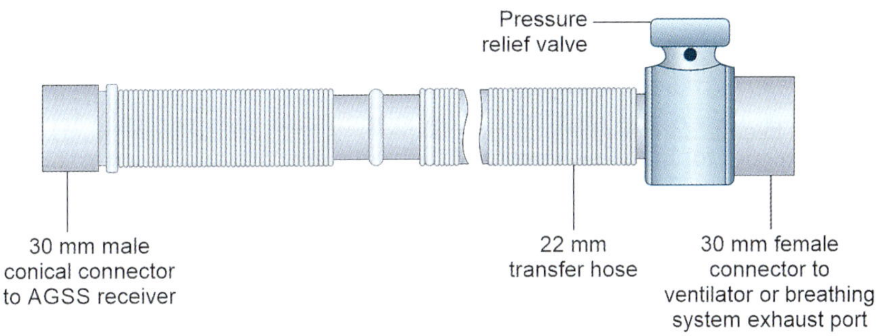

Fig. 12: Gas disposal in active scavenging. (AGSS: anesthetic gas scavenging system)

TABLE 3: Recommended trace concentrations of waste anesthetic gases (WAGs).

The recommended maximum accepted concentrations over a time-weighted average		
	UK (8 hours)	***US (1 hour)***
Nitrous oxide (ppm)	100	25
Isoflurane (ppm)	50	2
Halothane (ppm)	10	2
Other halogenated agents (ppm)		2

management of WAGs with a documented maintenance schedule for all anesthesia machines and the ventilation system in the operating room and postanesthesia care units.

Factors contributing to operating room pollution:

- Use of breathing systems with high-flow techniques
- Poorly fitting masks
- Failure to turn off gases at the end of anesthetic

- Filling anesthetic vaporizers without key systems
- Liquid agent spills
- Leaks in the machine and breathing systems
- Improper scavenging

The components of scavenging system are as shown in **Figure 11**. The waste gases are collected by suitable modification of adjustable pressure-limiting (APL) valves and ventilator relief valves and are transferred via special tubing to the scavenging interface. These tubes are of different size and appearance to prevent misconnection or direct connection to breathing systems (19 mm/30 mm—corrugated tubes used in breathing systems are 22 mm size). The interface protects the breathing systems from excessive positive or negative pressure. From the interface, the gases are conducted through collapse-proof tubing to the gas disposal assembly, which eliminates excess waste gas.

There are two types of gas disposable systems:

1. *Active:* This is the most common system and uses central vacuum. It provides for high flows but only slight negative pressure (*see* **Fig. 12**).
2. *Passive:* The pressure of the waste gas itself produces flow through the system and no vacuum is used.

Occlusion of scavenging systems can produce high levels of positive pressure in the breathing systems leading to barotrauma. In active systems, failure of the interface can transmit excess negative pressures to the patient.

SUGGESTED READING

1. Dorsch JA, Dorsch SE. Understanding Anesthesia Equipment, 5th edition. Philadelphia: Lippincott Williams & Wilkins; 2008.
2. Ehrenfeld JM, Areti YK. Medical gas supply, vacuum, and scavenging. In: Vacanti CA, Segal S, Sikka P, Urman R, Agarwala A, Aglio LS, et al. (Eds). Essential Clinical Anesthesia. New York, USA: Cambridge University Press; 2011. pp. 121-8.
3. Eisenkraft JB. Anesthesia delivery systems. In: Longnecker D, Brown D, Newman M, Zapol W (Eds). Anesthesiology. China: McGraw Hill Co.; 2008. pp. 767-820.
4. Gentile MA. The role of inhaled nitric oxide and heliox in the management of acute respiratory failure. Respir Care Clin. 2006;12:489-500.
5. Pajewski TN. Anesthesiology Pocket Guide. Philadelphia: Lippincott-Raven; 1997. p. 465.
6. Messer. Pamphlet P-1. Safe handling of compressed gases in containers: Compressed gas cylinder safety information and training. Compressed Gas Association, New York. [online] Available from https://specialtygases.messergroup.com/safe-handling-of-gases [Last accessed Oct., 2024].
7. Parbrook GD, Davis PD, Parbrook EO. Basic Physics and Measurement in Anesthesia, 2nd edition. Norwalk, Conn: Appleton-Century-Crofts; 1986.
8. Schumacher SD, Brockwell RC, Andrews JJ, Ogles D. Bulk liquid oxygen supply failure. Anesthesiology. 2004;100(1):186-9.

9. Scott L. Medical gas cylinders: physics, handling safety, pin indexing. In: Faust RJ, Cucchiara RF, Wedel DJ, Thomas Wass C, Rose SH (Eds). Anesthesiology Review, 3rd edition. Philadelphia: Elsevier Churchill Livingstone; 2001. pp. 210-2.

WEBSITES

1. http://www.osha.gov/SLTC/wasteanestheticgases/solutions. html. US Department of Labor, Occupational Safety & Health Administration (OSHA) website. Last accessed Oct., 2024.
2. http://www.bocmedical.co.uk/product_information/Cylinder_data_chart.pdf. Last accessed Oct., 2024.
3. http://www.scottecatalog.com/scotttec.nsf/74923c9ec562a6fb85256825006eb87d/8a6a71a802694ef2852572aa00614a. Airgas. Last accessed Oct., 2024.
4. http://www-safety.deas.harvard.edu/services/oxygen.html. Harvard Department of Chemistry and Chemical Biology. Last accessed Oct., 2024.
5. http://ecommerce.asahq.org/publicationsAndServices/wasteanes.pdf. Waste Anesthetic Gas Management. Last accessed Oct., 2024.

CHAPTER 3

Anesthesia Machine or Workstation

Yasodananda K Areti

INTRODUCTION

Since the first demonstration of ether anesthesia by WTG Morton in 1846, the apparatus to administer anesthesia have evolved from a simple Morton's inhaler to the present day sophisticated anesthesia workstations or anesthesia care stations. Major part of the 20th century saw anesthesia machines built around the prototype developed by Henry Edmund Gaskin Boyle (1875–1941) in 1917. An anesthesia workstation is described as a "system for administration of anesthesia to patients" and consists of:

- Anesthesia gas supply device
- Target controlled inhaled anesthesia
- Facility for total intravenous anesthesia
- Sophisticated anesthesia ventilators matching ICU ventilators suitable from neonates to adults
- Modular monitoring devices and monitoring recording systems
- Patient protection devices
- Data collection and communication facility.

Latest workstations, Ohmeda GE "Aisys", Dräger® "Zeus", and Maquette are very sophisticated **(Fig. 1)**. Zeus, according to Greek mythology, is the king of all Gods and is very powerful. The name "Zeus" is supposed to indicate the power that is packed into these machines.

In 1997, the American Society of Anesthesiologists conducted a closed claim analysis on 8,496 claims. Anesthetic mishaps due to machines are becoming a rarity due to the safety features that have been incorporated in the newer machines. 75% incidents were due to misuse of anesthesia equipment because of the lack of familiarity with the equipment, and inadequate preuse checking. Only 24% were due to actual equipment failure.

There are plenty of varieties of anesthetic machines. It is difficult to keep track of all the models; hence, it is advisable for all users to go through the machines and safety documents that come with it before using any equipment.

The head of the department is responsible for ensuring this.

Disadvantages of newer workstations include:

- Potential disruption of mechanical ventilation
- Potential disruption of gas delivery

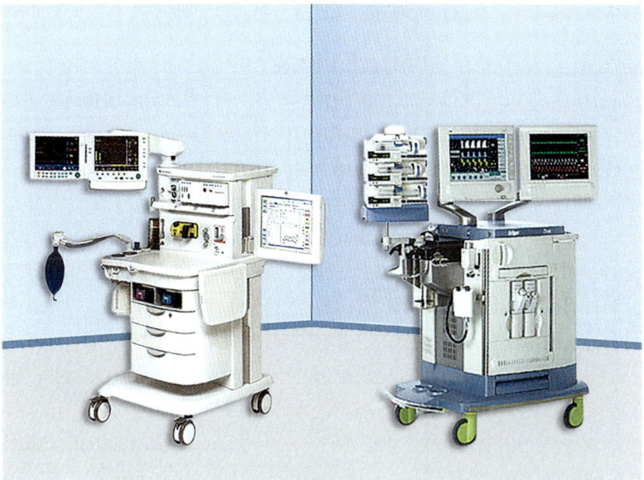

Fig. 1: GE "Aisys" and Dräger® "Zeus" workstation.

- Display failure
- Electrical failure, and
- Fires

STRUCTURE OF ANESTHETIC MACHINE

The machine itself can be divided into three sections **(Fig. 2)**:

1. *High pressure*: This part of the machine is exposed to the high pressures in the cylinders *(maximum pressure for N_2O is 745 psig and oxygen is 1,900 psig):*
    - Yoke
    - Pressure gauge, and
    - Pressure regulators
2. *Intermediate pressure:* This part of the machine is exposed to the pressures in the pipelines *(usual pressure 50–55 psi and 5 psi higher than reduced pressure from cylinder)*:
    - Pipeline connections
    - Oxygen fail-safe devices
    - Oxygen flush
    - Second-stage pressure regulator (*reduced to 26 psi for N_2O and 14 psi for oxygen*)
    - Ventilator gas outlets
    - Pressure gauge
    - Flowmeter needle valves
3. *Low pressure:* This part of the machine lies from needle valves of flowmeters to common gas outlet (CGO):
    - Flowmeters
    - Vaporizers back bar

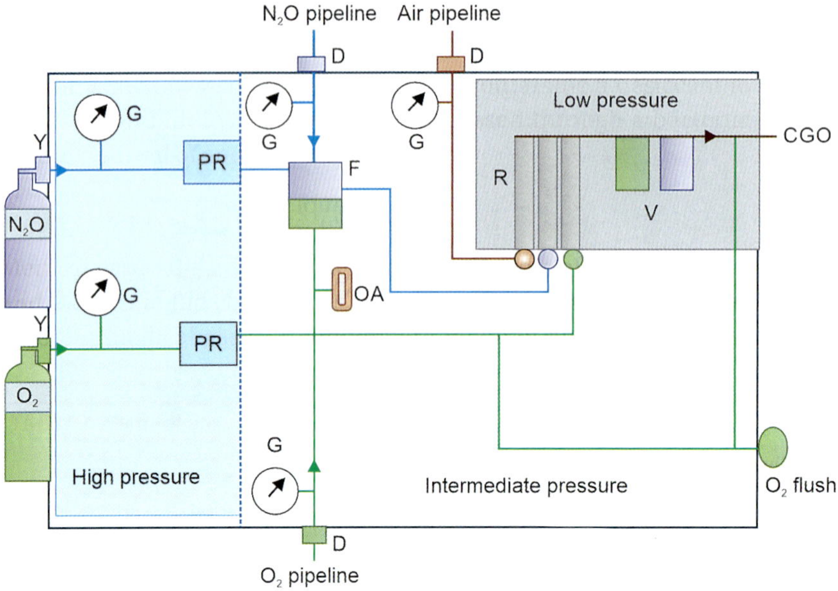

Fig. 2: Structure of anesthesia machine—schematic representation. [CGO: common gas outlet; D: diameter index safety system (DISS); F: oxygen fail-safe device; G: pressure gauge; OA: oxygen alarm; PR: pressure regulator; R: rotameters; V: vaporizer assembly; Y: Yoke]

- Vaporizer
- Pressure relief valve

This section should not be confused with the breathing systems, which are also referred to as low pressure systems.

COMPONENTS OF THE MACHINE

Power Supply (Figs. 3A and B)

Most modern machines' components are powered by electricity and the master switch should be turned on before using the machines. The master switch activates the flow of gases into the intermediate pressure pneumatic circuit of the machine. The emergency oxygen flush can be activated even when the power is off. An auxiliary oxygen flowmeter is provided in most workstations to enable the use of T-piece system in the event of power failure. The workstations also come with a backup battery system, which keeps getting charged when the machine is plugged in even though the master switch is in the off position. Once the power is turned on, the machines perform self-checks. In an emergency situation, the operator can bypass these checks. Some machines limit the number of consecutive times this bypass can be used. The machines are also equipped with visual and/or audible alarms to indicate loss of power.

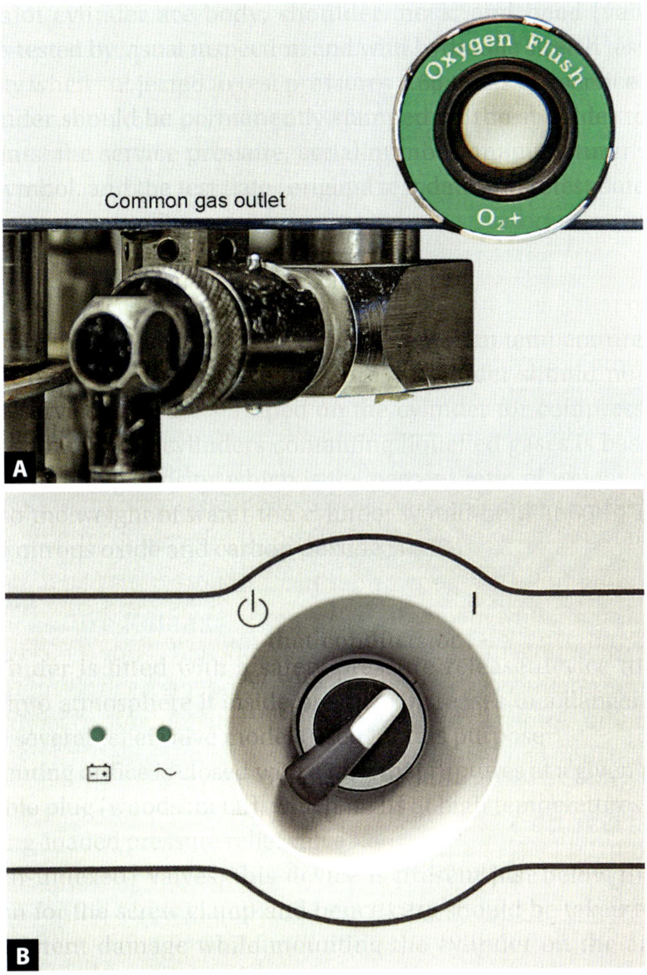

Figs. 3A and B: (A) No slip common gas outlet, and oxygen flush; (B) Power switch.

Medical Gas Inlets (Fig. 4)

The medical gases (oxygen, nitrous oxide, and air) are supplied through pipelines, which are connected to the machine through noninterchangeable connections. The standards for anesthesia workstation require that every anesthesia machine has a diameter index safety system (DISS) fitting for each pipeline inlet to prevent incorrect connections (*see* Chapter 2 for details of DISS).

All piped supplies have a backup cylinder supply (one or two "E" type cylinders). The outlet port of the cylinder is aligned with gas inlet nipple. A Bodok seal is placed between the cylinder and the yoke to ensure leak-free fitting. The assembly has PIN index safety system to prevent incorrect connection of gases. Two pins on the machine should be aligned with

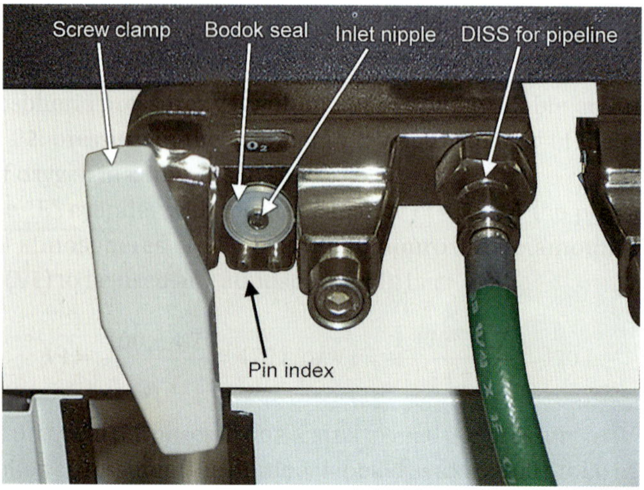

Fig. 4: Cylinder inlet yoke and pipeline inlet. (DISS: diameter index safety system)

corresponding holes in the cylinder head. Inadvertent placement of two Bodok seals may allow incorrect connections.

Before mounting, the cylinder should be opened gently (cracked) to blow away any dust in the port, and closed. The cylinder is securely mounted with a screw clamp. Applying soap water to the junction and observing for any bubble formation can detect presence of leaks in this area.

Pressure Gauge

All machines are equipped with Bourdon pressure gauges (patented in 1849) to monitor the pressure in the cylinders and the pipelines **(Fig. 5)**. A flexible tube (Bourdon tube) within this gauge straightens when exposed to gas pressure. This motion is transmitted to a pointer through a gearing mechanism. In the modern machines, these gauges are located at the front panel of the machine. The dials carry two types of units of measurement of pressure (psi and kPa × 100). Monitoring the pressure will ensure that there is adequate gas supply all times and the pressure in oxygen cylinder would give us an idea of the quantity of oxygen backup. The gauges on nitrous oxide cylinder do not give any indication of amount of N_2O in the cylinder as N_2O exists as a liquid.

Pressure Regulator

Each gas supplied from cylinders to the machine must have a pressure regulator **(Fig. 6)**. Pressure regulators not only reduce the pressure of gases from cylinders but also provide gases at a nearly constant reduced pressure to the flowmeters. Despite the changing pressures in the cylinders, the reduced pressure nearly remains constant. Since pressure is defined as force

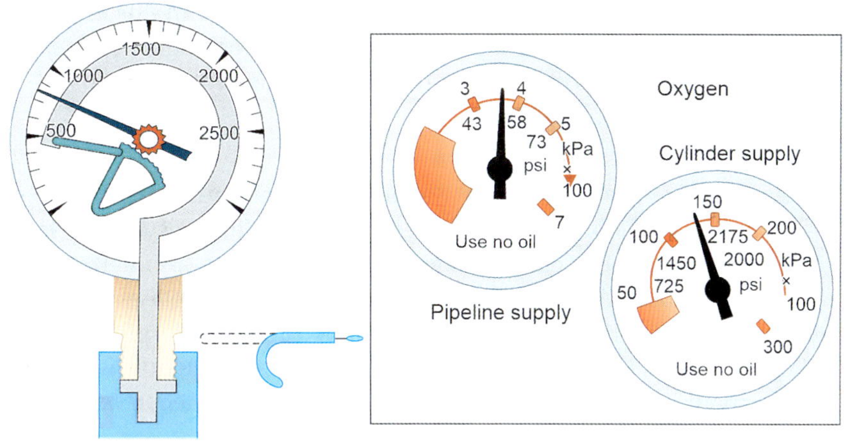

Fig. 5: Schematic diagram of Bourdon gauge and dials indicating pressure in cylinder and pipeline.

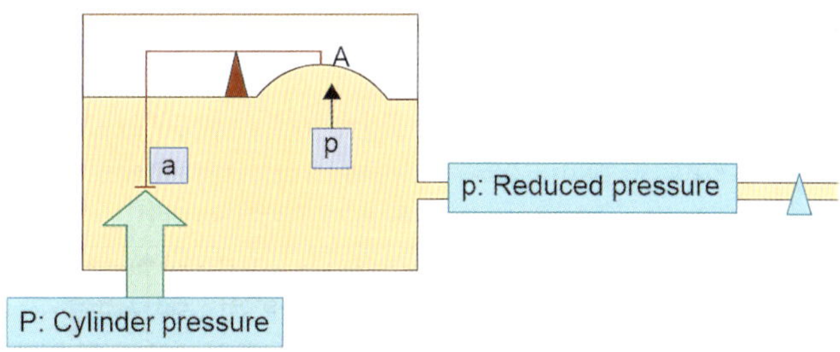

Fig. 6: Schematic representation of principle of "Pressure Regulator." P × a = p × A (high pressure acting on a small area is balanced by low pressure acting on a large area diaphragm).

per unit area, a high pressure acting on a small area can be balanced by a low pressure acting on a large area (large diaphragm in the regulator). A simple pressure reducing valve constructed using this principle will however result in decreasing reduced pressures as the cylinder contents empty. In order to smoothen the flow and keep the reduced pressure nearly constant, a set of high force springs are added in the regulator. The pressure regulators on the anesthesia machines are factory preset to reduce the high pressure in the cylinders to 300–350 kPa (45–50 psi). The pipeline pressures are supplied at a pressure of 350–400 kPa (50–55 psi) to ensure that the pipeline supply is used preferentially even if the cylinder is left open unintentionally. Some machines have second-stage regulators in the intermediate pressure section before the flowmeters and oxygen flush. The second regulator reduces the oxygen pressure further to approximately 20 psig for oxygen and 38 psig for nitrous oxide. This ensures lower pressure at oxygen flush, minimizes pressure fluctuation to the flowmeter, and hence maintains constant flow, and decreases the wear and tear of needle valves of the flowmeters. Two-stage regulators are also used in demand flow entonox apparatus.

Check Valves

Check valves are present on the yoke after the fresh gas entry port to prevent leaks during change of cylinders, and to prevent filling of cylinders from pipelines or the second backup cylinder even if the cylinders are inadvertently left in open position. These are also present at the entry of pipelines to prevent back flow into pipeline in the event of falling pressures in pipeline and backup cylinder is being used. A check valve is also present downstream of vaporizer bank, to ensure that back pressure is not transmitted to vaporizers, particularly when oxygen flush is activated.

Oxygen Fail-Safe Device

In Datex-Ohmeda machines, N_2O is always connected to its flowmeter through an oxygen fail-safe device. This device has a spring-loaded valve **(Figs. 7A and B)**. Oxygen pressure acts against the force of the spring and keeps this valve open so that N_2O can flow to its flowmeter. Once oxygen pressure drops below 30 psig (205 kPa), the unopposed force of the spring shuts the valve off and N_2O can no longer be administered.

In some machines, air supply also flows through a fail-safe device. However, some manufacturers allow air to be delivered directly to the flowmeter. This will enable the anesthesiologist to administer air in the event of oxygen failure. Modern machines incorporate an electronic switch, which will not allow air and N_2O to be used at the same time.

Oxygen Failure Protection Device

This device, used in Dräger® machines, proportionately decreases the N_2O pressure based on the oxygen pressure. In the oxygen fail-safe devices, the flow is "all or none." In the oxygen failure protection device, the flow is proportional and is variable and maintains a desired level of FiO_2. Only at extremely low oxygen pressure, the N_2O flow is cut off.

Proportioning Systems

Newer machines are equipped with proportioning devices, which ensure that a minimum FiO_2 is ensured all the time.

Datex-Ohmeda Link 25 (Figs. 8A and B)

The flowmeter control valves of oxygen and N_2O are mechanically linked with chains. Normally, both knobs can be operated independently.

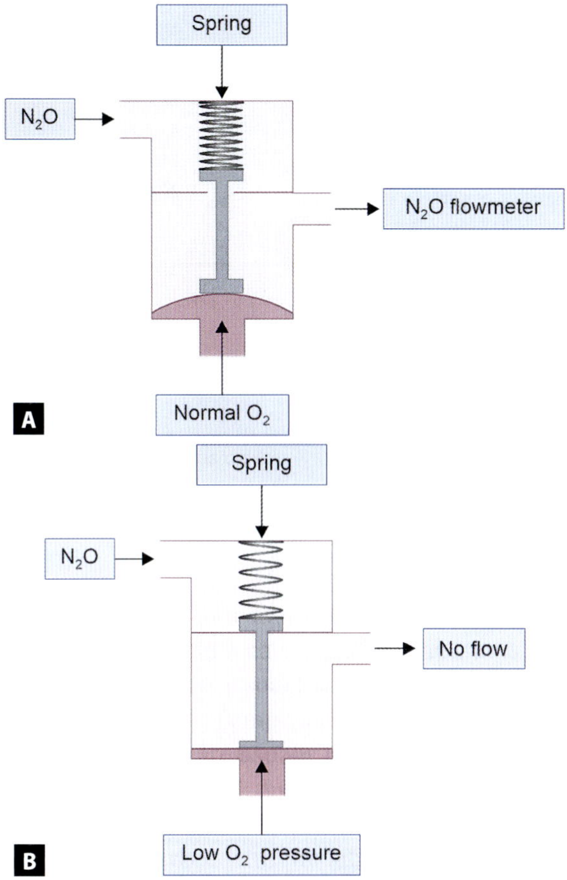

Figs. 7A and B: Oxygen fail-safe device. (A) Normal function; (B) N_2O cut off due to oxygen pressure failure.

Whenever the proportion oxygen approaches 25%, the gear engages and both control knobs get engaged simultaneously. This mechanical system is supported by pneumatic system whereby both the flowmeters operate at different pressures due to the differential setting in the respective second-stage pressure regulators. The resulting combination ensures a minimum FiO_2 of 25%.

Dräger® Oxygen Ratio Monitor Controller (Fig. 9)

The oxygen and N_2O are interlocked pneumatically to ensure a fresh gas O_2 concentration of at least 25% ± 3%. The pressures downstream of the flow control valves of N_2O and O_2 and upstream of the resistors before the flowmeter tubes are linked through pressure transducers. This system controls the slave control valve, which controls the N_2O inlet pressure.

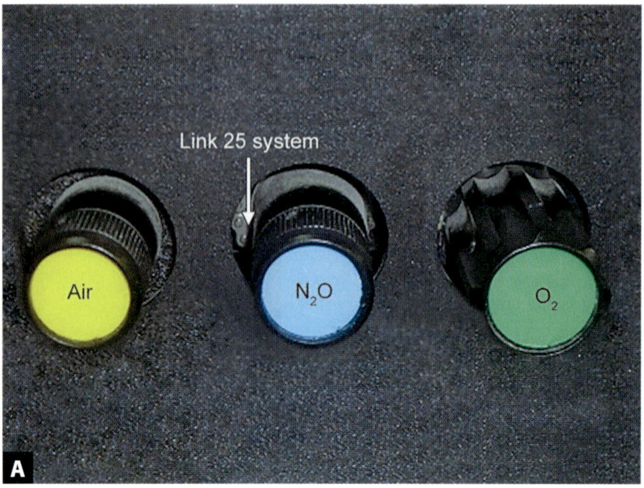

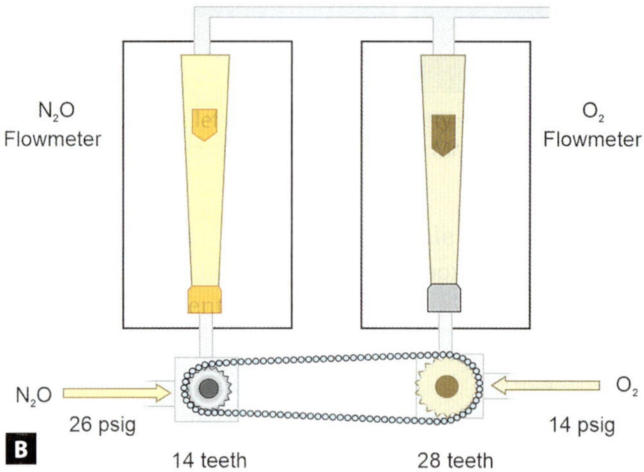

Figs. 8A and B: Color-coded and touch-coded flow control knobs. Link 25 proportionating system.

Oxygen Low-Pressure Alarm

The low pressure or oxygen supply failure alarm will go off when there is a significant increase or decrease of the O_2 supply pressure. This occurs when there is a sudden loss of cylinder or pipeline pressure or when the anesthesia machine is turned on or off. A commonly used mechanism utilizes a pressurized canister that is filled with oxygen when the anesthesia machine is turned on. The stream of oxygen that goes into the canister passes through a whistle, and a sound can be heard when the machine is turned on. If the oxygen pressure falls below a certain value, then this canister will empty and direct a reverse stream of oxygen through the whistle. This alarm may not be heard if the O_2 supply pressure drops very gradually over a long time.

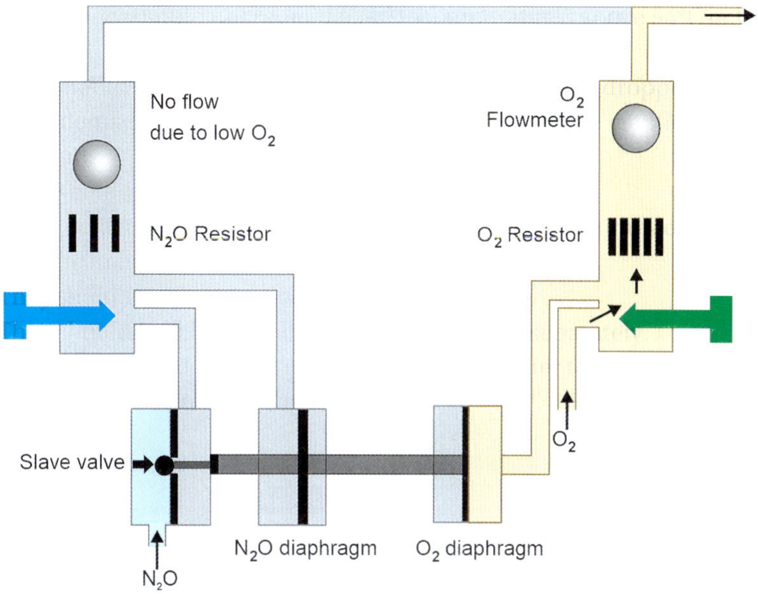

Fig. 9: Schematic representation of oxygen ratio control mechanism in Drager machines. Resistors have ratio of 1:3. The diaphragms and N_2O slave valve ensure that minimum FiO_2 is delivered.

Some machines have a visual alarm as well. The audible alarm should be activated within a few seconds after oxygen pressure drops below 200 kPa, and have a minimum noise level of 60 decibels at 1 meter. The alarm can be switched off only by restoring oxygen supply.

FLOWMETERS

The flow of oxygen, air, and nitrous oxide is measured by flowmeters and is supplied to vaporizers and CGO from fresh gas assembly. Presence of CO_2 and cyclopropane flowmeters in the machine is of historic interest only. Based on the control of flow and measurement of flow rate, they are classified into:

- Traditional (Ohmeda Excel, Astiva; Drager Narkomed, etc.)
- Hybrid (Datex ADU, Drager Fabius, etc.)
- Electronic (GE Aisys)

Traditional (Fig. 10)

A "needle valve" controls the flow of individual gases into the flowmeter. A needle valve has a relatively small orifice with a long, tapered, and conical seat. As the control knob is turned, the plunger is retracted and gases flow between the seat and plunger. Since it takes many turns of the fine-threaded screw to retract the plunger, precise regulation of the flow rate is possible.

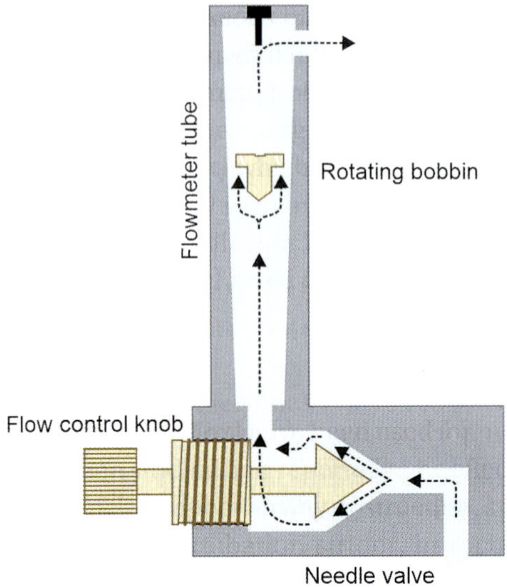

Fig. 10: Schematic diagram of traditional flowmeter containing needle valve and Thorpe tube.

In order to avoid damage to the seat, and preventing the stem from disengaging from the body, there are stops at the "OFF" and "MAXIMUM" flow positions. The control knobs are labeled clearly, color-coded, and touch-coded (*see* **Fig. 9**). The oxygen control knob is larger, protrudes farthest from the flowmeter assembly, and has fluted profile.

The actual flow is measured by cylindrical tubes with varying internal diameter (Thorpe tube). As per Hagen–Poiseuille equation, the laminar flow through tubes is directly proportional to the pressure difference across both ends, fourth power of radius, and is indirectly proportional to the length of the tube and the viscosity. As far as the flow through orifice is concerned, the flow is turbulent and is directly proportional to the square root of pressure difference across the orifice, square of radius, and indirectly proportional to the square root of density.

The flowmeters on a machine are traditionally called "rotameters" (a trade name adopted by the British Oxygen Company). They are variable orifice, fixed pressure difference devices. As the flow increases, the rotating bobbin raises in the flowmeter and the annular orifice around the cylindrical bobbin increases. The calibration is either etched on the flowmeter or written immediately to the right of the tube. One reads the flow at the top of the cylindrical bobbin and the center of the spherical bobbin. At low flows, the flow is laminar and viscosity influences the flow, whereas at high flows, the flow is turbulent and density influences the flow.

At low flows, the flowmeters are calibrated as mL/min (or in decimal fraction of L/min), whereas at high flows, they are calibrated in L/min.

In order to facilitate accuracy at low flows, there may be two tubes used to measure the flows for a single gas. One tube measures up to 1 L/min and the high flows are measured in the second tube. However, there is only one control knob and the flowmeter tubes are connected in series **(Fig. 10)**.

Flow tubes are equipped with float stops at the top and bottom of the tube. The upper stop prevents the float from ascending to the top of the tube and plugging the outlet. It also ensures that the float is visible at maximum flows instead of being hidden in the manifold. The bottom float stop provides a central foundation for the indicator when the flow control valve is turned off.

Traditionally, in a flowmeter assembly, oxygen is located upstream due to the fact that Boyle, inventor of the "Boyle's apparatus", is left-handed. This arrangement has a potential to deliver hypoxic mixture if a leak develops in other flowmeters. Hence, in most modern machines, the oxygen flowmeter joins downstream of all the flowmeters. In some machines (Penlon), the arrangement is not changed externally, but oxygen joins downstream due to presence of appropriate baffles inside the flowmeter assembly. However, damage to the oxygen flowmeter will result in hypoxic mixture if N_2O is also being used **(Figs. 11A to D)**. Continuous monitoring of the inspired oxygen concentration, with the associated alarms if hypoxic mixture is being delivered, is the only option to ensure that a hypoxic mixture is not delivered to the patient.

Hybrid

Most of the modern machines use conventional flow control and an electronic flow sensor. The flow may also be measured by adding small known volumes intermittently by the function of solenoid valves. The flow measured by the sensor is represented digitally and/or by simulated flowmeter on the anesthesia machine screen **(Fig. 12)**.

Electronic

These are more accurate and do not have the disadvantages of having multiple mechanical parts which are prone to leaks and breakages. The flow can be displayed either in digital or virtual form. The flow control is electronic and is measured by electronic sensors. Instead of adjusting the individual flowmeters, one has to adjust total fresh gas flow (FGF) and inspired oxygen concentration. Nitrous oxide and air cannot be administered at the same time.

An *auxiliary flowmeter* for oxygen is incorporated in modern workstations, which can deliver up to oxygen flow of 10 L/min without turning on the machine. This would enable the anesthesiologist to deliver oxygen therapy during regional anesthesia, and for emergency resuscitation.

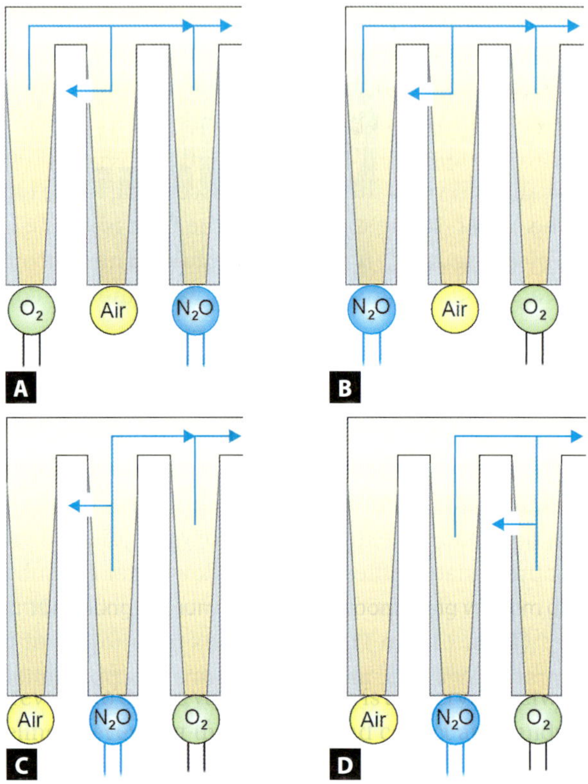

Figs. 11A to D: Flowmeter assembly. (A) Leak in air flowmeter leads to hypoxic mixture; (B) Assembly in Dräger® machine; (C) Assembly in Datex-Ohmeda machine. In B and C, a leak in air or N_2O flowmeter does not deliver hypoxic mixture; (D) Irrespective of the sequence of flowmeters, a break in O_2 flowmeter always leads to hypoxic mixture if N_2O is being used.

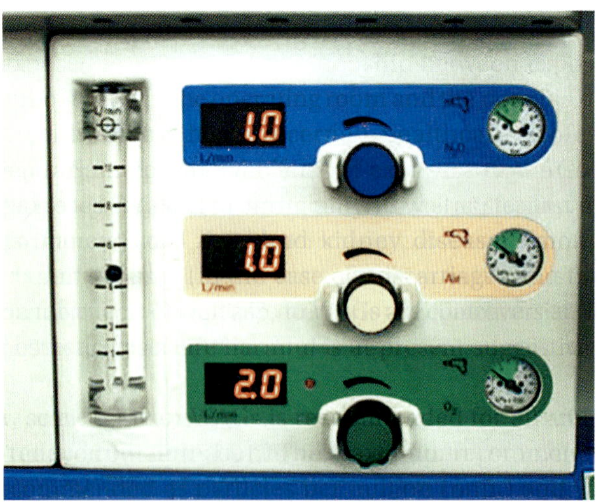

Fig. 12: Hybrid flowmeter assembly. Traditional flow control knobs. Digital flow rate display.

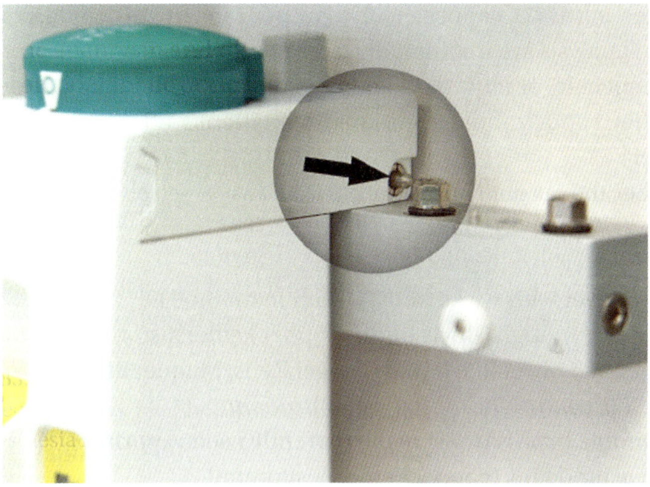

Fig. 13: Select-a-Tec vaporizer mounting indicating easy mounting back bar and mechanism which allows only one vaporizer to be used at a time.

The "Back Bar" (Fig. 13)

The back bar is a structure that supports the flowmeter block and vaporizers. This term is used to describe these supporting components and the gaseous pathways connecting them. Many machines use a system that allows the user to add or remove specific vaporizers quickly and easily, while maintaining a gas-tight system. Some machines have space for a single vaporizer only; others allow the attachment of two or more. However, only one vaporizer can be turned on at any given time. There are two popular interlock systems to achieve this, Select-a-tec (Datex-Ohmeda) and Dräger medical mounting system. Once a vaporizer is attached and turned on, gas flow is diverted from the back bar into the vaporizer to provide the required concentration of anesthetic vapor.

High-Pressure-Relief Valves

The anesthesia machines are also fitted with pressure-relief valves. In the intermediate pressure section, they are set to open at about 95–110 psig to protect against a defective pressure regulator. In the low-pressure section, they are set to open at about 40 kPa (6 psig). These relief valves protect the machine (not the patient) from high pressures. The patient should be protected from excessive pressures by relief valves within the breathing system.

VAPORIZERS

Vaporizers are devices used in anesthesia equipment, which convert volatile anesthetic liquid into its vapor and facilitate inhalational anesthesia. When one comes across a vaporizer, the points that need to be known in its functional analysis are traditionally termed as "classification."

- Agent specific, or multiple agents can be used (Goldman vaporizer)
- Whether vaporization is initiated by patient's effort (draw over; EMO inhaler)
- Whether the output concentration is known precisely (precision)
- *Method of vaporization:*
  - Flow over
  - Flow over with wicks (most common method)
  - Bubble through (Boyle bottle, copper kettle; historic importance only)
  - Injection of volatile liquid (Drager Zeus, Maquet FLOW-i vaporizer)
- *Method of controlling output concentration:*
  - Variable bypass (most of the currently used vaporizers)
  - Measured flow (copper kettle, desflurane)
- *Methods of controlling concentration despite changes in temperature:*
  - Thermostabilization (EMO ether inhaler, use of metal blocks in construction of modern vaporizers)
  - Temperature compensation by altering the bypass flow (bimetallic strip, or volatile agent filled bellows-Penlon)
- Effect of back pressure (pumping and pressurizing effects): Largely eliminated.
- *Flow compensation:* Most present-day vaporizers deliver near constant concentration at wide range of FGF.
- Vaporizer in circuit (VIC) or vaporizer outside circuit (VOC). Currently, most vaporizers are considered to be VOC. The dialed concentration is lower than the actual concentration inspired, when very low flows are used.

Functional Analysis of Vaporizers

All modern vaporizers are precise and are agent-specific. Color-coded filling systems are used to ensure that the vaporizers cannot be filled with incorrect agent. The currently used vaporizers are constructed to be on the machine and are not suitable to be used in the breathing system after CGO (VOC). They are calibrated at sea level and are flow and backpressure compensated. There are several types used in the modern machines.

Plenum Vaporizers

Sevoflurane, isoflurane, and halothane are administered using plenum vaporizers (e.g., Tec 5 and 7, Dräger® Vapor). The fresh gas stream is split into two streams, bypass stream and stream passing through the vaporizing chamber.

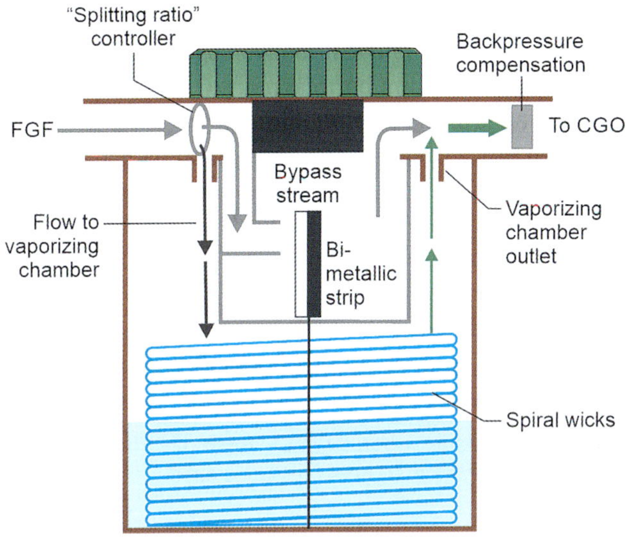

Fig. 14: Structure of variable bypass vaporizer.

The ratio of the two streams (splitting ratio) depends on the saturated vapor pressure (SVP) of the specific volatile agent and is controlled by the concentration dial **(Fig. 14)**.

Method of vaporization: The fresh gas passing through the vaporizing chamber picks up the vapor as it flows over the liquid agent (flow over or plenum). The gases flow over a spiral of wicks soaked with liquid agent, to increase time of contact and surface area of vaporization, thus improving the efficiency. The gas exiting the vaporizing chamber is fully saturated with the vapor and the amount of vapor picked will depend on the atmospheric pressure (ATP) and the SVP of the agent.

$$\text{Vapor } (mL) = \text{Fresh gas through vaporizing chamber } (mL)$$

$$= \frac{\text{SVP}}{\text{ATP} - \text{SVP}}$$

This equation is useful to understand the effect of changes in the ambient pressure and if the vaporizers are filled with incorrect volatile agent. The effect of ambient pressure on the output concentration of these vaporizers is variable and hence the American Society for Testing and Materials (ASTM) anesthesia workstation standards require that the effects of changes in ambient pressure on vaporizer performance be stated in the accompanying documents.

Regulating the output concentration: The control dial controls the flow through the vaporizing chamber; hence, they are termed as variable

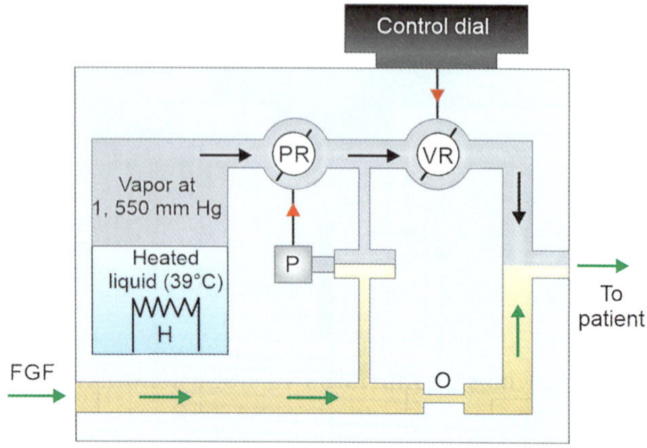

Fig. 15: Schematic desflurane vaporizer. (FGF: fresh gas flow; H: heating element; O: flow restriction orifice; P: a differential pressure transducer; PR: pressure regulator; VR: variable resistor)

bypass vaporizers. As the dial is turned to give higher concentration, the proportion of gas passing through the vaporizing chamber increases and the vapor output increases. Since the splitting ratio, which controls the output concentration, remains constant over wide range of FGFs, fairly reliable output concentration can be obtained even at very low FGFs.

Temperature compensation: As volatile liquid vaporizes, it consumes heat, known as latent heat of vaporization. This results in the cooling of the liquid and consequent change in the SVP, and hence a drop in the output concentration. This heat is supplied to some extent by the metal sink used in the construction (thermostabilization). In addition, either a bimetallic strip or liquid-filled bellows alters the bypass/vaporizer flow ratio so that the output remains constant even after long usage (thermocompensation).

Electronic Vaporizers

Desflurane vaporizer (Tec 6; ***Fig. 15****):* In view of the high SVP of desflurane, a special electronic vaporizer is required to administer this agent.

Method of vaporization: The desflurane vaporizer electrically heats the anesthetic in a sealed chamber to 39°C, creating a pressure of approximately 1,550 mm Hg. At this temperature and pressure, desflurane exists partly as liquid and partly as vapor. The vapor is added to the fresh gases in a controlled manner. There are heaters in the gas pathway to prevent condensation of vapor.

Regulating the output concentration: The FGF inlet pressure (varies with FGF) and the agent vapor pressure (varies with dial setting) are sensed by means of a pressure transducer (P). Based on the dial setting and FGF, required amount of vapor is added to get the desired output concentration. This can be considered as an addition of a measured amount of vapor to the FGF. A microprocessor control achieves this through integration of a pressure regulator (PR), a variable resistor (VR), and pressure transducer (P). The saturated agent flow and the FGF mix before their delivery to the CGO.

Temperature compensation: Since the liquid is heated to a constant temperature above the boiling point of desflurane, and a measured amount of vapor is added to the FGF, no additional temperature compensation is required.

Aladin vaporizing system: These vaporizers are designed for use in Datex-Ohmeda workstations (S5/ADU and Aisys; **Fig. 16**). They are designed for desflurane, sevoflurane, isoflurane, enflurane, and halothane. The cassettes are magnetically coded and are recognized by the machine as they are inserted into the slot. Only one cassette can be inserted into the machine at any given point of time. The electronic controls and the concentration dial are part of the anesthesia workstation, whereas the cassette contains the liquid anesthetic.

Method of vaporization: The fresh gas passing through the vaporizing chamber picks up the vapor as it flows over the liquid agent (flow over or plenum). The fresh gas passing through the vaporizer is fully saturated with vapor because it flows between the agent-soaked wicks and baffles.

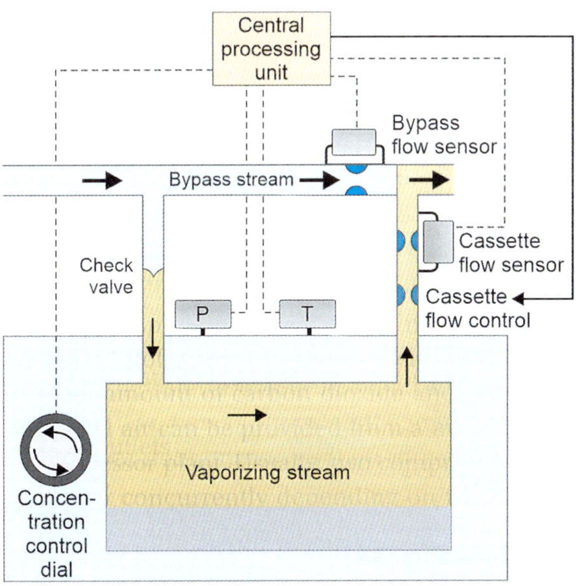

Fig. 16: Aladin vaporizer system.
(P: cassette pressure sensor; T: cassette temperature sensor)

Regulating the output concentration: These vaporizers perform similar to variable bypass vaporizers, but with electronic controls. The FGF is split into bypass flow in the machine and vaporizing chamber flow in the cassette and both flows are constantly monitored. A central processing unit (CPU) integrates the inputs from bypass flow sensor, cassette pressure sensor, cassette flow sensor, and the control dial setting to determine the ratio of bypass to the vaporizing chamber flow, and hence the outlet concentration, which is also constantly monitored.

Temperature compensation: Input from the cassette temperature sensor is integrated into the CPU and provides temperature compensation by adjusting the flow through the vaporizing chamber. The metal wicks and baffles provide thermostability. If the temperature falls below 18°C, a fan below is activated to facilitate heat transfer.

Direct Injection of Volatile Agents

Technological advances have led to innovative and reliable concepts of precise dosing of modern inhaled anesthetics. A calculated amount of volatile anesthetic agents is injected directly into heating chamber or the breathing system. When combined with a basal FGF in circle system, this technique enables rapid control of agent concentration as well as minimal consumption of anesthetic agent. Direct injection of volatile agents (DIVA) has been implemented in the Physioflex anesthesia machine, the Zeus anesthesia machine (both from Dräger®) and Maquet injection type vaporizer.

The DIVA in Drager unit comprises a reservoir unit, a dosing chamber, and a heating unit. The reservoir unit stores a quantity of liquid anesthetic in a tank and delivers it by means of automatic injection system. The agent is vaporized in a heated vaporizing chamber. The vapor is delivered to the breathing system via a heated pipe. The user can directly set the expiratory target concentration independent of FGF. A closed loop feedback mechanism is employed to achieve the target concentration. A circuit flow provided by a blower located in the inspiratory limb of the breathing system provides a homogenous agent concentration.

The Maquet injection type vaporizer is present exclusively on Maquet FLOW-i workstation. The liquid anesthetic is injected into heated vaporizing chamber. The agent, hence the vapor injected, will determine the output concentration, and depends on the concentration required and FGF set on the machine **(Fig. 17)**.

Oxygen Flush (see Fig. 3A)

The oxygen flush allows administration of 100% oxygen at rate of 35–75 L/min to the breathing system. The pressure downstream of pressure regulator

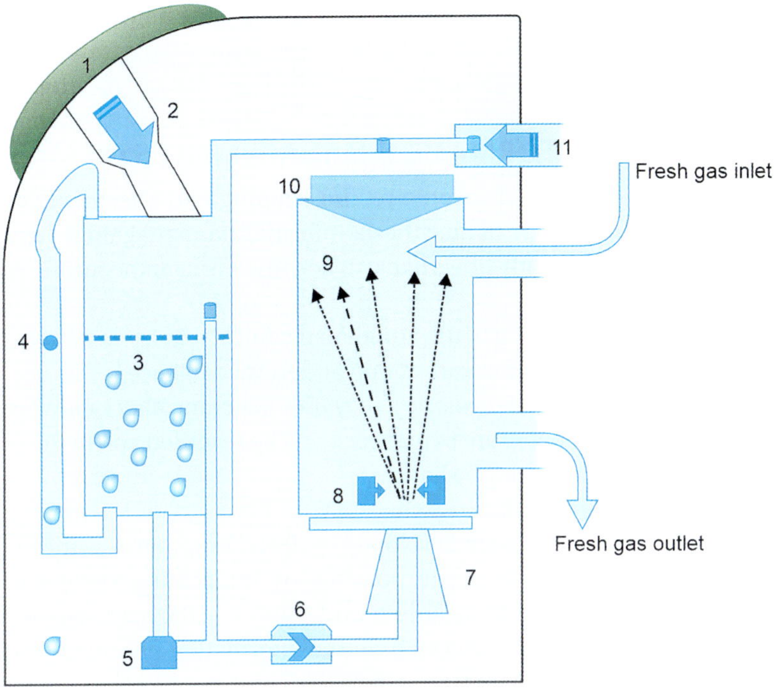

Fig. 17: Maquet liquid injection vaporizer. A heated surface within the vaporizing chamber facilitates evaporation of the anesthetic agent. Fresh gas flows through the chamber and is enriched with anesthetic gas.
Maquet vaporizer: (1) Lid and filler port, (2) Filling check valve, (3) Liquid anesthetic reservoir, (4) Level indicator, (5) Drain plug, (6) Safety valve, (7) Liquid anesthetic injector, (8) Injection sensor, (9) Evaporative surface, (10) Heater, and (11) Drive gas inlet.

is directly supplied to the flush valve. The oxygen joins downstream of the vaporizers. There is check valve to ensure that retrograde flow to the vaporizers is prevented when oxygen flush is activated. The flush is suitable for emergency jet ventilation in only a few models depending on the position of the check valve, hence it is not recommended for this purpose by the manufacturers. The flush works even if the main switch is not turned on. The valve is placed in a recessed position to prevent accidental activation. Overzealous intraoperative use can lead to awareness due to dilution of anesthetic agent. Accidental sticking or activating it during inspiration can lead to pulmonary barotrauma.

Common Gas Outlet (see Fig. 3A)

The mixture of gases and vapors exits the machine via a 22-mm male/15-mm female conically tapered pipe. Some machines may have no slip connection for breathing system. The connector is sometimes fixed, although some manufacturers provide a swiveling connector. The emergency oxygen flush is located close to the CGO, although this is not always the case in modern machines.

ANESTHESIA INFORMATION MANAGEMENT SYSTEM

Technology has enabled electronic record keeping and anesthesia workstation has become a part of anesthesia information management system (AIMS), and use of this software is likely to become norm of the future. AIMS is aimed at:

- Collection and recording of the automated clinical data
- Communication between workstation and AIMS database
- *Serves medicolegal and regulatory purposes:* Machine checks are logged and if automated checks are bypassed, it will be recorded and in the event of any accidents, one may be liable.
- Enables clinical audit for research.

The first paper records were developed in 1894. Computerized anesthesia record keeping (ARK) was made possible by integrating keyboards or proprietary keypads into the anesthesia workstations. ARK was used till mid-1990s. Since mid-90s, AIMS evolved into true information system leveraging on the explosion of healthcare technology.

Software

In order to use AIMS, several point-of-care software systems have evolved:

- Client-server architecture, where the client is referred is the workstation and the information database storage space is the server. This type of software poses challenges to the institution's information technology staff. Application from one vendor can adversely affect those from other vendors. Robust developments have evolved to prevent such errors.
- Web-based software uses web browsers to display functions and store information. Updating the software is quite easy.
- In order to utilize the power of the current handheld devices (iPhone, mobiles, notebooks, etc.) special dedicated software has to be devised and installed onto the workstations.

Hardware

Choosing the point-of-care hardware can be quite challenging and often ignored by the customers. The following aspects must be considered:

- Stationary and mounted hardware must be capable of being cleaned. The cleaning agents can harm the hardware. Hence, water resistance keyboards without crevices are essential. Otherwise, they become a source of nosocomial infections.

- Operating room temperature could vary outside the normal range of the workstations.
- They must be able to absorb the constant movements created during maintenance.
- The size should be small, as the machine already is cluttered. The positioning of the hardware (left or right) has to be considered carefully.
- The systems should be cost-efficient.

Integrating the physiological monitor and device data is a critical element of perioperative clinical information system. Artifacts due to clinical issues (cautery, automated BP measurements, etc.) could lead to recording of faulty data, which could be misleading in retrospective analysis. Although this is believed to lead to litigation, the evidence is contradicting, since inappropriate manual recording is worse.

SUMMARY OF SAFETY MECHANISMS TO PREVENT ADMINISTRATION OF HYPOXIC GAS MIXTURE

One of the devastating complications of administering anesthesia is the administration of hypoxic gas mixture. Though infrequent, the devastating effects of such incidents on patients, patients' families, and the involved anesthesiologists have been reported on several occasions. The incorporation of following standards in anesthesia workstation and its components has made these machines much safer:

- Color-coding of cylinders, pipelines, wall outlets, flow control knobs, and flow meter assembly
- Noninterchangeable threaded connection to the regulators of bulk cylinders
- Pipeline connections to wall outlet through noninterchangeable quick coupling or DISS
- Pin index safety system for cylinders mounted on the anesthesia machine.
- Pipelines connected to machine through DISS
- Oxygen fail-safe devices
- Fluted and protruding oxygen flow control knob
- Link 25 or oxygen proportion devices
- Oxygen being delivered downstream in the flowmeter assembly
- Incorporation of electronic flow control and flowmeter
- Safety mechanical or electronic switches to ensure that air and nitrous oxide cannot be administered at the same time.
- Appropriate calibration and monitoring of the *inspired oxygen concentration* delivered by the machine. Absence of this is one of the criteria used to decide machine obsolescence.

OPERATING ROOM PROTOCOL IN THE EVENT OF FAILURE OF PIPELINE OXYGEN SUPPLY

A planned preventive maintenance program can prevent potentially hazardous conditions. Several problems can occur due to lack of familiarity with the existing systems. Lack of communication between clinicians, maintenance department, and suppliers can lead to problems. Each department must formulate their protocols as the issues and systems are not universally uniform. Failure of oxygen supply is the most commonly reported issue. The following points should be considered:

- Disaster planning and evacuation if need be. This should be flexible and takes into account the possible local scenarios.
- Communication is crucial. The person detecting the problem must inform the telephone operator, who, in turn, should communicate with the operation room (OR) supervisor, head of surgery and anesthesia, maintenance department, and other units which depend on oxygen.
- No elective surgery should be started till the issue has been resolved.
- Conserve the existing backup and procure more backup oxygen.
    - Low flow anesthesia is preferable.
    - Gas-powered ventilators are not to be used, and manual ventilation is preferable.
- Supplies in recovery room should be checked.

SUGGESTED READING

1. Areti YK. Anesthesia machine. In: Vacanti C, Sikka P, Urman R (Eds). Essential Clinical Anesthesia. Boston: Cambridge University Press; 2011. pp. 129-37.
2. ASTM Standard F 1850, 2000 (2005). Standard Specification for Particular Requirements for Anesthesia Workstations and Their Components. ASTM International, West Conshohocken, PA; 2005.
3. Brockwell RC, Andrews JJ. Inhaled anesthetic delivery systems. In: Miller RD (Ed). Miller's Anesthesia, 6th edition. Philadelphia: Elsevier Churchill Livingstone; 2005. pp. 273-311.
4. Dorsch JA, Dorsch SE. Understanding Anesthesia Equipment, 5th edition. Philadelphia: Lippincott Williams & Wilkins; 2008.
5. Eisenkraft J. Anesthesia delivery system. In: Longnecker D, Brown D, Newman M, Zapol W (Eds). Anesthesiology. China: McGraw-Hill; 2007. pp. 767-820.
6. Meyer JU, Küllik G, Wruck N, Kück K, Manigel J. Advanced technologies and devices for inhalational anesthetic drug dosing. In: Schüttler J, Schwilden H (Eds). Modern Anesthetics (Handbook of Experimental Pharmacology). Berlin: Springer-Verlag; 2008. pp. 451-70.
7. Sandberg WS, Urman RD, Ehrenfeld JM (Eds). The MGH Textbook of Anesthetic Equipment. Philadelphia: Elsevier Saunders; 2011.

WEBSITES

1. http://www.frca.co.uk/article.aspx?articleid=100151. Schematic diagram of desflurane vaporizer. Last accessed Nov., 2024.
2. http://www.johnpowell.net/. Morton Inhaler & Clevedon Ventilator. Last accessed Nov., 2024.
3. http://medgadget.com/archives/2006/04/zeus_anesthesia.html. Zeus Workstation. Last accessed Nov., 2024.
4. http://www.udmercy.edu/crna/agm/. Flowmeters. Last accessed Nov., 2024.

CHAPTER 4

Anesthesia Breathing Systems

Yasodananda K Areti

INTRODUCTION

Anesthesia breathing system (formerly known as anesthesia breathing apparatus or anesthesia breathing circuit) is an interface between the anesthetic machine and the patient. They evolved over 160 years from the open systems used by Morton to the present day closed systems using carbon dioxide absorbents. The main purpose of these systems is to deliver the required oxygen and anesthetic gases, and maintain carbon dioxide homeostasis. In addition, they help us to assess, assist, or control ventilation, and condition temperature and humidity. Present day systems are constructed to facilitate scavenging of exhaled gases as well.

COMPONENTS

- *Connectors and adaptors* ***(Fig. 1)***: These connectors ensure quick connection between the breathing systems and masks or endotracheal tubes. Their sizes are universal and either male or female 15/22 mm connections. Some of them also incorporate gas-sampling ports.

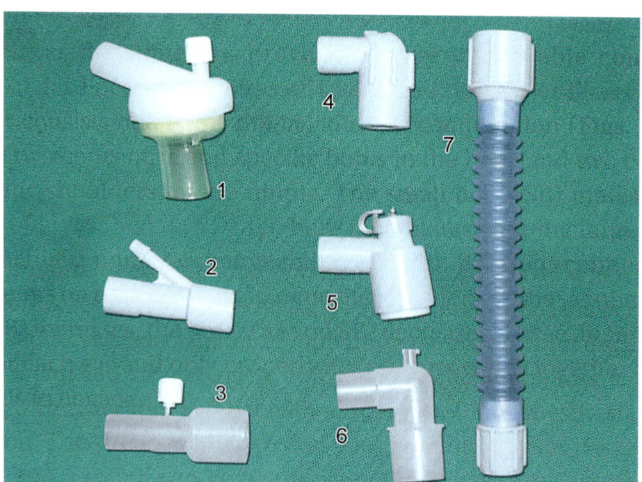

Fig. 1: Connectors. (1) Heat and moisture exchange filter with sampling port; (2) T-piece; (3) Straight connector with a side gas-sampling port; (4) Right angle connection; (5) Right angle swivel connector for insertion of a flexible fiberscope; (6) Right angle connector with gas-sampling port; (7) Flexible corrugated extension.

- *Reservoir bag (RB):*
    - Acts as a reservoir for gases to be stored during exhalation
    - Acts as a reservoir and ensures adequate supply of required flows during inhalation **(Fig. 2)**
    - Helps anesthesiologist to assess, assist, or control ventilation manually
    - Protects the patient from excessive pressure
- *Corrugated tubes:* Flexible, low-resistance, and lightweight connection from one part to other
- *Valves:*
    - *Adjustable pressure-limiting (APL) valves:* The APL valve is a user-adjustable valve that releases gases to a scavenging system. It is used to control the pressure in the breathing system.
    - *Unidirectional valves (UDVs)* ***(Fig. 3)****:* These valves ensure a required direction of flow in breathing systems.
    - *Nonrebreathing valves:* These valves are used more commonly in manual resuscitators.
- Carbon dioxide absorbent
- *Filters:*
    - *Bacterial filters:* These are meant to prevent transmission of infection to the patient or contamination of the equipment. The recommendations for their use vary for different countries. Generally, a new filter should be used for every patient or in the absence of a

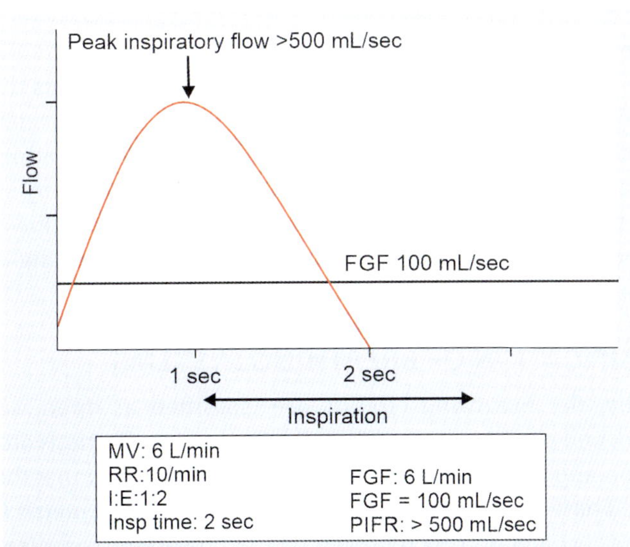

Fig. 2: Example to illustrate the function of reservoir bag (RB). RB supplies required flow during inspiration and stores continuously incoming gases during expiration. (FGF: fresh gas flow; MV: minute ventilation; PIFR: peak inspiratory flow rate; RR: respiratory rate)

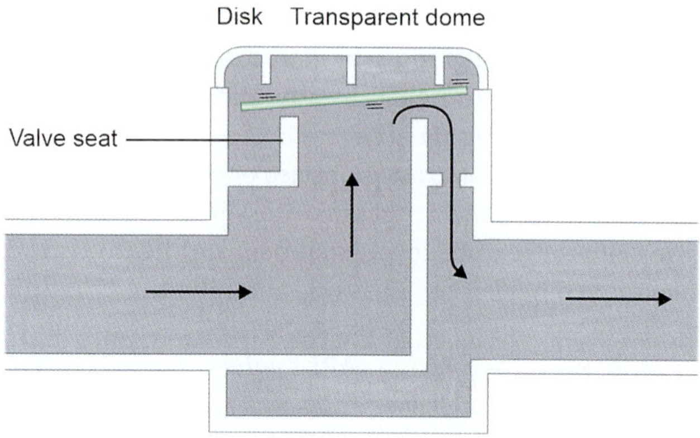

Fig. 3: Construction of unidirectional valves in circle system. A reciprocal arrangement ensures unidirectional flow in the patient circuit.

filter a disposable system should be used for every patient. Filters are generally not preferred for pediatric patients.

- *Heat and moisture exchange (HME) filters:* Administration of dry gases at room temperature could lead to heat loss and increased pulmonary complication. The function of the nose is to warm and humidify inhaled gases. When the nose is bypassed, it is advisable to use HME filters to achieve this objective. These devices also help to dehumidify the gases that are being sampled for analysis by sidestream devices.

APPARATUS DEAD SPACE

Some components that connect the breathing system to the patient act as an extension of patient's anatomical dead space. Since this dead space is imposed by a piece of apparatus, it is termed as apparatus dead space. *Apparatus dead space* can be defined as that part of the breathing system from which exhaled alveolar gases are rebreathed without any significant change in their carbon dioxide concentration. The volume of the apparatus dead space should be as small as possible or else rebreathing of carbon dioxide could result in hypercapnia.

CLASSIFICATION OF BREATHING SYSTEMS

Historically, the breathing circuits are classified as open, semiopen, semiclosed, and closed systems **(Table 1)**. These classifications are a source of confusion and inconsistency. Hence, it is recommended that the systems be classified based on CO_2 homeostasis in a four-quadrant matrix **(Table 2)**, i.e., whether exhaled CO_2 is removed by CO_2 absorbent, or eliminated by fresh gas inflow. One should also understand whether a system is efficient during spontaneous breathing, controlled ventilation or both, and whether it can be used for pediatric patients, adults or both. Among the CO_2 eliminators,

TABLE 1: Historic classification.

Type	*Inhalation*	*Exhalation to*	*Reservoir*	*Rebreathing*	*Example*
Open	Air + agent	Atmosphere	Nil	Nil	Open drop; T-piece
Semiopen	Air + agent from machine	Atmosphere	Small	Minimal	T-piece with small reservoir
Semi-closed	From machine	Atmosphere + machine	Large	Possible	• Magill attachment • Mapleson systems
Closed	From machine	Machine	Large	Yes + CO_2 absorbent	Circle system

TABLE 2: Classification of anesthesia breathing systems; four quadrant matrix.

	Unidirectional flow	*Bidirectional flow*
CO_2 absorption	Circle system	To-and-fro system
CO_2 elimination (no CO_2 absorbent)	• Nonrebreathing valves (use of Reuben valve, Ambu valve, etc.) • Self-inflating resuscitators	• Mapleson A-F, Humphrey A-D, Hafnia modifications • Afferent reservoir (ARS), junctional reservoir (JRS), efferent reservoir (ERS), and enclosed afferent reservoir system (EARS) • Ayre's T-piece systems

the three popular functional classes are Mapleson systems, Miller's classes, and T-piece systems based on Ayre's T-piece **(Table 3)**.

SYSTEMS WITH UNIDIRECTIONAL FLOW USING ABSORBENTS TO REMOVE CO_2 (CIRCLE SYSTEM)

These systems were developed to conserve gases, to save costs, minimize pollution, and to some degree retain heat and moisture. All the exhaled gases are rebreathed except the carbon dioxide which is removed by different formulations of carbon dioxide absorbents (soda lime, Lithsorb, Baralyme, Amsorb®, Drägersorb®, etc.).

Fresh gases are added to the system based on the leaks in the system, uptake of oxygen and inhalational anesthetic agents by the body, arrangements of various components of the system, and clinical state and duration of anesthesia. The CO_2 from exhaled gases combines with water to become a weak acid, carbonic acid, which reacts with a strong alkali (calcium hydroxide, lithium hydroxide, etc.) producing a carbonate and water. This reaction of neutralization is exothermic and steps are as follows:

Functional Analysis

Fresh gas flow: The system is classified into three functional types based on the FGF.

- *High flow:* FGF greater than or equal to patient's alveolar ventilation. In an ideal arrangement, this results in selective elimination of all the exhaled gases from the patient and hence there is no rebreathing of alveolar gases. The inspired concentration of oxygen and anesthetic agents will be the same as that are set on the machine. Some authors refer to this as open technique. The system can be used without soda lime. This technique is usually recommended:
  - At induction
  - Intermittently during a long anesthetic
  - Whenever patient's depth of anesthesia needs to be changed rapidly, and
  - During recovery
- *Low flow:* FGF $\leq$ patient's alveolar ventilation (but not basal). These flows result in conservation of part of the exhaled gases. This technique allows for a bit of flexibility, requires less sophisticated technology, and lessens the effects due to accumulation of compound A and CO.
- *Closed system or basal flow:* The use of very low FGF makes these systems economical and exciting. FGF supplies only the consumed oxygen and anesthetic agents by the patients. The requirements for this technique are:
- *Anesthesia machines:* Currently available sophisticated workstations (such as Dräger Zeus and GE Aisys) make this technique practically easy to master and use. Ideal features of these workstations are:
  - Leak should not be >100 mL/min
  - Fresh gas controls should be precise and flow meters calibrated for low flows
  - Precision, pressure, temperature, and flow-compensated vaporizers
  - Ventilators must be capable of compensating tidal volumes (V_T) for FGFs
- Monitoring of following parameters is essential.
  The gas should be sampled between the Y-piece and the patient.
  - Inspired oxygen concentration
  - End-tidal CO_2
  - End-tidal inhaled agents
  - Airway pressures
- Clinically, a constant end-expiratory position of RB indicates lack of leaks.
- Prolonged use of basal flow system could lead to accumulation of breakdown products. Hence, FGF should be increased intermittently.

Factors influencing alveolar concentration during basal flow:

Inspired concentration: Higher the inspired concentration, faster the wash-in. Historically, the vaporizers are used either in the circle (VIC), or outside the circle (VOC). The present day vaporizers can only be used as VOCs. During the use of basal flow, the inspired concentration at the patient is much lower than the dialed concentration. Rapid rise in inspired concentration can be obtained by injection of volatile agents into the circle system [digitally injected volatile agents (DIVAs)]. Vaporizers with high minimum alveolar concentration (MAC) multiple (highest dial setting ÷ MAC) allow one to dial high concentration and consequently faster wash-in.

Fresh gas flow and the circuit volume: Higher the FGF in relation to circuit volume, faster the wash-in.

Techniques using low FGF demonstrate slower wash-in. This principle depends on the time constant (time taken for a process to complete provided the reaction speed is constant). Approximately 96% change occurs in three time constants. In order to facilitate faster wash in, one should use high FGF technique, whenever a rapid change in alveolar concentration is required, and also larger changes in inspired concentration.

Advantages and Disadvantages of Circle System

The main advantages of circle system include economy, reduced pollution, and conservation of heat and humidity. The disadvantages include the need for more vigilance, good equipment, need for extensive monitoring of inspired gases, and accumulation of byproducts of anesthetic agent degradation.

SYSTEMS WITH BIDIRECTIONAL FLOW USING CO_2 ABSORBENT

Waters to-and-fro System (Fig. 5)

Ralph Waters (anesthetist in Kansas City) in 1921 described the clinical use of a canister filled with soda lime. Patients exhaled through the canister (placed close to the patient's airway) into a RB and inhaled them during the next breath, free of CO_2, from the RB, passing again through the canister (i.e., a to-and-fro canister). This revolutionary innovation meant that inhalation anesthesia could be given without dilution by room air. High concentrations of oxygen could be given, heat was conserved, and pollution of the operating room air was avoided (pollution was considered to be a problem even in 1926). This system is no longer used.

UNIDIRECTIONAL SYSTEMS USING NONREBREATHING VALVES FOR CO_2 ELIMINATION

A nonrebreathing valve facilitates FGF to be breathed in. All the exhaled gas including exhaled CO_2 is eliminated out. These systems have largely

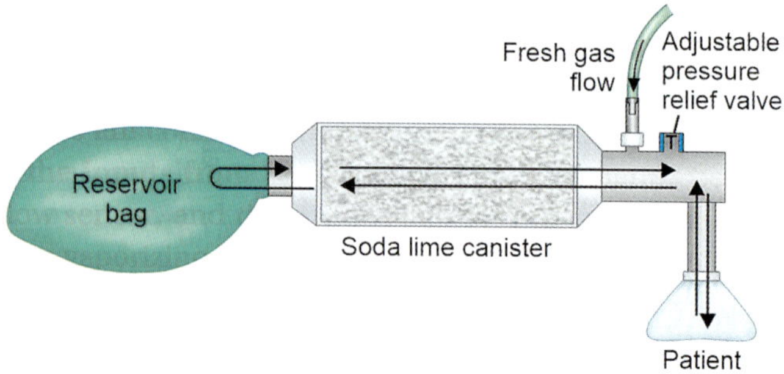

Fig. 5: To-and-fro system.

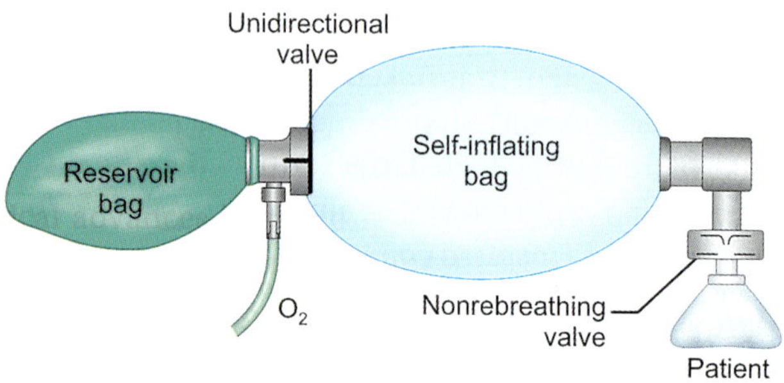

Fig. 6: Schematic diagram of self-inflating resuscitator.

disappeared from anesthetic practice, mainly due to bulky and noisy valve, and repeated FGF adjustments to match the minute ventilation.

However, manual resuscitators **(Fig. 6)** are used commonly in the medical practice. Self-inflating bags with nonrebreathing valves (Ambu bag is one of the common names) are principally used for transport of patients and for resuscitation of patients by paramedics, emergency room staff, critical care staff, and the operating room personnel. The nonrebreathing valve allows the gases from the bag to be delivered to the patient and prevents any exhaled gases to enter the self-inflating bag and thus prevent CO_2 rebreathing. The bag is filled with oxygen-enriched air through another set of UDVs. The inspired oxygen concentration depends on the oxygen flow and size of the reservoir. A positive end-expiratory pressure (PEEP) valve can be added to the system at the patient exhalation port to optimize gaseous exchange. A pressure monitoring and limiting valve is also added to prevent any barotrauma. These units are available in different sizes to suit different patient populations. Patients breathing spontaneously will either breathe ambient air or oxygen-enriched ambient air. The equipment is portable and simple to use. However, failure to familiarize oneself with the available equipment can lead to adverse outcomes.

CO_2 ELIMINATION SYSTEMS WITH BIDIRECTIONAL FLOW (NO CO_2 ABSORBENT)

Mapleson Systems (Fig. 7)

The Magill attachment has been in use since 1928. In 1954 on the advice of William Mushin, Mapleson analyzed the relation between FGF, relative positioning of fresh gas inflow, reservoir, APL valve, and minute ventilation, and reported on the functional analysis to eliminate rebreathing. Mapleson systems AE were thus born and system F (Jackson Rees modification of T-piece) was added to the analysis in 1975. Mapleson never made any attempt to classify the breathing systems. The Mapleson A, B, and C systems are rarely used today, but the D, E, and F systems are commonly used.

Lack system **(Fig. 8)** is a coaxial modification of Mapleson A (1972).

As per Miller's functional analysis, Mapleson A is termed as afferent reservoir systems, Mapleson B and C are termed as junctional reservoir systems, and Mapleson D, E, and F are termed as efferent reservoir systems.

Bain Circuit (Fig. 9)

The Bain circuit is a modification of the Mapleson D system and was introduced in 1972. It is a coaxial circuit in which the FGFs through a narrow inner tube within the outer corrugated tubing. Traditionally, the length of the system is 1.8 meters. The length can be increased by adding additional

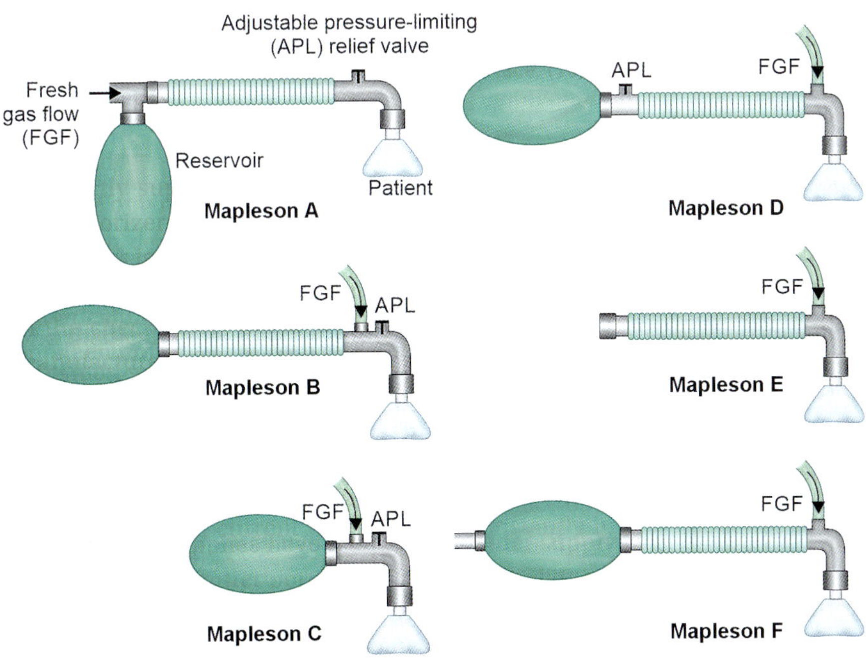

Fig. 7: Mapleson systems.

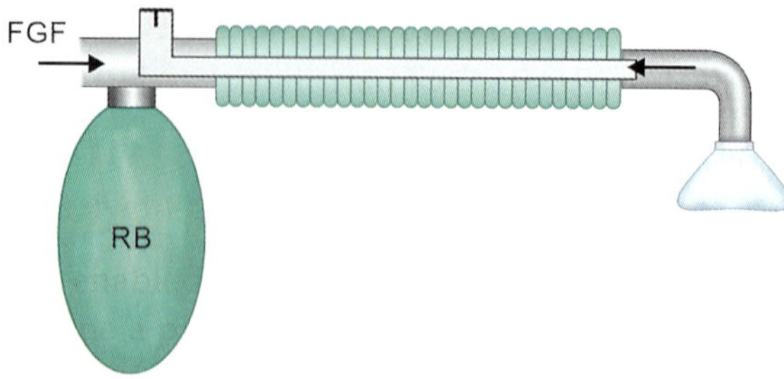

Fig. 8: Lack system (coaxial Mapleson A). (FGF: fresh gas flow; RB: reservoir bag)

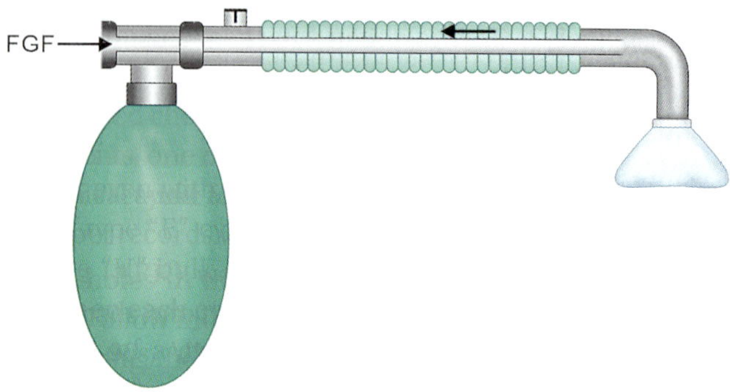

Fig. 9: Bain circuit. (FGF: fresh gas flow)

corrugated tube at the machine end without altering its functionality. This may be of particular benefit for remote anesthesia as in magnetic resonance imaging units.

Advantages of Bain's: It is lightweight, convenient, easily sterilized, and reusable. Scavenging of the gases from the expiratory valve is facilitated because the valve is located away from the patient. Exhaled gases in the outer reservoir tubing add warmth to inspired fresh gases.

Hazards of Bain's: Kinking, leakage, or disconnections in inner tube can cause severe hypercapnia. Hence, the outer tube should be transparent to allow inspection of the inner tube. The integrity of the inner tube should be checked by the following tests:

- Set a low flow on the oxygen flow meter and occlude the inner tube (with a finger or the barrel of a small syringe) at the patient end while observing the flow meter indicator. If the inner tube is intact and correctly connected, the indicator will fall slightly.
- Activate the oxygen flush and observe the bag (Pethick test). A Venturi effect caused by the high flow at the patient end will create a negative pressure in the outer exhalation tubing, and this will cause the bag to deflate. If the inner tube is not intact, this maneuver will cause the bag to inflate slightly.

T-piece Systems

Ayres introduced T-piece systems. They are simple, contain no valve, light weight, and low-resistance systems. Jackson Rees modification is popular for children, and head and neck surgery.

Enclosed Afferent Reservoir System

Enclosed afferent reservoir system (EARS, 1987) is represented in **Figure 10**. In this system, APL and RB are enclosed in a second system. Alternately, the entire Mapleson A is enclosed. It works efficiently both during spontaneous and controlled breathing.

Functional Analysis

The amount of carbon dioxide rebreathing associated with each system is multifactorial, and variables that dictate the carbon dioxide homeostasis are as shown in **Box 1**. The FGF in various systems is summarized in **Table 4**. Functional analysis of Mapleson A to F is shown in **Figure 11**.

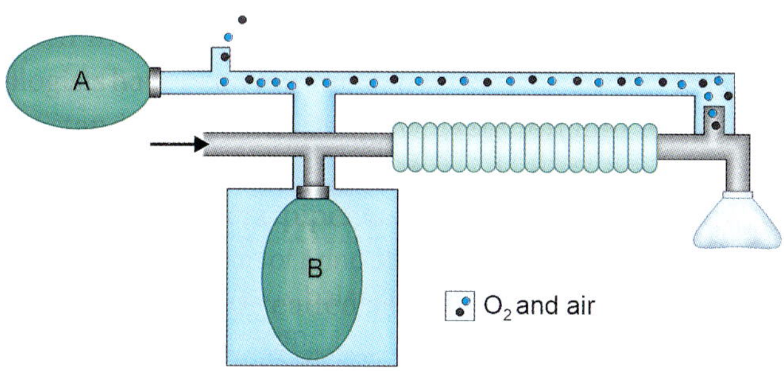

Fig. 10: Enclosed afferent reservoir system (enclosed Magill's) (light blue and black dots represent exhaled gases).

BOX 1: Factors affecting CO_2 rebreathing.

- The fresh gas inflow rate
- The minute ventilation
- The mode of ventilation (spontaneous or controlled)
- The tidal volume
- The respiratory rate
- The inspiratory to expiratory ratio
- The duration of the expiratory pause, the peak inspiratory flow rate
- The volume of the reservoir tube
- The volume of the breathing bag
- Ventilation by mask
- Ventilation through an endotracheal tube
- The carbon dioxide sampling site

TABLE 4: Fresh gas flow in different systems.

		Fresh gas flow	*VE controlled by*
Mapleson A	Spontaneous Controlled	~ VA or VE > Twice VE	Patient Operator
Mapleson B and C	Spontaneous Controlled	2 times VE 2–2.5 times VE	Patient Operator
Mapleson D	Spontaneous Controlled	1.5–2 times VE 70 mL/kg/min for normocapnia 100 mL/kg/min for mild hypocapnia	Patient Operator (150 mL/kg/min)
Mapleson E	Spontaneous Controlled	> Twice VE (Time for one breath/ inspiratory time) * VE (Intermittent expiratory limb occlusion)	Patient Operator
Mapleson F Jackson Rees	Spontaneous Controlled	1.5–2 times VE 1.5–2 times VE	Patient Operator
During spontaneous ventilation, the order of efficiency is A > DFE > CB During controlled ventilation, the order of efficiency is DFE > BC > A.			
EARS, 1987	Spont/Cont	~ VA or VE	Patient/operator
Nonrebreathing	Spont/Cont	= VE = Gas uptake by body (basal flow)	Patient/operator
To-and-fro circle	Spont/Cont	< VA and > basal flow (low flow) > VA (high flow)	Patient/operator

(EARS: enclosed afferent reservoir system; VA: alveolar ventilation; VE: minute ventilation)

Mapleson A (Magill attachment, 1928): This is the most efficient system during spontaneous respiration. FGF equaling minute ventilation eliminates rebreathing **(Fig. 12)**, while partial pressure of arterial carbon dioxide ($PaCO_2$) is determined by the patient's minute ventilation. The functional analysis assumes plug type movement of gases from various compartments, and no mixing of gases occurs at various interfaces. The apparatus dead space in this system extends from the APL valve to the patient.

During spontaneous ventilation, the APL valve is kept in the fully open position; however, it remains closed till its opening pressure is exceeded. As the patient exhales, the dead space gases followed by alveolar gases enter the corrugated tube and travel toward the RB. Simultaneously, the fresh gas also flows into the bag. Once the bag is full, the pressure in the system rises and the APL valve opens. From this point, the alveolar gases from the patient are vented through APL valve. The fresh gas entering the corrugated tube forces the alveolar gases in the corrugated tube out through the open APL

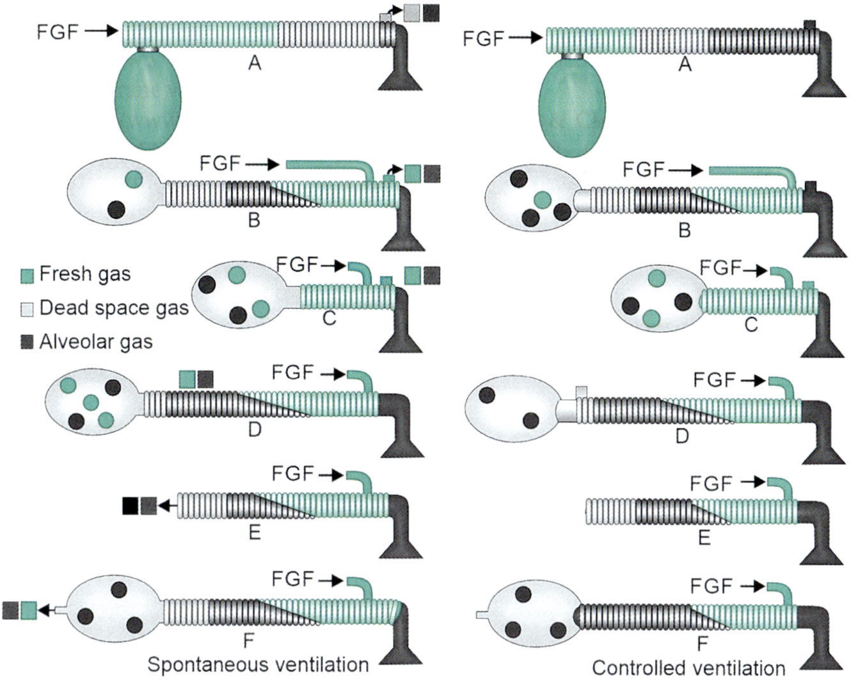

Fig. 11: Gas disposition at end expiration during spontaneous (left) and controlled (right) ventilation in circuits A through F. (FGF: fresh gas flow).

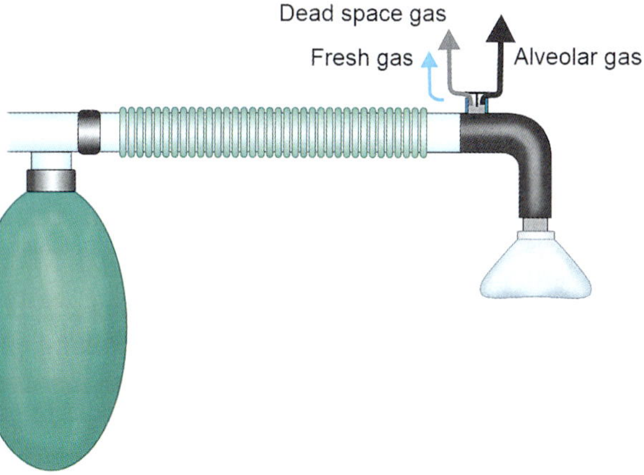

Fig. 12: Disposition of gases at the end of spontaneous exhalation when fresh gas flow equals or slightly more than minute ventilation. During next inspiration, patient breathes gases from apparatus dead space and fresh gas.

valve. If the FGF is equal to or higher than patient's minute volume, all the alveolar gases and the dead space gases will be vented through APL valve **(Fig. 12)**. At the beginning of next inspiration, patient inhales alveolar gases from apparatus dead space followed by fresh gases from the corrugated tube.

If the FGF is equal to the alveolar ventilation then the gas from the dead space that entered the corrugated tube will be conserved **(Fig. 13)**. Since these gases do not contain any CO_2, rebreathing of these dead space gases will not result in CO_2 accumulation in the patient.

However, if the FGF were to be less than the alveolar ventilation then significant rebreathing of CO_2 containing alveolar gases could result in hypercapnia **(Fig. 14)**.

During controlled ventilation, the Mapleson A is the least efficient system **(Fig. 15)**. The APL valve has to be partially closed to inflate the lungs. Hence, the opening pressure of the APL valve is high and the gases are not vented out of the system during exhalation. At the end of exhalation, the patient end

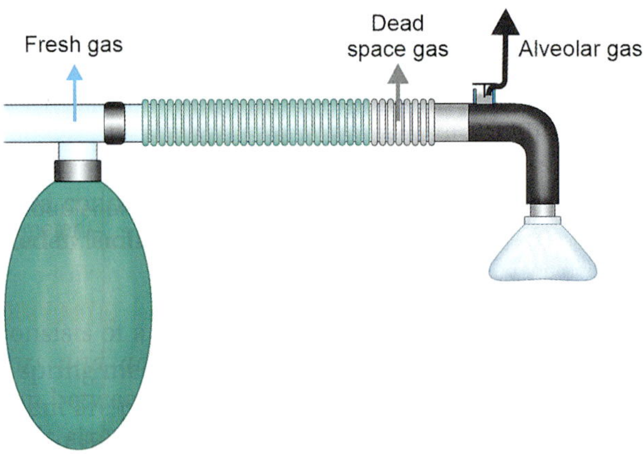

Fig. 13: Disposition of gases at the end of spontaneous exhalation when fresh gas flow equals alveolar ventilation. During next inspiration, patient breathes gases from apparatus dead space, dead space gas, and fresh gas.

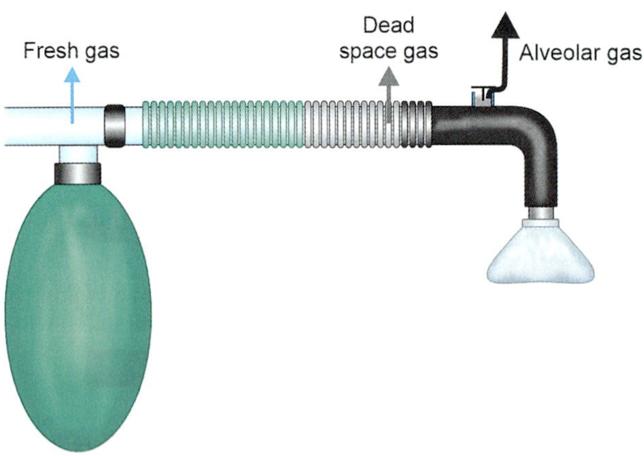

Fig. 14: Disposition of gases at the end of spontaneous exhalation when fresh gas flow is less than alveolar ventilation. During next inspiration, patient breathes alveolar gas, dead space gas, and fresh gas.

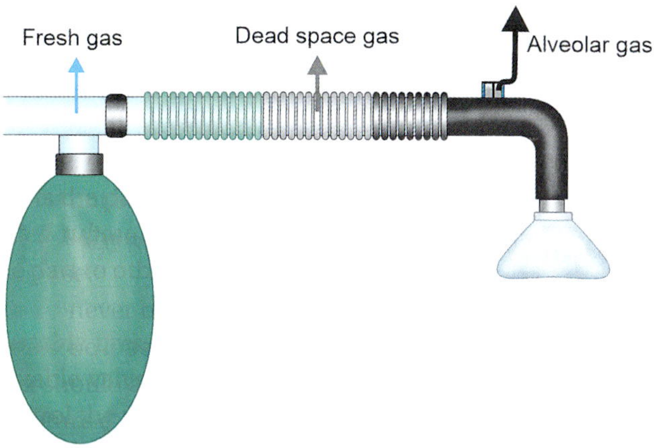

Fig. 15: Disposition of gases at the end of exhalation (controlled ventilation). During next inspiration patient is ventilated with alveolar gas, dead space gas, and fresh gas. There will be significant wastage of fresh gas.

of the corrugated tube is filled with alveolar gases. The RB and the machine end of the corrugated tube contain fresh gases. During the early part of the next inspiration, a portion of the alveolar gases enters the patient and some is vented out through the APL valve. During the latter part of inspiration, fresh gases enter the patient's lungs and some are vented out. This results in wastage of fresh gases and significant rebreathing of alveolar gases making this system inefficient.

*Mapleson B and C (see **Fig. 11**):* During spontaneous breathing, APL valve is kept open and during controlled ventilation, APL is partially kept open. At the end of exhalation, the reservoir contains fresh gas, dead space gas, and alveolar gas. During inspiration, there will be rebreathing of alveolar gas and during exhalation there will be wastage of fresh gas. Hence, the FGF should be high and hence the system is considered inefficient. Prior to the Mapleson's analysis, these systems were popular due to several misconcepts. Since 1954, the Mapleson A system had become routine on anesthetic machines.

In EARS, the RB and APL valve are enclosed. The system functions as Mapleson A in spontaneously breathing patient. Even during controlled ventilation, the enclosed APL remains closed during inspiration and opens during expiration when the system pressure becomes higher than the opening pressure of APL. Hence, the EARS makes is efficient both during spontaneous breathing and controlled ventilation.

Mapleson D: The Mapleson D, E, and F systems function as T-piece systems. The apparatus dead space in these systems extends from the patient to the point of entry of FGF.

All through the exhalation, the dead space gases and alveolar gases mix thoroughly with fresh gases and collect in the RB and corrugated tubing.

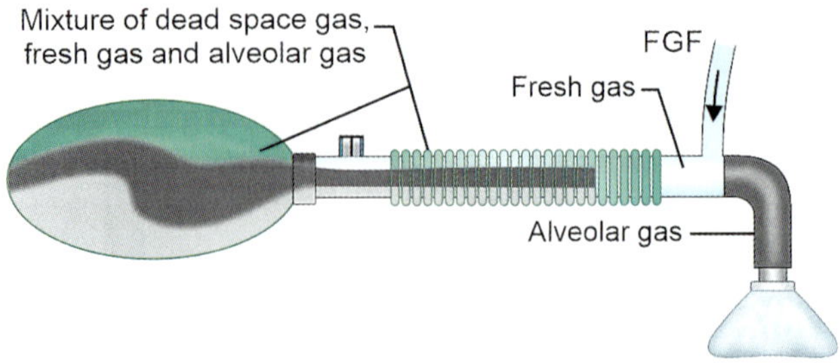

Fig. 16: Disposition of gases at the end of exhalation in Mapleson D and similar systems. (FGF: fresh gas flow)

During the expiratory pause, the fresh gases collect at the patient end of the corrugated tube **(Fig. 16)**. During the next inspiration, the fresh gas flowing from the machine and fresh gas in the corrugated tube enters the patient first. The contribution of this to the tidal volume will depend upon the FGF and the expiratory pause. During latter part of inspiration, the mixture of fresh gas, dead space gas, and alveolar gas enters the patient. Some of these gases remain in the anatomical dead space of the patient, hence minimizing the effect of rebreathing. The functional analysis is similar in both spontaneous and controlled ventilation. Hence, this system can be used safely during both spontaneous and controlled ventilation. FGF of 1.5–2 times the minute ventilation of the patient was reported to produce adequate $PaCO_2$, which depends primarily on the minute ventilation.

The system is slightly more efficient during controlled ventilation because of the control over the expiratory pause. When high FGF (>2 times the minute volume) is used, there is no rebreathing and the minute ventilation determines the arterial CO_2 levels. This principle is commonly employed in pediatric population.

The adult patient is hyperventilated (minute volume >150 mL/kg/min with normal to low respiratory rate) and CO_2 levels are controlled by adjusting FGF and hence the rebreathing. Studies using Bain circuit have demonstrated that a FGF of 70 mL/kg/min maintains normocapnia, whereas a FGF of 100 mL/kg/min maintains mild hypocapnia.

T-piece Systems

Ayre's T-piece was introduced in 1937. The resistance was considered to be lower than systems containing valves. Numerous modifications of the T-piece system were made. The Jackson Rees modification is widely used in pediatric anesthesia. In this system, the APL valve is replaced by open-ended RB.

Functionally, the Jackson Rees attachment performs like Mapleson D. Rebreathing is prevented by using FGF about two times the minute ventilation. This system is used in children for both spontaneous and controlled ventilation. The T-piece systems are widely used for pediatric anesthesia, oxygen therapy, pediatric and neonatal resuscitation, and in pediatric ventilators.

MONITORING

Inspired Oxygen Concentration

The current recommendations require that all modern machines must have inspired oxygen concentration monitoring along with low O_2 and high O_2 alarms. Most units incorporate oxygen concentration monitor either at the common gas outlet (CGO) or in the inspiratory limb of the circle system to ensure that hypoxic mixtures are not delivered. In addition, inspired oxygen concentration is also monitored at the patient end using paramagnetic analyzers. Causes of inadequate O_2 concentration in the breathing system include:

- Hypoxic gas being delivered via the pipeline or tanks
- Disconnected fresh gas hose during use of a hanging bellows ventilator
- O_2 flow control valve turned off
- Failure of oxygen failsafe system
- Proportioning system failure
- O_2 leak in the low pressure system of the machine
- Closed system with inadequate O_2 inflow rate

Airway Pressure

Airway pressure monitoring warns the user about high pressures, low pressures and disconnections. Many traditional anesthesia breathing systems incorporate an analog pressure gauge, as well as an electronic pressure monitoring and alarm system. Most currently used anesthesia machines incorporate low pressure, high pressure, sustained pressure, or disconnection alarms. Airway pressure monitoring can give us an approximate idea of changes in airway resistance and lung and thoracic compliance. The modern anesthesia machine can give us real-time pressure tracing plotted against time. During volume controlled ventilation, when inspiratory pause is used, changes in plateau pressure indicate changes in lung and thoracic compliance; whereas changes in the peak to plateau pressure gradient indicate changes in airway resistance provided there are no alterations in tidal volume.

Spirometry

Spirometry is used to monitor the tidal volume, compliance, resistance, and breathing system integrity. These values provide valuable information regarding changing pulmonary mechanics during anesthesia. The ventilator bellows are marked to give us an approximate idea of tidal volume. In traditional anesthesia machines, monitoring of expired tidal and minute volumes is achieved using a spirometer placed in the vicinity of the expiratory UDV. The modern machines use flow sensors (D-Lite flow sensor, heated wire anemometer, ultrasonic flow sensor, etc.) between the patient and breathing system, and give an accurate idea of minute volume, compliance, and resistance. These modules enable us to monitor flow-volume and pressure-volume loops as well.

Capnography

It is interesting and essential to have a good understanding of functional analysis of breathing systems. However for all practical purposes, one depends on capnography to maintain CO_2 homeostasis. Monitoring partial pressure end-tidal carbon dioxide ($PETCO_2$) levels gives us an estimate of $PaCO_2$, and hence the FGF and minute ventilation can be manipulated to maintain desired CO_2 levels. Evaluation of the inspiratory phase of the capnogram gives us an idea of rebreathing of exhaled CO_2 **(Fig. 17)**. The ideal site to sample gases is between the patient and the elbow adaptor after the breathing system.

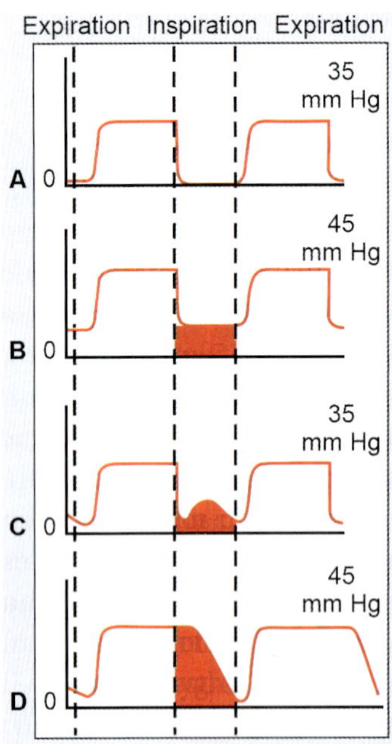

A. Normal capnogram. $PETCO_2$ is normal

B. Exhaustion of soda lime. Base line is elevated above zero indicating rebreathing (shaded area during inspiration). $PETCO_2$ is increased

C. Camel hump during inspiration indicating rebreathing of mixed gas (alveolar and fresh) during later part of inspiration. This is typical of Mapleson D in controlled ventilation. The $PETCO_2$ may remain normal despite rebreathing

D. Rebreathing during controlled ventilation with Mapleson A or malfunctioning inspiratory unidirectional valve in circle system. The expiration appears prolonged due to rebreathing of alveolar gases without any change in CO_2 content. $PETCO_2$ is increased

Fig. 17: Capnography and rebreathing.
($PETCO_2$: partial pressure end-tidal carbon dioxide)

SUGGESTED READING

1. Brockwell RC, Andrews JJ. Inhaled anesthetic delivery systems. In: Miller RD (Ed). Miller's Anesthesia, 6th edition. Philadelphia: Elsevier Churchill Livingstone; 2005. pp. 273311.
2. Collins VJ. Principles of Anesthesiology. Philadelphia: Lea & Febiger; 1966.
3. Dorsch JA, Dorsch SE. Understanding Anesthesia Equipment, 5th edition. Philadelphia: Lippincott Williams & Wilkins; 2008.
4. Eisenkraft JB. Hazards of the Anesthesia Workstation. Philadelphia: Wolters Kluwer Health; 2008.
5. Mapleson WW. Editorial I: Fifty years after—reflections on 'The elimination of rebreathing in various semiclosed anaesthetic systems'. Br J Anaesth. 2004;93(3):31921.
6. Miller DM, Miller JC. Enclosed afferent reservoir breathing systems. Description and clinical evaluation. Br J Anaesth. 1988;60:46975.
7. Wang J, Vacanti C. Anaesthesia breathing apparatuses. In: Vacanti C, Sikka P, Richard U, Segal S (Eds). Essential Clinical Anesthesia, 1st edition. Boston: Cambridge university press; 2010.

WEBSITES

1. http://www.asevet.com/resources/circuits/index.htm. Last accessed November, 2024.
2. http://www.capnography.com/Circuits/Breathingsys/ravi. htm. Last accessed November, 2024.
3. http://www.anesthesia2000.com/physics/Chemistry_ Physics/physics14.htm. Last accessed November, 2024.

CHAPTER 5

Anesthesia Ventilators

Yasodananda K Areti

INTRODUCTION

The earliest delivery of anesthesia in 1846 used a simple vaporization chamber that required spontaneous ventilation by the patient to inhale oxygen and diethyl ether. Boyle's anesthesia machine, 70 years later, incorporated a breathing circuit and reservoir bag that contained the anesthetic gases and finally allowed the clinician to ventilate the patient, though this did require manually squeezing the reservoir bag. Blease's eventual invention of the "pulmoflator" (a simple bellows ventilator), in 1945, enabled automatic positive-pressure ventilation for patients undergoing surgery. This was followed by continued refinement with the Bird and Bennett ventilators two decades later.

Currently, more challenging patients are being taken up for surgery and anesthesia, and the newer ventilators should ensure adequate intraoperative gas exchange. In order to facilitate this process, the anesthesia ventilators match the precision and sophistication of intensive care unit (ICU) ventilators. Some of these ventilator options can be particularly useful for patients requiring extremes of ventilation, such as neonates with very low tidal volumes and patients with stiff or resistive lungs due to diseases such as acute respiratory distress syndrome (ARDS).

The contemporary anesthesia ventilators on the anesthesia workstations by Dräger, Datex-Ohmeda, Maquet, and other companies have integrated many advanced ICU-type ventilation features and are capable of providing ventilation for the most challenging patients brought to the operating room. These anesthesia ventilators have sophisticated computerized controls, have several modifications to the circle breathing system, and are able to provide advanced types of ventilatory support such as synchronized intermittent mandatory ventilation (SIMV), pressure-controlled ventilation (PCV), positive end-expiratory pressure (PEEP), and pressure support ventilation (PSV) in addition to the conventional controlled mechanical ventilation (CMV). A basic understanding of the mechanics of these ventilators and the modifications to the breathing circuits is critical for every anesthetist to use this complicated techniques safely.

MODES OF VENTILATION IN THE ANESTHESIA VENTILATORS

Volume Control Ventilation

Most commonly used mode of ventilation during anesthesia is the volume-controlled ventilation (VCV), also called volume-targeted or volume-limited ventilation. In the VCV, the ventilator attempts to deliver a specified tidal volume by delivering a constant inspiratory flow for the programmed inspiratory time **(Figs. 1A and B)**.

The pressure versus time in VCV is shown in **Figure 2**. The peak inspiratory pressure (PIP) represents the airway resistance and total compliance (chest wall and lungs). The plateau pressure (P_{plat}) measured during inspiratory pause, represents the total compliance. Thus, the airway resistance is reflected by the difference between PIP and P_{plat}, whereas the difference between P_{plat} and PEEP, or baseline zero pressure represents total compliance.

The airway pressure will rise throughout inspiration as the lung volume steadily increases. The rate of airway pressure rise depends on the inspiratory flow rate, and the total compliance of lung and chest wall. The tidal volume is delivered despite a decrease in the total compliance at the cost of increased airway pressures.

Disadvantages of Volume-controlled Ventilation

The high PIP generated due to decreasing thoracic compliance, exposes the patient to *barotrauma*. In order to minimize the risk of barotrauma, a

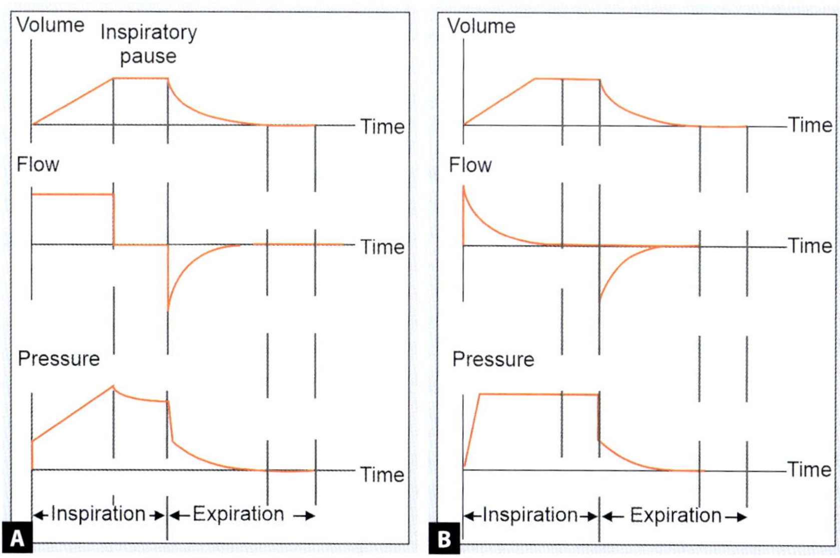

Figs. 1A and B: Relation between tidal volume, flow, and pressure: (A) Volume-controlled ventilation; (B) Pressure-controlled ventilation.

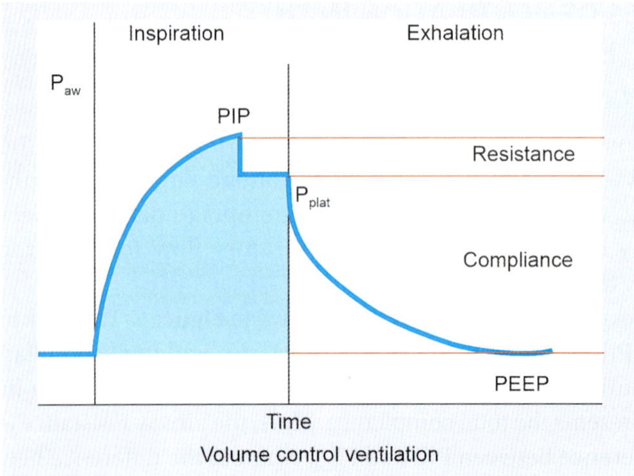

Fig. 2: The components of mechanical ventilation inflation pressures. (P_{aw}: airway pressure; PEEP: positive end-expiratory pressure; PIP: peak airway pressure; P_{plat}: plateau pressure)

pressure limit is usually set and once this pressure is reached, the ventilator no longer delivers the set tidal volume. The traditional use of large tidal volumes during ventilation in ICU is also being linked with *volutrauma* and current recommendations suggest that low volume, PCV may be superior. Gas distribution in the lungs may not be optimal during VCV, as difficult to fill alveoli may not fill until late in the inspiratory time, leaving less time for gas exchange. VCV may not be the ideal ventilation mode for patients with lung disease or for pediatrics.

Very small airways, and the small bore endotracheal (ET) tubes and laryngeal mask airways (LMAs) encountered in pediatric anesthesia may cause high airway resistance. The combination of constant flow and high resistance can produce very high inspiratory pressures. In addition, uncuffed ET tubes may cause airway leaks around the ET tube, leading to *delivery of inadequate tidal volume.*

Pressure Control Ventilation

In PCV, or pressure-limited ventilation, the controlled parameter is the airway pressure during inspiration. The ventilator will vary the inspiratory flow rate to generate the specified inspiratory airway pressure **(Figs. 1A and B)**. This will tend to produce larger tidal volumes at lower pressures, and so is very useful when lung compliance is low, e.g. laparoscopy, obesity, ARDS, and pregnancy. In PCV, the risk of barotrauma is less. In patients with lung disease, there is some evidence that PCV may result in better matching of ventilation and perfusion. Every patient can be ventilated using this mode.

Disadvantages of Pressure-controlled Ventilation

As with VCV, PCV is also a time-cycled method of ventilation. The inspiration terminates at the end of the set inspiratory time (as set by respiratory rate and I:E ratio). Because the inspiratory flow rate varies, the total volume delivered at the end of the inspiratory time varies depending on the overall lung and system compliance at the time of each inspiration. This can sometimes result in wide swings of resultant tidal volumes. If the compliance of the lungs and breathing circuit are constant, the volumes delivered will tend to be constant. If the lung compliance decreases, e.g., with abdominal insufflation, external pressure on the chest, and a momentary contraction of the diaphragm (as with a cough), the airway pressure will increase. The ventilator will decrease the inspiratory flow in order to maintain the set airway pressure; consequently, the volume delivered will decrease. Conversely, when there is a sudden increase in lung compliance, such as release of abdominal pressure at the end of a laparoscopy, the subsequent tidal volume will increase significantly unless the set inspiratory pressure is immediately decreased.

Pressure-controlled Ventilation with Volume Guarantee (Fig. 3)

This is one of the recently introduced modes in anesthesia ventilation, combining the advantages of VCV and PCV. A preset tidal volume is delivered with a decelerating flow at the lowest possible PIP during a preset inspiratory time, at the preset respiratory rate, thereby enhancing and facilitating patient ventilation. SmartVent 7900 uses this mode. This mode with decelerating flow

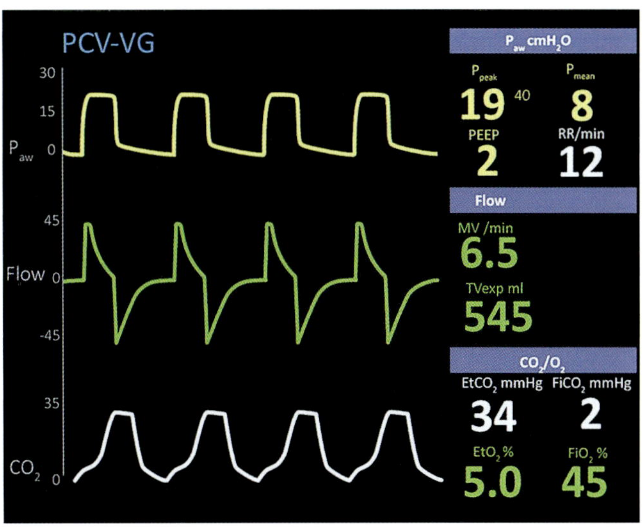

Fig. 3: Redrawn screen shot of Aisys workstation. Volume preset pressure control ventilation or pressure control ventilation with volume guarantee (PCV-VG).

provides better gas exchange at lower airway pressure. The system monitors changes from breath to breath and compensates for changes in compliance. Safety features are included to warn the user of dramatic increase in pressures or inadequate volume delivery.

The main parameters that have to be set in the earlier mentioned modes are shown in **Table 1**.

Synchronized Intermittent Mandatory Ventilation

Synchronized intermittent mandatory ventilation was initially introduced as a weaning mode; however, it has become a standard mode of ventilation from the initiation to the weaning. The ventilator delivers a preset number of breaths and allows patient to breathe spontaneously in between the ventilator breaths **(Fig. 4)**. If a spontaneous breath is initiated during a window prior to the time when a controlled breath is due, the controlled breath is synchronized with the spontaneous breath, preventing the "stacking" of machine delivered breath on patient's spontaneous breath. The total respiratory rate includes the machine breaths and the spontaneous additional breaths. SIMV has found application in the operating room to facilitate emergence from anesthesia as the patient transitions from controlled to spontaneous ventilation.

TABLE 1: Main parameters for different ventilator modes.

	VCV	*PCV*	*PCV-VG*
Tidal volume	Set in mL		Set in mL
Inspiratory pressure	Changes based on resistance and compliance	Set in cmH_2O	Ventilator determines the inspiratory pressure from breath to breath
Respiratory rate	Breaths per minute—set by the operator		
Cycling time from inspiration to expiration PEEP	Ratio of inspiratory time to expiratory time (I:E) cmH_2O	Inspiratory time in sec. or I:E ratio cmH_2O	I:E ratio cmH_2O
Maximum inspiratory pressure (P_{max})	Pressure limit (cmH_2O) Set tidal volume not delivered	Maximum airway pressure, at which time the ventilator will alarm and end inspiration	Pressure limit (cmH_2O)
• Inspiratory pause • Rise rate	0–50% of inspiratory time	The rate at which the ventilator will reach the targeted airway pressure	The rate at which the ventilator will reach the targeted airway pressure

(PCV: pressure control ventilation; PCV-VG: pressure control ventilation-volume guarantee; VCV: volume control ventilation)

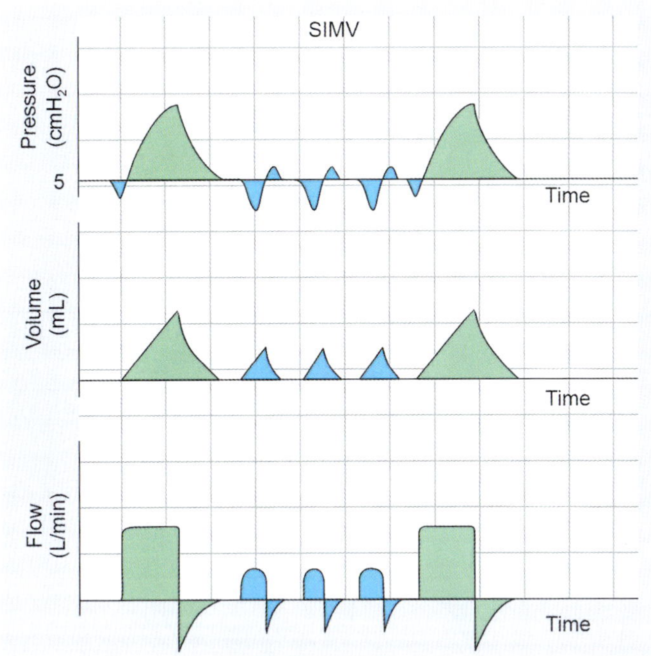

Fig. 4: The pressure, volume, and flow to time waveforms for synchronized intermittent mandatory ventilation (SIMV).

Pressure Support Ventilation

In PSV, the ventilator supports patient's effort by providing programmed pressure assistance throughout the breath. Low values of pressure support will primarily overcome the resistance of the ET tube or LMA, and the ventilator circuit, thus decreasing patient's work of breathing. The patient's own ventilatory musculature provides the remainder of the work to generate the tidal volume. The level of support can be increased to provide the desired tidal volume after each breath initiation.

Pressure support can be used for induction, maintenance and emergence. It is no longer necessary to squeeze the bag at any stage of the anesthetic, keeping both hands free for other things. The use of LMAs has led to a dramatic increase in spontaneous ventilation in the operating room. PSV is a useful adjunct in such techniques. During transition from muscle relaxation, a combination of SIMV and PSV may be used **(Fig. 5)** or only PSV can be used.

In strict PSV, all breaths are patient-initiated. The most sensitive inspiratory triggers use inspiratory flow sensors, the sensitivity of which can be adjusted to avoid false triggering on the heartbeat. A good machine can trigger a 5 kg child on an adult circuit and do a better job in supporting their respiration at 40 breaths/minute than we could with a T-piece!

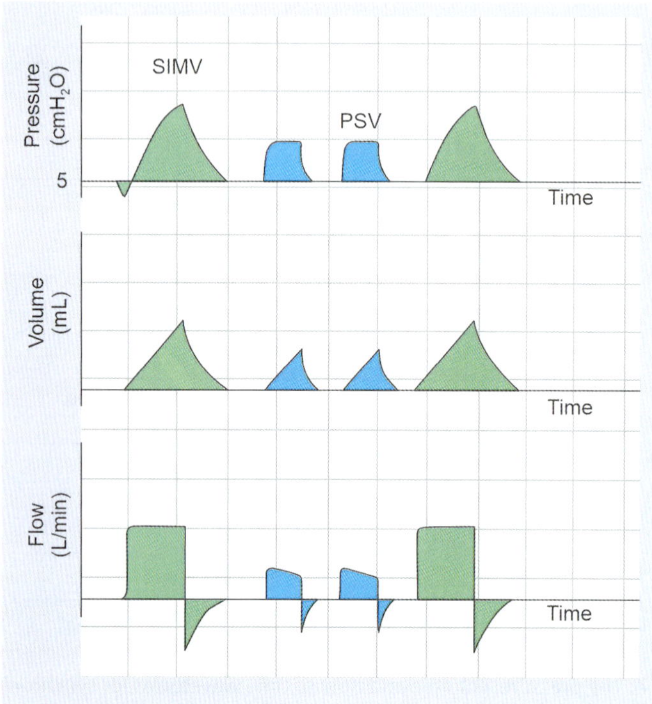

Fig. 5: The pressure, volume, and flow to time waveforms for synchronized intermittent mandatory ventilation (SIMV) with pressure support ventilation (PSV).

If the trigger is inadequate to initiate a breath, the ventilator will not cycle. Hence, with many ventilators, pressure support includes a "backup", or safety mode. If the patient does not initiate a breath within a certain period, the machine defaults to a mode of controlled ventilation to ensure adequate ventilation.

Traditional hand bagging gives us visual feedback by watching the chest move and tactile feedback from squeezing the bag. In pressure support, the bag is not held, so that useful tactile information is no longer available.

Positive End-Expiratory Pressure

General anesthesia and positioning during surgery decreases functional residual capacity and increases closing capacity. In addition, techniques using denitrogenation will remove airway splinting. These factors could lead to pulmonary atelectasis and intraoperative pulmonary shunting resulting in hypoxemia. The magnitude of shunt is correlated with the formation of pulmonary atelectasis, which appears within minutes after induction of anesthesia in 85–90% of all patients. Application of PEEP has the obvious advantage in such situations instead of using very high-inspired oxygen concentration, which by itself predisposes to atelectasis. In addition, PEEP would be essential for patients on ventilator therapy in ICU coming for surgery and anesthesia. Application of PEEP is also known to reduce the incidence of atelectasis in obese patients undergoing general anesthesia. Application of continuous positive airway pressure (CPAP) during preoxygenation is also well tolerated and has been shown to prevent atelectasis and deoxygenation during induction even in morbidly obese patients. Application of CPAP to the unventilated lung has also been used to improve oxygenation during one lung anesthesia. A small PEEP of around 3 cmH_2O is inherent in ascending bellows ventilator. PEEP valves are available for increasing PEEP as required. However, most modern ventilators provide electronic flow-controlled PEEP or CPAP.

CLASSIFICATION OF ANESTHESIA VENTILATORS

Anesthesia ventilators can be classified based on mechanism of tidal volume delivery, the design of breathing circuit, ventilator drive mechanism, cycling, and compensation for fresh gas flow (FGF) and compliance changes. The users must understand the *functional analysis* of the ventilator they use, as per the following classification to ensure safe ventilation during anesthesia.

- *Mechanism of tidal volume delivery:*
  - Expiratory limb occluders (T-piece systems)
  - Minute volume dividers (Manley, Ohmeda 7100)
  - Bag squeezers (bag-in-box arrangement)
  - Piston ventilators
  - TurboVent blower (Dräger Zeus)
  - Volume reflectors (VRs) (Maquet FLOW-i workstation)
- *Breathing circuit design:*
  - Double circuit (bellows-in-box)
  - Single circuit (piston, TurboVent)
- *Ventilator drive mechanism:*
  - Pneumatic (oxygen or air)
  - Electrical (piston)
  - Intermittent blowers (electronic computer-controlled)
- *Cycling:*
  - Volume
  - Pressure
  - Time
  - Flow
  - Patient
- *Fresh gas coupling:*
  - FGF compensation (SmartVent 7900)
  - Fresh gas decoupling (Dräger piston ventilators)
  - FGF interruption

CHALLENGES SPECIFIC TO ANESTHESIA VENTILATORS

- Use of inhalational anesthetic agents
- Use of low-flow techniques
- Driving the ventilators
- Effect of FGF on tidal volume
- Changes in total compliance in patients, effect of breathing system compliance, and leaks around ET tubes or LMAs
- Ability to switch from manual to mechanical ventilation
- Use of oxygen flush
- Anesthetizing and ventilating patients of different sizes and ages
- Scavenging of waste anesthetic gases
- Difficulty in applying PEEP/CPAP

Several modifications are required to overcome these issues in modern ventilators.

Low-flow Inhalational Anesthesia

Inhalational anesthesia requires administration of known concentration of oxygen, volatile agent vapor, and nitrous oxide. Low flows are used to save costs and to minimize pollution. This necessitates use of breathing circuits with carbon dioxide absorption techniques. Traditionally, spontaneous breathing is largely unassisted (manual assistance is done if required) and controlled ventilation is achieved by partially closing the adjustable pressure-limiting (APL) valve and squeezing the reservoir bag.

The traditional ventilators achieved mechanical ventilation with all the earlier mentioned objects by enclosing the reservoir bag (bellows replaced reservoir bag) in a rigid box, which is pressurized intermittently mimicking the intermittent squeezing of the reservoir bag. This resulted in two circuits; one with inhalational agents connected to patient and the other one where the driving gas pressurizes the rigid box, hence the name double-circuit technology. These ventilators are also known as "bag-in-bottle" or "bellows-in-box" ventilators. These bellows could be hanging bellows (descending) or more commonly standing bellows (ascending) based on whether the bellows descend or ascend during expiratory filling **(Fig. 6)**. The descending bellows have the disadvantage of creating negative pressure during expiration or filling with gases from the box if there is a leak in the bellows.

Driving the Ventilator

Gas-driven

The driving gas in the anesthesia ventilators could be compressed air, oxygen or a venturi device delivering mixture of oxygen and air. If oxygen is the driving gas, one must switch to manual ventilation in the event of failure of pipeline supply necessitating the use of oxygen from "type-E" cylinder.

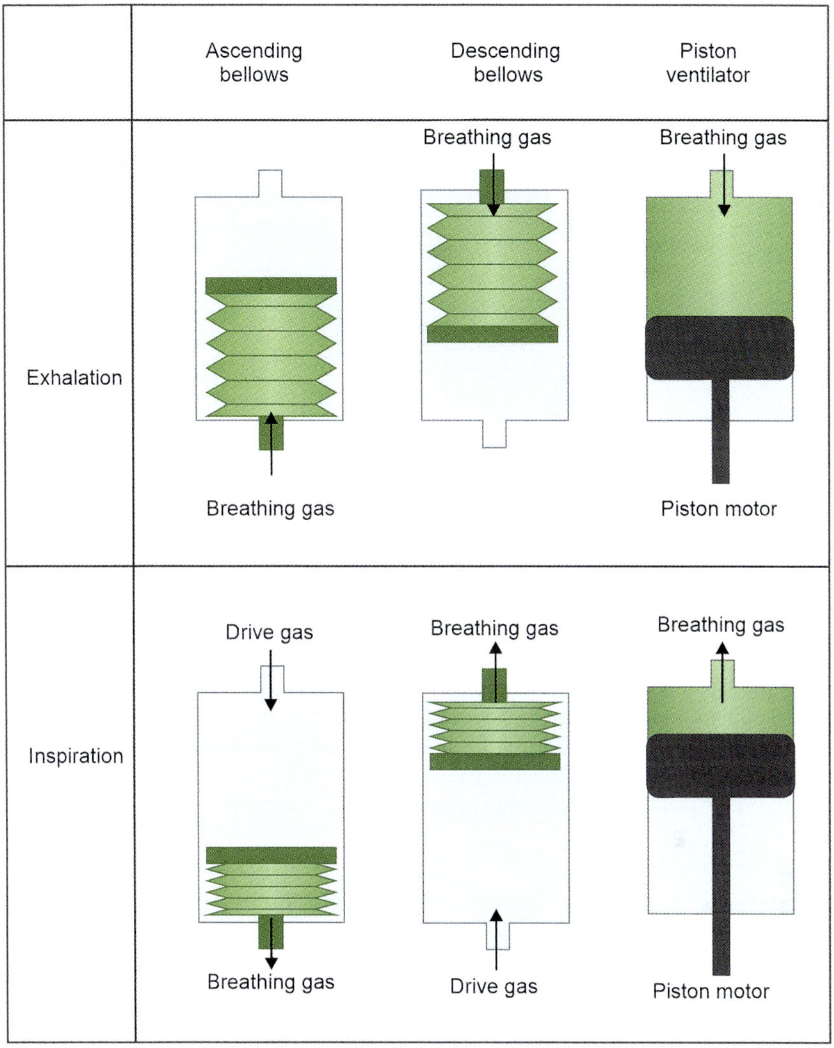

Figs. 6: Three types of ventilator drive mechanisms during exhalation and inspiration. Breathing gas is bluish and ventilator drive gas is gray.

Piston Ventilators

In some modern ventilators (Dräger), there has been a resurgence in the use of mechanical devices like a piston to drive these ventilators **(Figs. 6 and 7)**. These piston type ventilators use a computer-controlled stepper motor, instead of compressed drive gas, to actuate gas movement in the breathing system. In these systems, instead of having dual circuits with gas for the patient in one and the drive gas in another, there is a single gas circuit for the patient. They are classified as *piston-driven, single-circuit ventilators*. The piston operates much like the plunger of a syringe to deliver the desired

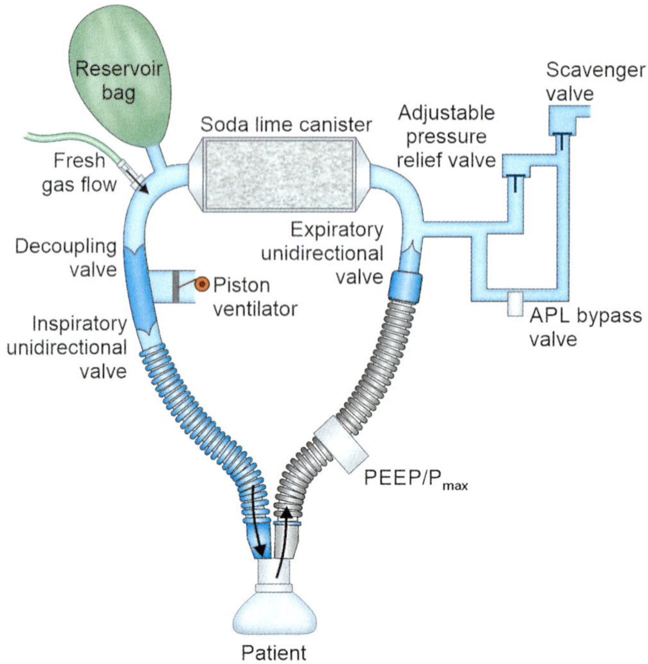

Fig. 7: Modifications in circle-breathing system using piston ventilator to achieve fresh gas decoupling (Dräger). There is a decoupling valve. The ventilator is located between decoupling valve and inspiratory unidirectional valve. Manual and ventilator relief valves are modified and connected to scavenging system. (APL: adjustable pressure-limiting; PEEP: positive end-expiratory pressure; P_{max}: maximum inspiratory pressure)

tidal volume or airway pressure to the patient. The major advantage of the piston ventilator is the ability to deliver tidal volume accurately to all patients under a large variety of clinical conditions. There is no oxygen cost of driving gas, and the loss of tidal volume due to internal compliance of bellows is eliminated. However, since they are electrically operated, one has to depend on the limited battery backup (about 30–90 minutes) in the event of power failure.

TurboVent

The latest in the anesthesia ventilation is the use of TurboVent, a revolutionary closed-system ventilator (Dräger Zeus®). The ventilator consists of an electronic driven and controlled compressor turbine placed in the inspiratory limb. The compressor turbine is dynamically driven by a brushless direct current (DC) motor, enabling high flow of gases in patient circuit. This type of ventilator results in:

- Buildup of the breathing pressure and deliver the corresponding flow to the patient during inspiration, and

- Delivery of circuit flow that is required to mix the gas within the breathing system independently from patient inspiratory effort.

This ventilator allows spontaneous respiration in all breathing modes and with virtually unlimited inspiratory flow. TurboVent is suitable for all forms of ventilation, even those required in intensive care.

Volume Reflector Technology

FLOW-i takes advantage of Maquet innovation called the Maquet VR. This unique system uses SERVO-controlled platform with unique VR device that allows partial rebreathing of exhaled gases. *The VR is oxygen-driven by design. It is a double-circuit ventilator.* All the gas modules use *feedback loop-controlled, solenoid-actuated, pneumatic valves* similar in function those found in a SERVO-controlled ICU ventilator. The VR is a coiled, 3.6 m plastic channel with an approximate 1.2 L capacity, which serves as reservoir for exhaled gases.

Effect of Fresh Gas Flow on the Delivered Tidal Volume

Traditionally, the FGF is delivered directly into the breathing system (circle system). This flow is added to the tidal volume delivered by the ventilator and is termed as fresh gas coupling. If the FGF is low, this contribution will be small. If FGF is high, it significantly contributes to ventilation. For example, if FGF is set at 6 L/min (100 mL/s) then approximately 100 mL of FGFs into the circuit every second. If the ventilator is set to deliver a tidal volume of 600 mL in 2 seconds then 200 mL of fresh gas will be added to this volume resulting in a total inspiratory tidal volume of 800 mL. If the FGF is low at 1 L/min then the additional volume is only about 33 mL, with a total inspiratory volume being 633 mL, a minor contribution. Hence, the fresh gas coupling could be particularly hazardous to infants and small children when FGF is altered.

Fresh Gas Decoupling or Fresh Gas Compensation

The aim in the contemporary anesthesia ventilator is to ensure that tidal volume is not affected by FGF. There are several approaches to dealing with the problem of changing tidal volume with changes in FGF.

Fresh gas decoupling: The Dräger Julian, Narkomed 6000 and Fabius GS use fresh gas decoupling, i.e., the fresh gas is not added to the delivered tidal volume. Thus, fresh gas decoupling helps ensure that the set and delivered tidal volumes are equal. These machines use piston ventilators that are usually located in the *inspiratory limb* (*see* **Fig. 7**). The action of the piston closes a one-way *decoupling valve*, diverting the FGF to the manual breathing bag during the inspiratory cycle. A series of electronically controlled valves must work in concert with the ventilatory phase to accomplish this decoupling.

In machines where the ventilator is present in the inspiratory limb, because of this decoupling valve, there would be no back pressure to close the expiratory unidirectional valve. Hence, a *PEEP/*P_{max} *valve* is interposed between the patient and the expiratory unidirectional valve.

The visual appearance of the reservoir bag during this type of decoupling is unusual:

- The manual breathing bag, normally quiescent during mechanical ventilation, moves with each breath.
- The manual breathing bag movement is opposite to the movement seen in a mechanical ventilator bellows: The manual-breathing bag *inflates* during inspiration (due to FGF) and *deflates* during expiration as the contents empty into the ventilator. If the reservoir bag were to be removed, atmospheric air will be entrained and the ventilator functions without activating any alarms; hence, the anesthesiologist must be aware of this potential problem.

Fresh gas compensation: This is utilized in the Aestiva, S/5 ADU, and Aisys. The volume and flow sensors provide feedback, which allows the ventilator to adjust the delivered tidal volume so that it matches the set tidal volume, in spite of the total FGF. These measurements may be done in the first few breaths and compensation is instituted from subsequent breaths, which may result in high tidal volumes during the first few breaths. The sensors also compensate for breathing system compliance and leaks around ET tube.

Fresh gas interruption: This approach is used in Dräger Julian to minimize the effects of FGF on tidal volume. The FGF is measured and reported electronically and the computer controls interrupt the flow during inspiration. The machine works as intermittent flow machines.

Effect of Compliance and Leaks on Delivered Tidal Volume

During intermittent positive pressure ventilation (IPPV), a part of the tidal volume gets compressed in the breathing system, leading to the decrease in the delivered tidal volume. This is known as the internal compliance of the breathing system, which is approximately 5–10 mL/cmH_2O. The traditional ventilators do not have any compensation for this loss and anesthesiologist has to depend on chest expansion, spirometry, and end-tidal CO_2 to ensure that the ventilation is adequate and not to rely on the volume indicated on the box. Compliance compensation is incorporated in some of the modern ventilators (Datex-Ohmeda 7900-SmartVent™, Dräger Fabius, etc.). During the preuse test, the ventilator assesses the internal compliance and makes the appropriate changes to ensure that the set tidal volume is delivered. One has to repeat the self-tests if the circuit is changed between patients in a surgical list. Alternately, some machines (SmartVent) monitor the volumes and flow at both inspiratory limb, and the expiratory limb of the breathing system, and ensure that the set tidal volume is delivered through a servo-feedback loop.

Presence of small leak around uncuffed ET tubes or LMAs results in loss of tidal volume, which is not detected by preuse check. This can only be compensated by measuring the inspiratory and expiratory flows and making the necessary adjustments to deliver the set tidal volume.

Ability to Switch from Mechanical to Manual Ventilation

During induction of anesthesia patients are transitioned through spontaneous breathing to manual ventilation followed by CMV. The opposite occurs during recovery. The isolation of patient circuit from the ventilator circuit helps us to achieve this object. Adjusting the pressure relief valve helps us to transition from spontaneous to manual ventilation. A manual switch is incorporated in the circuit to switch between the reservoir bag and the ventilator bellow (Chapter 4). The relief valve in the ventilator circuit is distinct from the APL valve. It relieves excess gas from the patient breathing circuit at the end of *exhalation*, contrary to the APL valve during manual ventilation, which relieves excess patient gas during *inspiration*. The relief valve in the ventilator is kept sealed during inspiration.

Use of Oxygen Flush

A more significant problem with fresh gas coupling can result from activation of the oxygen flush valve during the inspiratory phase of the ventilator. As with FGF, this additional flow (35–75 L/min) will add to the inspiratory flow. This translates to over 1,000 mL of flow per second and leads to build up of excessive pressures in the circuit with a possibility of barotrauma or volutrauma. In contemporary workstations, the pressure limit set by the user minimizes this risk. Some machines may also have a factory preset pressure limit of 60 cmH_2O to minimize the risk of high pressure. In machines featuring fresh gas decoupling, the decoupling valve directs the excess oxygen flush flow away from the patient during IPPV and thus maintains stable volume and pressure (*see* **Fig. 7**).

Pediatric Ventilation

The loss of tidal volume due to breathing system compliance and leaks around the uncuffed ET tubes has maximal effect in pediatric patients. Hence, appropriate breathing systems are chosen for pediatric subjects. In the bellows-in-box arrangement, smaller ventilator bellows have to be used to be able to deliver small tidal volumes accurately. The new piston and turbine ventilators allow the clinician the flexibility of delivering wide range of tidal volumes more accurately and obviate the need to change bellows.

Waste Anesthetic Gas Scavenging (see Fig. 7)

The exhaled gases in ICU ventilators are vented out to the atmosphere. However, anesthesia ventilators should be able to vent the exhaled gases to the waste gas scavenging systems of the operating rooms in order to eliminate operating room pollution. Both the APL valve in the circle system and the relief valve in the ventilator are suitably modified to achieve this.

Application of Positive End-expiratory Pressure

Application of PEEP would be an obvious solution to counter the effects of anesthesia on pulmonary system. In the past, PEEP valves were used for this purpose. Because of the dangers of mounting them incorrectly, they are no longer recommended. The modern ventilators incorporate electronic PEEP control. In standing bellow ventilators, there normally is an end-expiratory pressure of +2.5 cmH_2O because of the PEEP effect of the ventilator relief valve. Application of PEEP could result in loss of tidal volume set on the ventilator. The position of the PEEP valve varies in different models of anesthesia ventilators. The Datex-Ohmeda SmartVent applies PEEP at the ventilator relief valve and result in no loss of tidal volume. Any deviation from the tidal volume set would be sensed by the inspiratory flow transducer and a correction would be made via the SmartVent compensation system.

COMMONLY USED CURRENT MODELS OF ANESTHESIA VENTILATORS

Dräger Divan Ventilator (Piston and Bellows)

The Dräger Divan ventilator is a modern ventilator, offering features such as pressure control mode, SIMV, correction for compliance losses, and integrated electronic PEEP. The piston driven bellows are inconspicuous and are horizontally mounted.

The ventilator has automatic adjustments to deliver the set tidal volume despite:

- *FGF changes:* Fresh gas decoupling.
- *Patient compliance changes:* Dynamic measurement of patient compliance in the first few breaths and automatic compensation, if changes occur during the course of anesthesia.
- *Breathing system compliance changes:* A pressure transducer within the ventilator measures compliance losses; appropriate adjustments are made by the ventilator microprocessor to ensure that the set tidal volume is delivered to the patient.
- *Detecting leaks:* By automatically checking for leaks in the total breathing circuit (absorber head and corrugated limbs) and hoses, the ventilator helps to ensure minimal airway leakage and automatically compensates to deliver constant tidal volume.

E-Vent plus Piston Ventilator (Primus IE, Fabius GS; Figs. 8 and 9)

This is electrically powered, electronically controlled, high-speed piston ventilator. It delivers peak flows comparable with ICU ventilators with full range of volume and pressure-oriented modes. It consumes no drive gas.

An adjustable flow trigger helps reduce respiratory work, and PEEP can be applied regardless of ventilator mode. It is capable of PSV and volume AutoFlow ventilation for patients with pulmonary obstruction. This ventilator has clear advantages for pediatric (including neonates) and critical care patients.

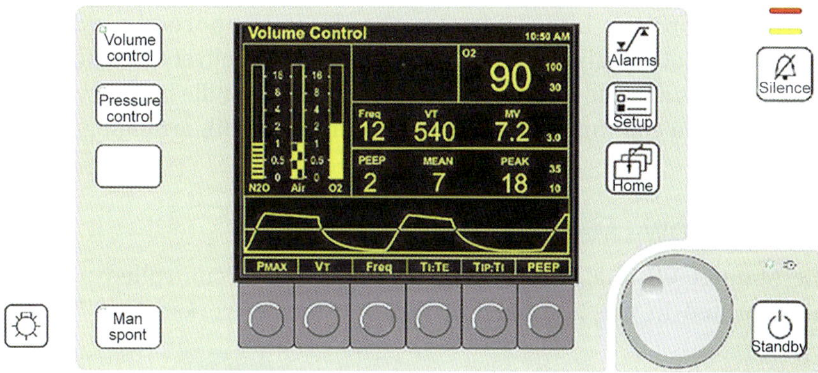

Fig. 8: Fabius GS ventilator controls.

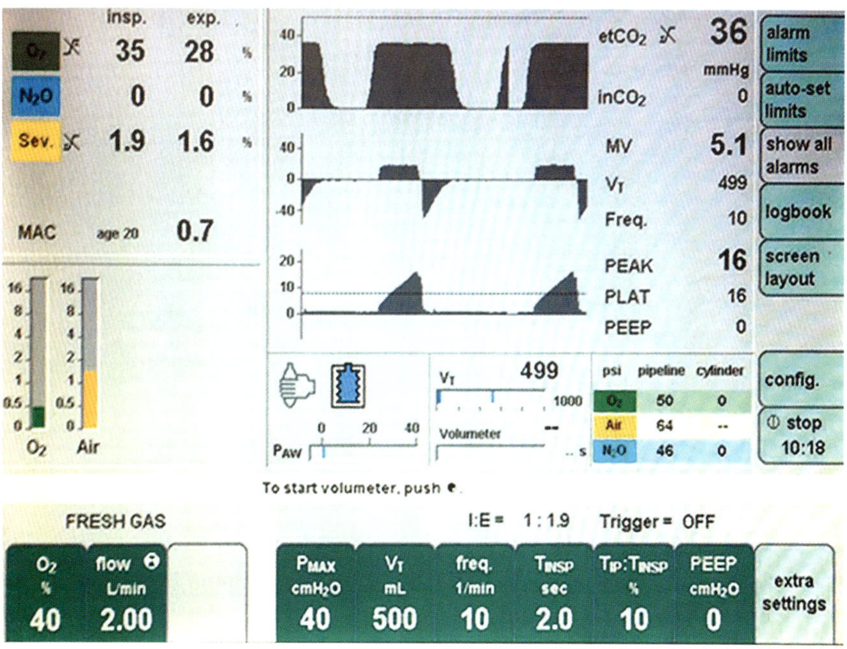

Fig. 9: Dräger Primus screen display with ventilator controls.

Fresh gas decoupling is achieved by diverting the fresh gas to a reservoir bag during inspiration. Compliance compensation is achieved by checking the circuit compliance during preuse check. Leaks in the reservoir bag can lead to air dilution and no alarms sound. This could be a possible cause awareness.

Zeus TurboVent®

The Zeus Infinity Empowered (IE) gives you high quality ventilation in the operating room and is ideally suited for use in adults, children and neonates alike. The innovative, turbine-driven TurboVent ventilation provides unlimited inspiratory flow, regardless of the ventilation mode.

The TurboVent blower-driven ventilator supports spontaneous respiration in all breathing modes and can be used to deliver newer modes of ventilation. As a result, anesthetists can confidently handle hard to ventilate patients, while eliminating the headaches involved with arranging for ICU ventilators.

Maquet FLOW-i Machine (Fig. 10)

The Maquet VR is a unique system using SERVO-controlled platform incorporated in the Maquet FLOW-i anesthesia workstation. The VR

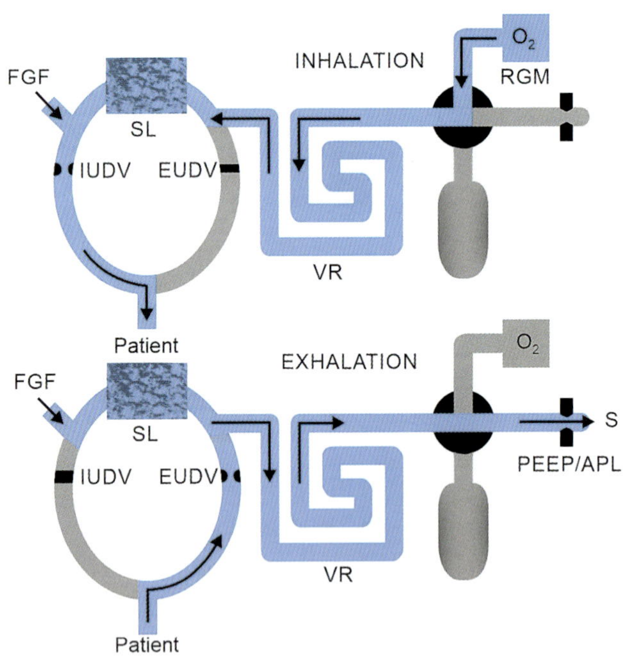

Fig. 10: Schematic representation of volume reflector technology. [APL: adjustable pressure-limiting; EUDV: expiratory unidirectional valve; FGF: fresh gas flow; IUDV: inspiratory unidirectional valve; PEEP: positive end-expiratory pressure; RGM: reflector gas module; S: scavenging; SL: soda lime canister; VR: volume reflector module (air piston)]

technique is able to optimize pressure and flow and enable fast, powerful interventions. A low internal volume in combination with a powerful flow and pressure generator achieve this. Less internal volume also enables rapid changes in gas concentrations when needed.

FLOW-i has the capability to deliver the set tidal volume in spite of high abdominal and thoracic pressure. It has the capability to deliver high inspiratory flow both peak and continuously and thus adapt to individual patient demands. The fast rise time, low expiratory work of breathing and a high performance trigger facilitate PSV even in pediatric patients. FLOW-i controls the pressure drop during expiration very fast. This gives quick and accurate PEEP control, minimizing the risk for auto-PEEP at higher respiratory rates.

Ohmeda 7000 Bellows Ventilator (Fig. 11; Ohmeda Excel)

These are electrically powered, double-circuit, pneumatically driven, ascending bellows, time-cycled, and electronically controlled ventilators. This is a minute-volume preset ventilator (unique among current ventilators). Tidal volume *cannot* be set directly but is calculated from settings of minute volume and respiratory rate. Inspiratory flow stops when driving gas equivalent to the set tidal volume has been delivered to the driving circuit side of the bellows chamber or if pressure >65 cmH_2O is attained. The ventilator can work with adult bellows and pediatric bellows.

Datex-Ohmeda 7100 Bellows Ventilator (Aespire, Aestiva Machines)

The 7100 ventilator is a microprocessor-based, electronically controlled, pneumatically driven, with built-in monitors for inspired oxygen, airway pressure, and exhaled volume. Sensors in the breathing circuit compensates for compression losses, FGF changes, and small leakages in the breathing system. PEEP is generated electronically; however, CPAP is not available.

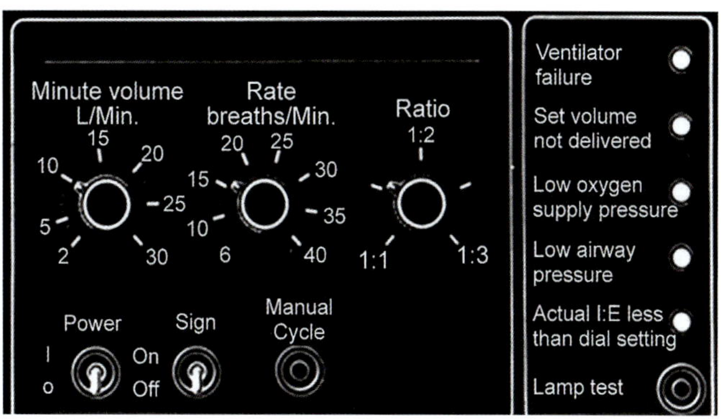

Fig. 11: Minute volume divider.

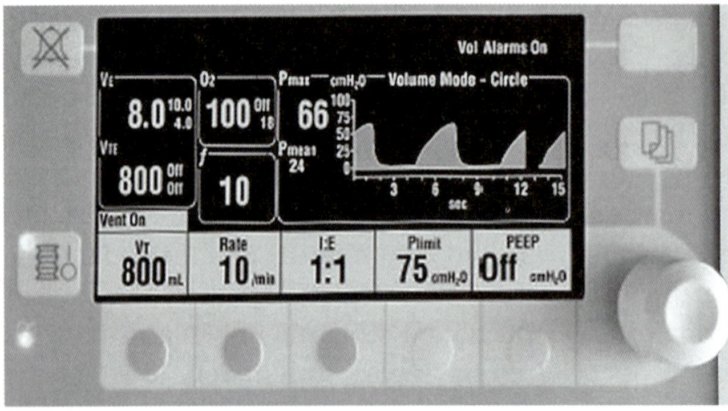

Fig. 12: SmartVent 7900.

Ohmeda 7900 "SmartVent" Bellows Ventilator (Fig. 12)

SmartVent is a pneumatic, double-circuit, and ascending bellows ventilator. Microprocessor control delivers the set tidal volume in spite of changes in FGF, small leaks, and breathing system or bellows compliance losses proximal to the sensors. The flow sensors are placed between corrugated plastic-breathing circuit and the absorber head, in both limbs. These are connected to pressure transducers in the ventilator. It offers such desirable features as integrated electronic PEEP control and PCV mode. It has been reported that the sensors can be quite sensitive to humidity, causing ventilator inaccuracy or outright failure; hence, use of heat and moisture exchanger (HME) filters are recommended.

Datex-Ohmeda S/5 ADU Bellows Ventilator

This is a microprocessor-controlled pneumatic, double-circuit, and ascending bellows ventilator. This ventilator has several unique features. Single switch activation (setting the bag/vent switch to "Auto") is all that is needed to start mechanical ventilation. FGF is located between the inspiratory unidirectional valve of the circle system and the patient. Delivered tidal volume is adjusted to compensate for changes in FGF, and total breathing circuit compliance losses through the *D-Lite sensor* at the Y-piece. The ventilator can utilize either oxygen or air as a driving gas, and will switch automatically from one to the other if pipeline pressure is lost. Volume control, pressure control, and SIMV modes are offered, along with integrated electronic PEEP.

TYPICAL VENTILATOR ALARMS

All current gas machines have volume, pressure, and oxygen monitoring built in the breathing circuit. Most have agent monitoring as well. Some have spirometry and capnography. It is important to understand the alarms and set the limits appropriately so that the operators are not distracted with false alarms. Though not mandatory, these alarms usually set around 20% beyond the normal values.

These alarms typically are:

- High pressure
- Pressure below threshold for 15–30 seconds (apnea or disconnect)
- Continuing high pressure
- Subatmospheric pressure
- Low tidal or minute volume
- High respiratory rate
- Reverse flow (may indicate incompetence of expiratory unidirectional valve in the breathing circuit)

Low Inspired Oxygen

Machines without this monitoring are generally considered for machine obsolescence.

Apnea/disconnect alarms may be based on:

- *Chemical* monitoring (lack of end-tidal carbon dioxide)
- *Mechanical* monitoring:
  - Failure to reach normal inspiratory peak *pressure*, or
  - Failure to sense return of tidal *volume* on a spirometer
- *Visual* monitoring:
  - Failure of standing bellows to fill during mechanical ventilator exhalation
  - Failure of manual breathing bag to fill during mechanical ventilation (machines with fresh gas decoupling: the Apollo, Fabius GS, and Narkomed 6000)
- *Auditory* monitoring:
  - Lack of breath sounds in precordial
  - Lack of sound from ventilator cycling, etc.
- *Optic* monitoring:
  - Failure of the hanging bellows to fill completely (the "garage door" electronic eye sensor on the Julian)

SUGGESTED READING

1. Areti YK. Anesthesia ventilators. In: Vacanti C, Sikka P, Richard U, Segal S (Eds). Essential Clinical Anesthesia. Boston: Cambridge University; 2011.
2. Badgwell M, Swan J, Foster AC. Volume-controlled ventilation is made possible in infants by using compliant breathing circuits with large compression volume. Anesth Analg. 1996;82:719-23.
3. Brochard L, Rua F, Lorino H, Lemaire F, Harf A. Inspiratory pressure support compensates for the additional work of breathing caused by the endotracheal tube. Anesthesiology. 1991;75:739-45.
4. Eisenkraft J. Anesthesia delivery system. In: Longnecker D, Brown D, Newman M, Zapol W (Eds). Anesthesiology. China: McGraw-Hill; 2008.

5. Gajic O, Dara SI, Mendez JL, Adesanya AO, Festic E, Caples SM, et al. Ventilator-associated lung injury in patients without acute lung injury at the onset of mechanical ventilation. Crit Care Med. 2004;32:1817-24.
6. Gammon RB, Shin MS, Buchalter SE. Pulmonary barotrauma in mechanical ventilation: Patterns and risk factors. Chest. 1992;102:568-72.
7. Klemenzson GK, Perouansky M. Contemporary anesthesia ventilators incur a significant "oxygen cost". Can J Anesth. 2004;51(6):616-20.
8. Nathan SD, Ishaaya AM, Koerner SK, Belman MJ. Prediction of minimal pressure support during weaning from mechanical ventilation. Chest. 1993;103:1215-9.
9. Stayer SA, Bent ST, Campos CJ, Skjonsby BS, Andropoulos DB. Comparison of NAD 6000 and Servo 900C ventilators in an infant lung model. Anesth Analg. 2000;90:315-21.
10. Tobin MJ. Medical progress: advances in mechanical ventilation. N Engl J Med. 2001;344:1986-96.

WEBSITES

1. Dosch MP. The Anesthesia Gas Machine. https://healthprofessions.udmercy.edu/academics/na/agm/08.htm. Last accessed November, 2024.
2. Amanullah S, Beaulieu KA, Talavera F, Rice TD. Ventilator Graphics, CME article. http://emedicine.medscape.com/article/305120-overview#aw2aab6b5. Last accessed November, 2024.
3. http://emedicine.medscape.com/article/304068-over-view#a1. Last accessed November, 2024.

CHAPTER 6

Equipment for Airway Maintenance

Aruna Parameswari, Akilandeswari Manickam, Archana Areti

ENDOTRACHEAL EQUIPMENT

Airway management is an important aspect of anesthesia care and resuscitation. Several devices are used for the management of the normal and difficult airway. Over the last few decades, many new devices with different designs have been introduced. The utility of these advantages and disadvantages over other devices are highly variable. Knowledge of the available equipment and the indications for use and their limitations are necessary in choosing the right and safe technique of airway management in a particular patient.

DEVICES FOR NORMAL AIRWAY MANAGEMENT

FACE MASK

This allows administration of oxygen and anesthetic gases and vapor from the breathing system to the patient in a noninvasive manner, by creating a low-pressure airtight seal around the face. Face mask is also used to provide continuous positive airway pressure (CPAP) and noninvasive ventilation. It can be made of rubber, plastic, silicon, neoprene, or polycarbonate. The parts include a body, a seal, and a connector.

Parts of the Face Mask

Body

This is the main part of the mask and can be opaque or transparent **(Figs. 1A and B)**. When transparent, it allows the visualization of secretions, vomit, and blood. Monitoring of spontaneous respiration by visualization of condensation during exhalation is also possible with a transparent mask.

Seal (Edge)

This is the portion of the mask that is in contact with the patient's face and establishes the low-pressure seal and a snug fit. It can be of the cuff or the flap type. The pad, cuff, or the cushion type requires inflation of the seal with air or some other material while the flap is just an extension of the body that is

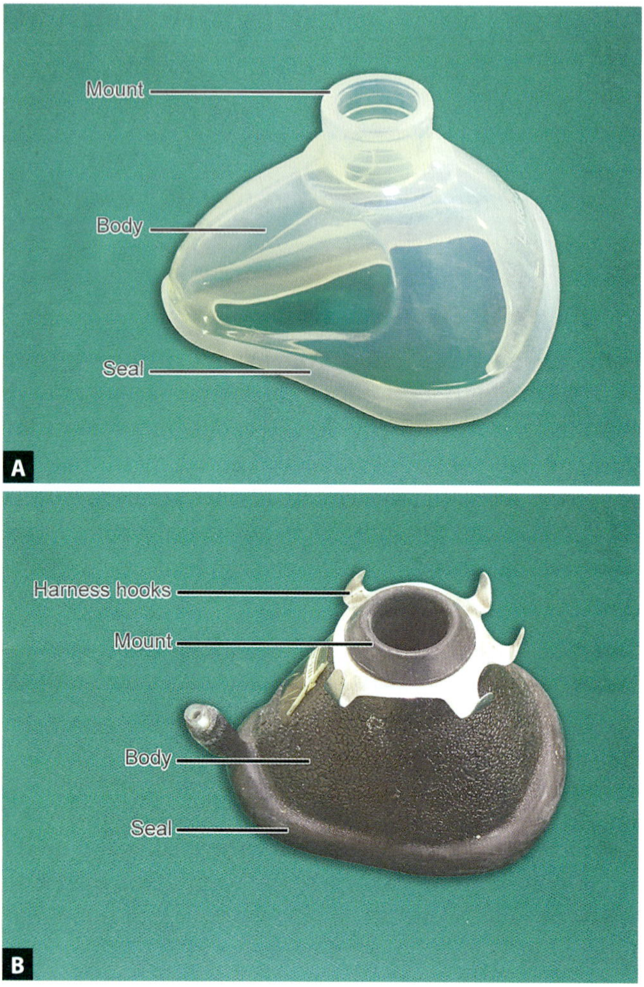

Figs. 1A and B: Parts of a face mask: (A) Laerdal silicone face mask with a transparent body and a seal of the flap type and (B) Black anatomical face mask with an opaque body and a seal of the cuff type.

flexible and takes the contour of the face. A good seal is essential to prevent dilution of administered gases by room air during spontaneous respiration and also to provide positive pressure ventilation without gas leak.

Connector (Mount)

This is the portion of the mask on the opposite side of the seal, which has a standard internal diameter (ID) of 22 mm for connection to the breathing system. It is made of thickened rubber, plastic, or metal. It has a ring with hooks for attachment of a harness or mask strap.

Types of Face Masks

Masks are of different types depending on the shape and the type of material from which they are made. These include black rubber anatomical face masks, transparent anatomical face masks, transparent round face masks, Rendell-Baker Soucek face masks, endoscopic face masks, etc. **(Fig. 2)**.

Sizes Available

It is important to have all available sizes of face masks on the airway or intubation trolley as one size would not fit all faces. Masks come in sizes 00 to 6 **(Fig. 3)**.

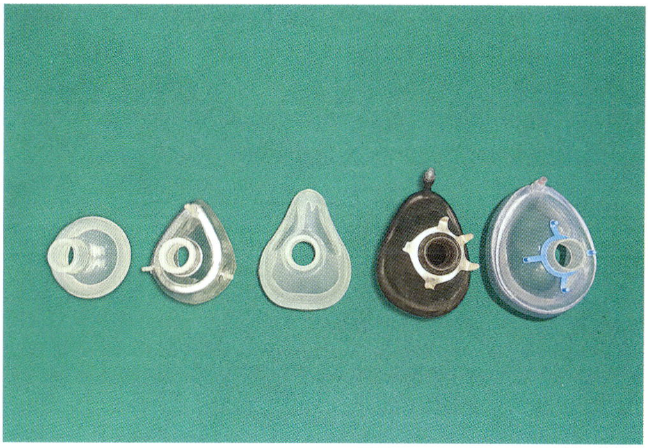

Fig. 2: Different types of face masks.

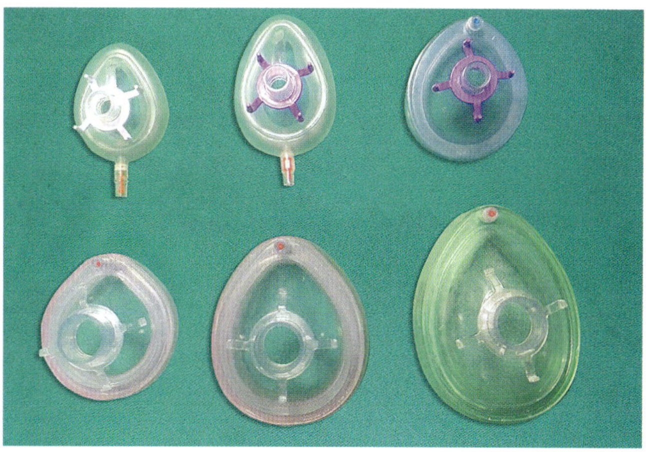

Fig. 3: Different sizes of face masks (from size 0 to size 5). Sizes 00 and 6 are not shown in this picture.

Dead Space

The mask contributes to the apparatus dead space that can assume significance in neonates and infants. The dead space can be reduced by using a smaller mask, increasing the pressure on the mask, or by changing the volume of the cushion. The dead space of an adult face mask can range from 80 to 200 mL.

Technique of Use

In the one-hand technique, the thumb and the index finger of the left hand should be placed over the body of the mask on either side of the connector with downward pressure to create a seal **(Figs. 4A and B)**. The other three fingers of the left hand are placed over the mandible. It is important to avoid pressure on the eyes. In the two-hand technique, the thumbs are placed on either side of the connector and the fingers of both the hands are placed on the angles of the mandible to lift the mandible. Another person is needed to provide positive pressure by squeezing the reservoir bag.

Advantages of Face Mask

- Lower incidence of sore throat
- Lesser anesthetic depth needed for use
- Cost-effective

Disadvantages of Face Mask

- Anesthesia provider's hands have to be used continuously leading to user's fatigue.

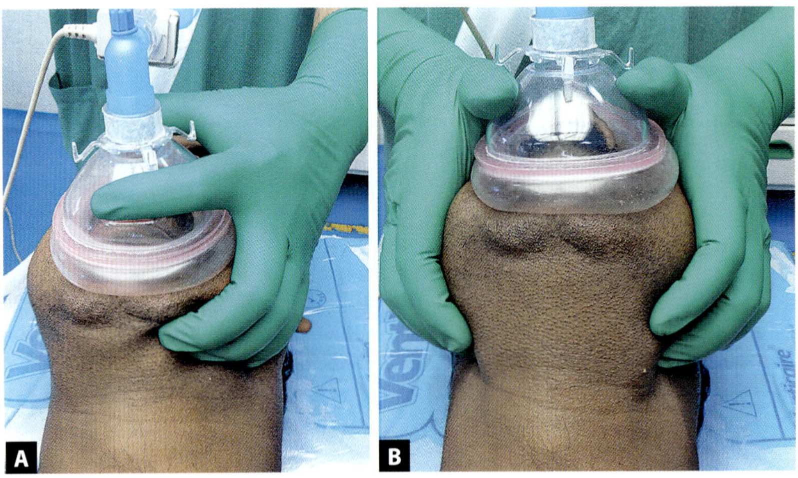

Figs. 4A and B: Technique of holding the face mask. (A) One-hand technique; (B) Two-hand technique.

- Gas leak leading to environmental pollution and gas wastage (due to higher fresh gas flows)
- It does not protect airway against aspiration.
- This can lead to gastric inflation with positive pressure ventilation.
- It is difficult to use in situations where airway access to anesthesiologist can be difficult (MRI).
- More intraoperative airway manipulations are needed to maintain the airway.
- It can cause injuries to the eye, skin, and nerves.

ARTIFICIAL AIRWAYS

The maintenance of an open airway is important for gas exchange. In unconscious and anesthetized patients, loss of muscle tone leads to upper airway obstruction at the level of the tongue, soft palate, and epiglottis as these structures fall against one another or against the posterior pharyngeal wall. Artificial airways are adjuncts used to open the natural airway and maintain its patency, when maneuvers such as head tilt, chin lift, and jaw thrust have failed to open the natural airway. These can be inserted through the mouth (oropharyngeal airways) or through the nose (nasopharyngeal airways).

Oropharyngeal Airways

These are inserted through the mouth and maintain airway patency by pushing the tongue and the epiglottis away from the posterior pharyngeal wall.

Description

They can be made of plastic or elastomeric material. The parts of the oropharyngeal airway include the flange, the proximal buccal end, the bite portion, the curved portion, the air channel, and the distal pharyngeal end **(Fig. 5)**. The flange at the buccal end prevents the airway from slipping deeper into the mouth and helps in fixation. The bite portion is the rigid part that lies between the teeth and is the straight portion of the airway. It prevents the patient from closing the lumen of the airway by biting. The curved portion of the airway lies between the tongue and the palate. The pharyngeal end of a correctly placed airway should lie at the posterior part of the tongue above the epiglottis. The air channel extends from the buccal to the pharyngeal end.

Specific airways include the Guedel airway, the Berman airway, the Patil Syracuse airway, the Ovassapian fiberoptic intubating airway, the Williams airway intubator, the Berman intubating airway, etc.

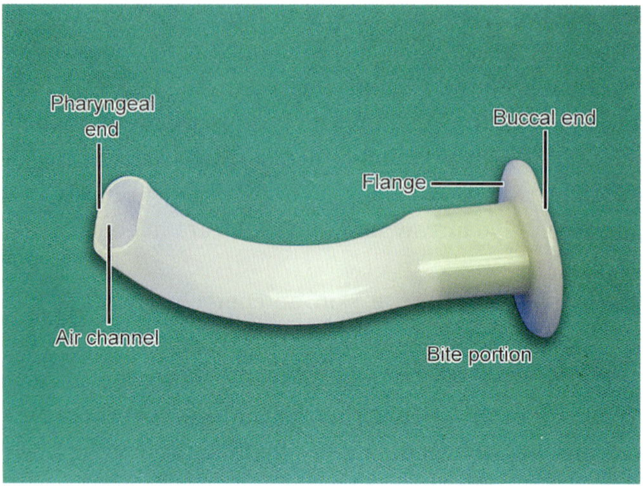

Fig. 5: Parts of the Guedel oropharyngeal airway.

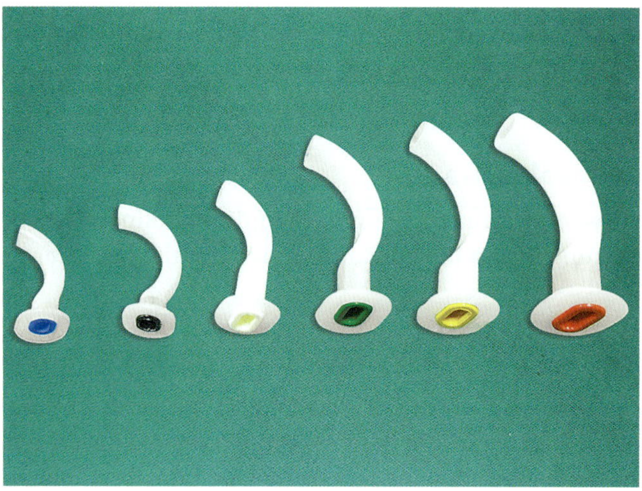

Fig. 6: Sizes of Guedel oropharyngeal airway.

Sizes

Airways come in different lengths and diameters for patients of different sizes, and they are color- and number-coded according to standards **(Fig. 6)**. The correct size of the Guedel's airway is chosen by placing the unstraightened airway between the lips and the tragus of the patient. If it is not inserted deep enough, it can cause the tongue to fold back and worsen airway obstruction. If the airway is inserted too deep, it may push the epiglottis and worsen airway obstruction or irritate the laryngeal inlet leading to laryngospasm.

Technique of Insertion

After extending the head and opening the mouth, the airway is inserted with its concave surface facing toward the upper lip and hard palate and advanced till the bite portion reaches the incisors, at which point it is rotated 180° so that the concave surface now faces the tongue. Jaw thrust can be used to overcome any resistance during insertion. Alternately, it can also be inserted with the concave side facing the tongue, using a tongue depressor and then advanced.

Complications

- Airway obstruction by the airway if an inappropriate-sized airway is used.
- Trauma to the teeth and oropharyngeal structures
- Edema, ulceration, and necrosis of the tongue with prolonged use
- Coughing and laryngospasm, if it is inserted in a light plane of anesthesia

Nasopharyngeal Airways

These are used for relief of airway obstruction at the level of the nares, nasopharynx, tongue, and soft palate.

Description

They are soft and made of rubber, plastic, or polyurethane. They have a curved body (like a short tracheal tube) and a fixed or adjustable flange at the proximal end to prevent loss of device into the nose. The tip is beveled and atraumatic.

Size

They are available in different sizes **(Fig. 7)** from 2 to 9 mm, described by the ID in millimeter. The correct length of the airway is estimated by measuring the distance from the tip of the nose to the tragus of the ear. The correct size is determined by the size of the nostrils.

Insertion Technique

The lubricated nasopharyngeal airway is inserted through the external nares with the bevel facing the septum and advanced over the floor of the mouth till the tip lies in the oropharynx below the base of the tongue and above the epiglottis. The proximal end can be connected to a breathing circuit using a 15-mm tracheal tube connector for oxygenation, CPAP, and to maintain anesthesia during fiberoptic intubation. They are better tolerated than oropharyngeal airways.

Their use is contraindicated in fractures of the skull base, coagulopathy, and sepsis or deformity of the nose.

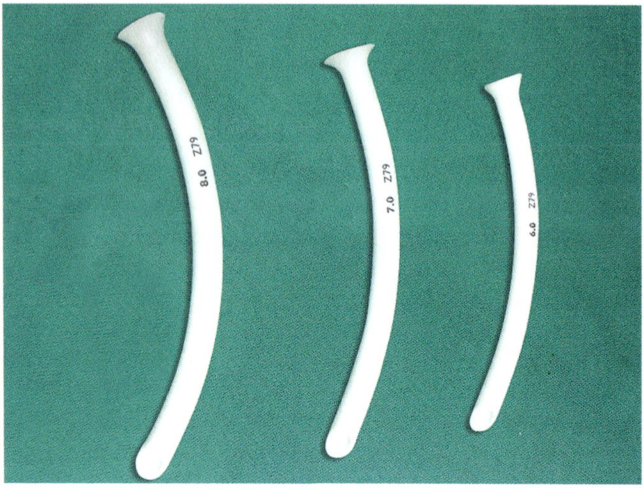

Fig. 7: Different sizes of nasopharyngeal airways.

Complications

- Bleeding from the nose
- Stimulation of laryngeal reflexes if inserted too deep.

LARYNGOSCOPES

These are devices that are used to visualize the larynx to facilitate endotracheal intubation, and they can be rigid or flexible.

History

The first direct laryngoscopy was performed by Alfred Kristein in 1895 using an esophagoscope that he had modified for this purpose and it was called the autoscope. In 1913, Chevalier Jackson popularized the use of direct laryngoscopy further. But, the use of the laryngoscope for visualization of the vocal cords for intubation was popularized by Sir Robert Reynolds Macintosh and Sir Ivan Magill in the 1940s.

Parts of a Rigid Laryngoscope

The parts of the rigid laryngoscope include the handle and the blade **(Fig. 8)**, which can be detachable or attached as a single piece. When the blade and handle are detachable, there is usually a hook on connection between them. This is the part that is held in the user's hand and it has a rough surface to provide a good grip. It houses the power source in the form of disposable or rechargeable batteries. Handles are either made of surgical stainless steel or hardened aluminum (in the newer laryngoscopes), which makes the handle lighter.

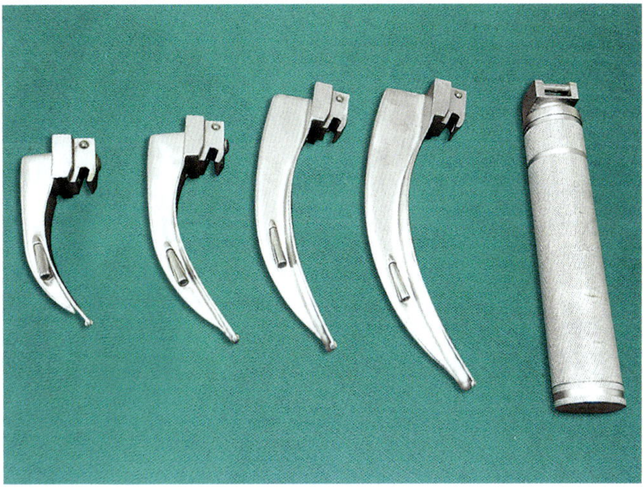

Fig. 8: Macintosh curved blade laryngoscope with blades of four sizes (1, 2, 3, and 4) and handle.

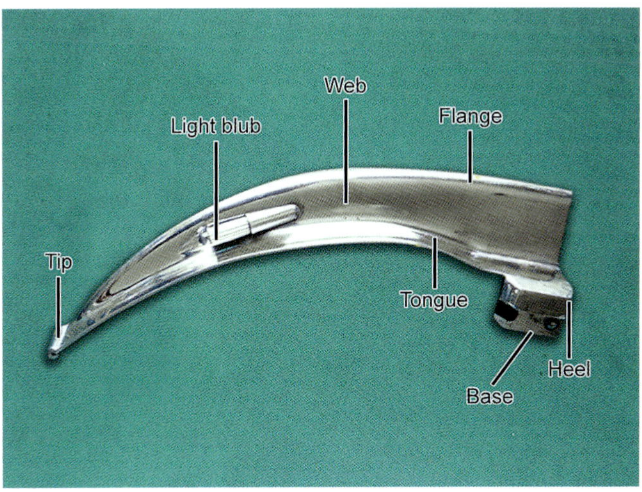

Fig. 9: Parts of the Macintosh curved blade.

Blade

This is the portion of the laryngoscope that is inserted into the patient's mouth during direct laryngoscopy. It consists of the base, heel, tongue, flange, web, tip, and the light source **(Fig. 9)**. The base is the part of the blade that comes in contact with the handle through a hinge connection. It has a slot to accommodate the hinge pin of the handle. The end of the base is the heel. The tongue is that part of the blade that is used to deflect the patient's tongue and other oropharyngeal structures. It can be curved or straight, based on which the laryngoscope is classified as a curved- or straight-blade laryngoscope. The distal end of the blade is the tip that is in contact with the vallecula or epiglottis and is made blunt to avoid trauma. The flange is the portion of the blade that projects from the side of the tongue. The web is the part of the blade between the tongue and the flange that has the electrical connections and the bulb.

The angle between the handle and the blade is usually 90°, but it can be made more obtuse or acute, by using an adapter between the blade and the handle.

Light Source

The light source is either an incandescent bulb located in the blade with the power source located in the handle or the bulb in the handle with the light transmitted to the blade through a fiberoptic bundle **(Figs. 10A and B)**.

When the bulb is located in the blade, it is usually at one-third distance from the tip of the blade and is of the screw on type. The electrical connection is completed when there is metallic contact between the handle and the blade, which happens when the blade is opened for use. The socket for the bulb can get soiled by fluids during laryngoscopy causing the light to fail.

The advantage of the fiberoptic bundle **(Figs. 11A and B)** is that there is no risk of the bulb getting detached and lost during laryngoscopy and there is also a decreased incidence of burns. Cleaning and sterilization are easier. These laryngoscopes are marked by a green dot in the heel for identification, as per the ISO standards **(Figs. 12A and B)**.

Newer laryngoscopes use light-emitting diodes (LEDs) in the handle instead of halogen bulbs, which provide white and brighter light. The LED light source is also energy efficient providing longer-lasting power.

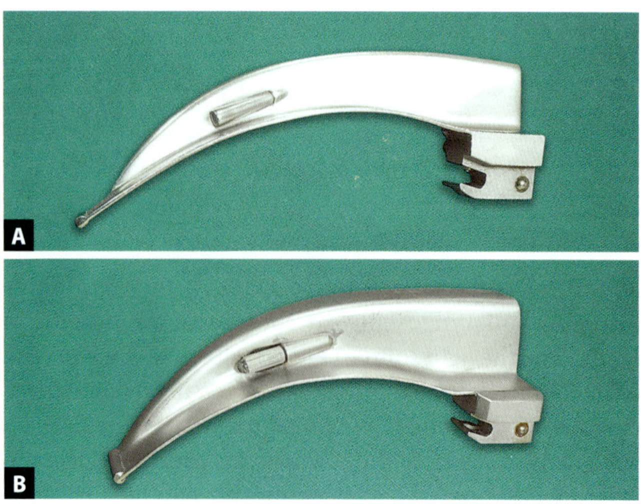

Figs. 10A and B: (A) Blade with a bulb of the screw type in a socket with light source in the handle; (B) Blade with fiberoptic light guide with light source in the handle.

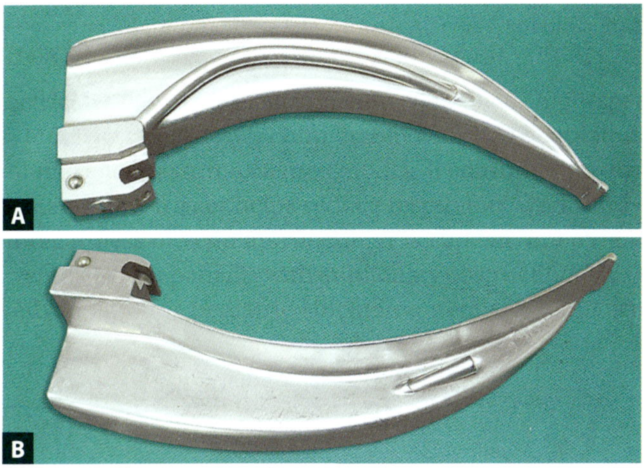

Figs. 11A and B: Fiberoptic guide as light source in Macintosh curved-blade laryngoscope. (A) Light guide is seen emerging from the base of the blade and extending along the web; (B) Light guide is seen emerging on the tongue of the blade.

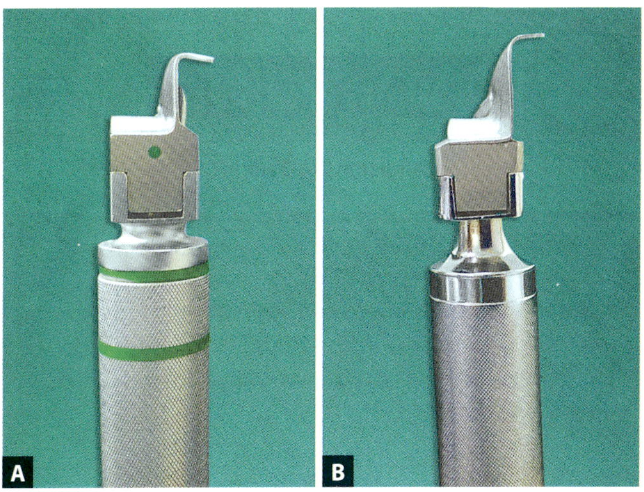

Figs. 12A and B: Fiberoptic laryngoscope identification. (A) Fiberoptic laryngoscope having green circular bands in the handle and a green dot in the heel of the blade; (B) Conventional laryngoscope without a fiberoptic light source with no green mark on the handle or blade.

Sizes of Laryngoscopes

Laryngoscopes are sized according to the blade size. They come in eight sizes as per the ISO standard from 000 for the small premature infant to size 5 for the extra-large adult **(Table 1)**. The blades and handles from different manufacturers are interchangeable and there are two ISO standards, the green system (ISO 7376/3) and the red system (ISO 7376/1) that allow this,

TABLE 1: Different sizes of laryngoscope blades with the age for intended use.

Size of the laryngoscope blade	*Age for intended use*
000	Small premature neonate
00	Premature neonate
0	Neonate
1	Small child
2	Child
3	Adult
4	Large adult
5	Extra-large adult

the difference between the two being the position of the light source and the dimensions of the hinges.

Types of Blades

There are different types of blades. Some of the commonly used ones include:

Macintosh

This is the standard curved-blade laryngoscope that is most commonly used. The tongue, flange, and the web form a reverse "Z" on cross-section. A curved blade is more suitable for adults and also for children with macroglossia.

Miller

This is a straight-blade laryngoscope that is commonly used in children **(Figs. 13A and B)**. The tongue of the blade is straight except for a gentle upward curve near the tip. In cross-section, the tongue, flange, and the web form a flattened "C" **(Fig. 14)**.

McCoy

This is a modified Macintosh blade in which the tip can be flexed by pressing a lever attached to the handle. The flexible tip allows further elevation of the vallecula and the epiglottis, thus improving the laryngoscopic view **(Fig. 15)**. However, movements are limited to the last 25 mm from the tip.

Polio

This is a modification of the Macintosh blade where the angle between the handle and the blade is more obtuse (135° instead of the usual 90°). It is useful in situations like large breasts, barrel chest, and restricted neck mobility.

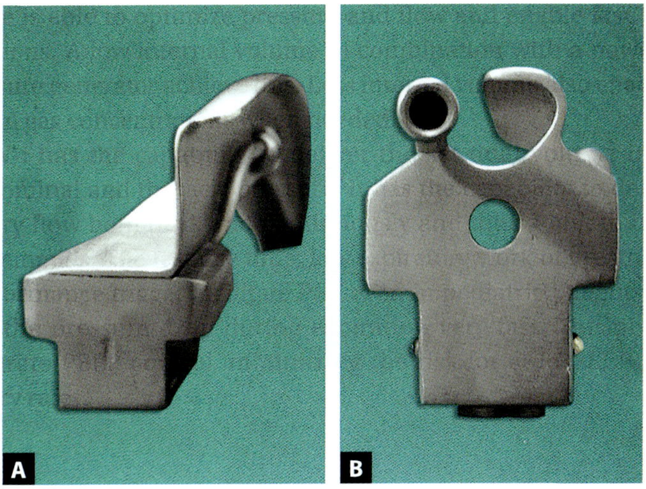

Figs. 13A and B: (A) Reverse "Z" configuration of the Macintosh blade and (B) flattened "C" configuration of the Miller blade-port for oxygen insufflation also is seen.

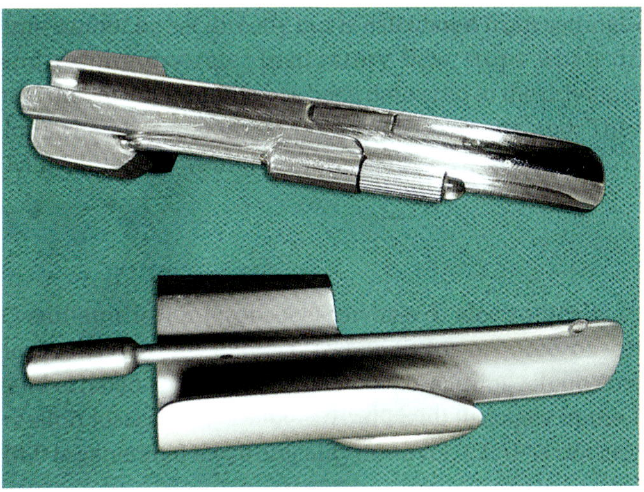

Fig. 14: Two different types of Miller blades. Top panel shows Miller blade without fiberoptic guide and port for oxygen and bottom panel shows Miller blade with port for oxygen insufflation.

Flexiblade

This combines a dynamically bending yet instantaneously rigid blade. It has a rigid front and rear portion with a flexible intermediate portion segmented by six slots. It resembles the Macintosh blade in the unflexed position. It has a lever attached to the handle, which when squeezed, allows the blade to be flexed at these hinges and become more curved.

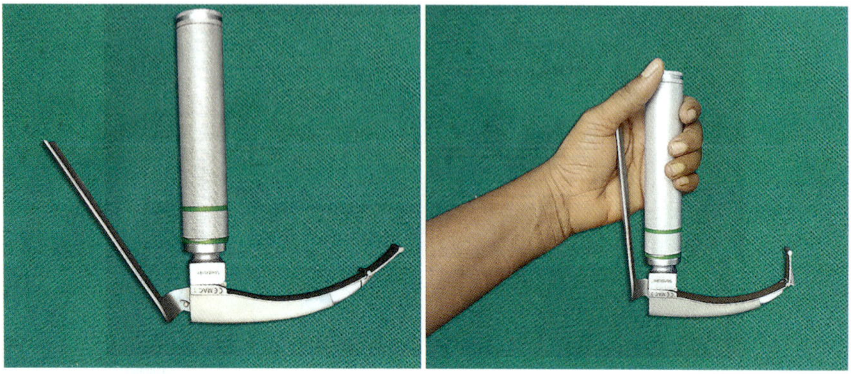

Fig. 15: The McCoy blade with a lever to flex the distal 25 mm of the tip.

Single-Use Blades

These disposable blades eliminate the risk of cross-contamination and are meant for single patient use. The blades are made of metal or plastic.

Technique of Laryngoscopy

The patient's head and neck have to be properly positioned to provide flexion at the lower cervical spine and extension at the atlanto-occipital joint (Magill's position or "sniffing the morning air" position). The laryngoscope is inserted from the right corner of the mouth and is advanced inside to deflect the tongue and other soft tissues that are pushed into the mandibular space. It is then further advanced till the epiglottis is visualized and the tip of the blade is at the vallecula. Traction is then applied along the handle at right angle to the blade. This movement pulls the base of the tongue and the epiglottis forward to provide an uninterrupted line of sight to the laryngeal inlet.

With a straight-blade laryngoscope, the epiglottis is lifted so that the tip of the blade is posterior to the epiglottis. This is especially useful in children, where the epiglottis is floppy and falls over the laryngeal inlet. It is also useful for adults with a large epiglottis or a small mouth.

If the laryngeal view is not good, the backward, upward, and rightward pressure ("BURP") maneuver can be used to improve the visualization. This involves BURP on the thyroid cartilage by an assistant to push the laryngeal structures into the line of sight.

Complications

- Trauma to the oropharyngeal and laryngeal structures
- Cervical spine injury due to positioning
- Burns
- Foreign body aspiration (bulb)
- Failure of light
- Infection due to cross-contamination

TRACHEAL TUBES

A tracheal tube is a device that is inserted into the trachea through the larynx to allow passage of gases and anesthetic vapor to and from the lungs and to protect the lungs from aspiration. It is considered the gold standard for securing the airway.

History

The first report of orotracheal intubation anesthesia was by William Macewan in 1878 and was a blind and digital intubation. New York physician, Joseph O'Dwyer in subsequent years, developed metal tubes to relieve airway obstruction in children suffering from diphtheria. Hans Kuhn modified the O'Dwyer's tube by creating a flexometallic tube. During World War I, Sir Ivan Magill and Stanley Rowbotham performed several intubations in patients for head and neck surgeries and Magill introduced the tracheal tube with inflatable cuff. Magill also developed the technique of blind nasal intubation.

Design

The tracheal tube consists of a proximal or machine end, a distal or tracheal end, and a cuff system. The tube is circular in cross-section and has a preformed curve to approximate the anatomical curve of the airway. The radius of curvature varies from 12 to 16 cm. There is a radiopaque marker along the entire length of the tube or at the top to facilitate the confirmation of tube position by radiography.

The distal end has a bevel facing to the left to facilitate visualization of the tube being passed between the vocal cords. The angle between the longitudinal axis of the tube and the bevel is called the angle of the bevel and is approximately 38°. The side opposite the bevel can have a hole called "the Murphy's eye" to provide an alternate pathway for the flow of gas if the distal end of the tube is obstructed. In tubes without the Murphy's eye, the cuff can be placed closer to the tip of the tube.

The proximal end receives the tapered 15-mm male connector for attachment to the breathing system **(Fig. 16)** and this end can be cut to shorten the tracheal tube.

Cuff System

This is present in cuffed tracheal tubes and includes the inflatable cuff and the inflation system that includes the inflation tube, the inflation lumen, the pilot balloon, and the inflation valve.

Cuff

The inflatable cuff lies proximal to the tip of the tube and its function is to seal the space between the tube and the wall of the trachea to prevent gas leaks

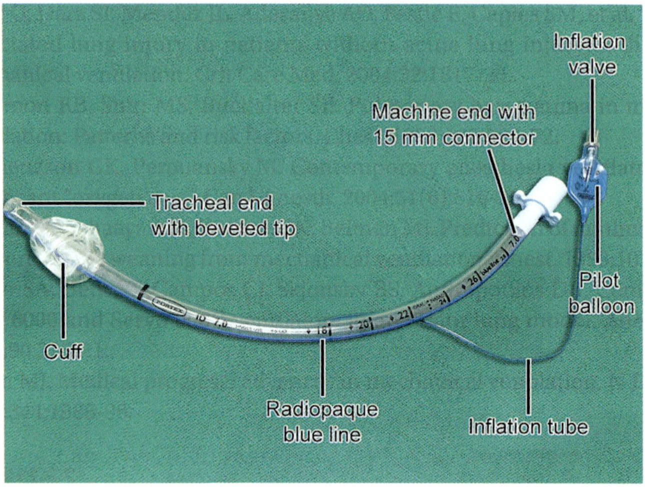

Fig. 16: Parts of an endotracheal tube.

during positive pressure ventilation and also prevent aspiration. The cuff also ensures the tube stays in the center of the trachea. The cuff should be made of a soft and pliable material that is also resistant to tear. Cuffs can be made of rubber, polyvinyl chloride (PVC), or polyurethane.

Cuff can be of low-volume, high-pressure type or the high-volume, and low-pressure type. With the low-volume, high-pressure cuff, the residual volume is low, the cuff has a smaller diameter at rest and a higher intracuff pressure is required to provide a seal with the trachea. The cuff is made of thick material and the area of contact with the trachea is small leading to increased risk of ischemic damage to the tracheal mucosa with prolonged duration of use. The high-volume low-pressure cuff has a higher residual volume and diameter. It seals the tracheal without stretching the tracheal wall. The area of contact between the cuff and the tracheal wall is large leading to lower intracuff pressure. This allows prolonged use of these tubes without risk of tracheal mucosal damage as long as the cuff is not overinflated. The cuff is made of very thin material with many folds. These microfolds can allow pharyngeal contents to pass through resulting in micro aspiration and an increased risk of ventilator-associated pneumonia.

Inflation Lumen

This is the portion of the inflation system that is located within the wall of the tracheal tube and connects the external inflation tube to the cuff.

Inflation Tube

This is the portion of the inflation system that is external to the tube with an external diameter not exceeding 2.5 mm.

Pilot Balloon

This is located close to the inflation valve and indicates the distention of the cuff. Inflation valve is a one-way valve that allows the cuff to be inflated with air with a syringe. Gas cannot escape from the cuff until it is aspirated through a syringe.

Cuff Pressure

It is desirable to keep the cuff pressure below 30 cmH_2O so that it is below the tracheal capillary perfusion pressure, which is 35 mm Hg, to avoid mucosal ischemia. Cuff pressure can be monitored using a manometer that can be attached to the pilot balloon to maintain the desired level of pressure. There are also integrated pilot pressure monitors available. Diffusion of nitrous oxide into the cuff can further increase the cuff pressure, the extent of diffusion depending on the surface area of the cuff, the permeability of the cuff material and the inspired partial pressure of nitrous oxide. The equilibration takes place in 20 minutes and hence the cuff pressure can be checked at this time to prevent over distention and complications. There are devices to limit the cuff pressure like the Lanz and the Brandt device.

Markings on the Tube

These include:

- Internal and external diameter of the tracheal tube
- Tube size is specified according to the ID, as this determines the resistance to breathing offered by the tracheal tube. In tubes smaller than 6 mm, the external diameter has to be specified. The difference between the internal and external diameter of the tube indicates the wall thickness and may vary depending on the type of tracheal tube and the manufacturer. For example, laser tubes have a greater wall thickness compared to regular tracheal tubes of the same internal diameter.
- Graduated markings to show distance in centimeters from the tip of the tube, to know the depth of insertion
- Whether it is oral or nasal
- Name of manufacturer
- A radiopaque line along the length of the tube
- A horizontal black mark several centimeters proximal to the cuff to indicate the distance the tube should be placed beyond the vocal cords. The tube should be inserted till the horizontal black line is at the level of the vocal cords. If there are two black lines, the tube should be placed so that the vocal cords are between the two black lines. This mark is to ensure inadvertent deep insertion and endobronchial intubation but ultimate confirmation by auscultation is mandatory.

- Markings for implantation testing (Z79-IT) and CE marking (Conformite Europeene) to denote compliance with the essential requirements of the Medical Devices Directive.

Construction Material

Originally, endotracheal tubes (ETTs) were made from red rubber or natural latex. The disadvantages with these tubes include:

- They are opaque and hence obstruction of the tube by secretions due to inadequate cleaning or foreign bodies could be overlooked.
- As these tubes are reused, repeated cleaning and sterilization could lead to damage and degradation.
- They have poor resistance to kinking.
- They do not soften at body temperature.
- They cannot be used in patients with latex allergy.

These days ETTs are made of plastics like polyvinyl chloride or polyurethane and silicone rubber (polymethylsiloxane). PVC tubes are transparent, inexpensive, meant for single use, become soft at body temperature and, hence, confirm to the shape of the airway and are also compatible with tissue. Polyurethane is softer than PVC but is also more expensive. Silicone rubber is also soft and can be reused as it can withstand autoclaving, but is more expensive. Chemicals called plasticizers can be added to the PVC tubes during manufacturing, to make them softer. The most commonly used plasticizers are the phthalates, but there are concerns about carcinogenicity and mutagenicity with their use.

The material used for the construction of the tracheal tube is tested for its nonirritant nature by implantation in the paravertebral muscle of anesthetized rabbits for 70–144 hours, after which the implant sites are assessed for evidence of inflammation. The number marked on the tube "Z79-IT" denotes this implant testing according to the American National Standards Institute.

Size

It is important to choose the right size of tracheal tube for a given patient as a smaller tube, though easier to insert can result in increased resistance and difficulty in passing suction catheters and a larger tube can result in increased incidence of postoperative sore throat.

There are several scales for the tube size. The Magill scale in which tubes were from size 0 for an infant to size 10 for a large adult is the oldest scale of tube sizes. The French scale uses the French catheter gauge (FCG), which is approximate outer circumference of the tube and is three times the external diameter of the tube in millimeter. As per current standards, tube size is based on the ID in millimeter. A 7 or 7.5 mm ID tracheal tube is suitable for most adult females and an 8 or 8.5 mm ID tracheal tube is suitable for most adult males. The tube size is marked on the tracheal tube and sometimes also on the pilot balloon.

The length of the tracheal tube increases with the increase in internal diameter.

For children, there are several formulae to determine the tracheal tube size based on age, height, or weight and the use of cuffed or uncuffed tubes.

Formula for Uncuffed Tubes

Cole's formula:

Tube size (French Gauge) = age (years) + 17

Morgan and Steward's modification of Cole's formula:

Tube size (mm ID) = [age (years) + 16]/4

Penlington formula:

Children <6 years of age: Tube size (mm ID) = age (years)/3 + 3.5

Children older than 6 years: Tube size (mm ID) = age (years)/4 + 4.5

Formula for Cuffed Tubes

For children ≥2 years, ID (mm) = age/4 + 3.5

For children 1–2 years of age, ID (mm) = 3.5

For neonates ≤3 kg and infants, ID (mm) = 3

Khine formula for cuffed tubes: Tube size (mm ID) = age/4 + 3

Motoyama formula for cuffed tubes: Tube size (mm ID) = age/4 + 3.5

Technique of Intubation

The tracheal tube can be inserted through the mouth or the nose, using direct laryngoscopy, videolaryngoscopy, blindly or by using flexible fiberoptic bronchoscopy.

Oral Insertion by Direct Laryngoscopy

Before use, the tube has to be examined and the cuff checked for leaks. After direct laryngoscopy, the tracheal tube should be inserted from the right corner of the mouth toward the laryngeal inlet with the bevel parallel to the vocal cords. The passage of the tube through the vocal cords should be observed and this is the direct method of confirming endotracheal intubation. The tube should be inserted 2–2.5 cm beyond the vocal cords in adults. As a general guide, the depth of insertion should be till the 21 cm mark in females and the 23 cm mark in males is at the level of the incisors.

Nasal Intubation by Direct Laryngoscopy

The tracheal tube is inserted through the most patent nostril with the bevel facing the septum to avoid injury to the turbinates. It is then advanced along

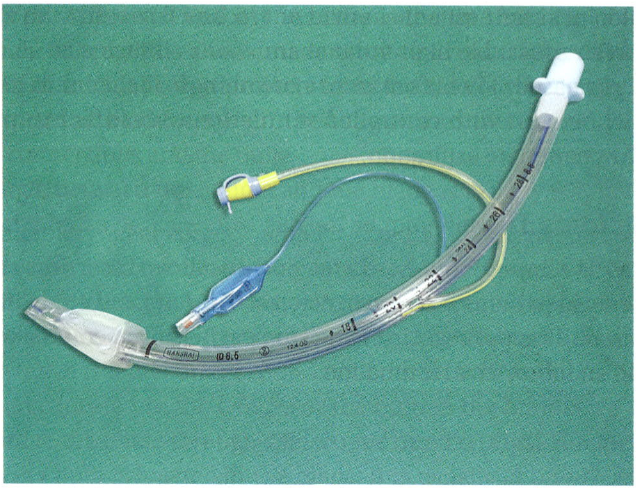

Fig. 22: The "SACETT"—Suction above the Cuff Endotracheal Tube: Endotracheal tube with a separate suction channel that is colored yellow for identification.

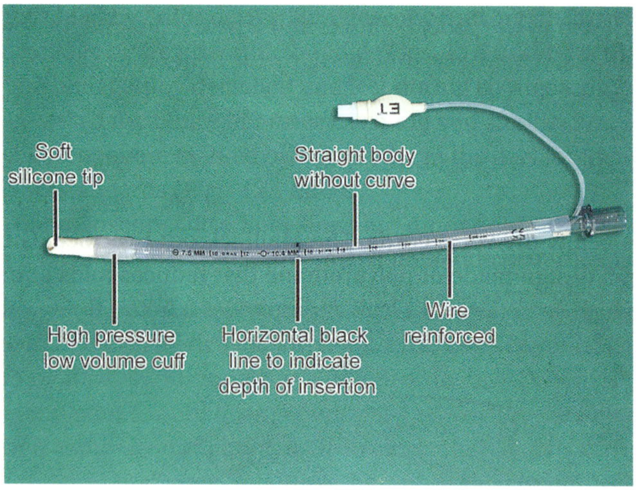

Fig. 23: The endotracheal tube for intubating laryngeal mask airway.

It is available in five sizes of 6-, 6.5-, 7-, 7.5-, and 8-mm ID, and is meant for insertion through the ILMA. It prevents the holdup of the tracheal tube at the level of the arytenoids and can also be used with fiberoptic intubation.

Tubes for Lung Isolation

Separation of the two lungs and one-lung ventilation is required in some situations like infection and hemorrhage to avoid contamination of the other lung to control the distribution of ventilation as in bronchopleural fistula or giant unilateral lung cyst and for unilateral bronchopulmonary lavage. It is also a relative indication for some surgeries like pneumonectomy, lobectomy, thoracoscopy, thoracic aortic aneurysm repair, esophageal surgery, and spine surgery.

Double-Lumen Tubes

Double-lumen tubes (DLTs), as the name suggests, have two lumens. This is because they are made by bonding together two tracheal tubes of the same diameter but of different length. After correct placement, the distal end of the shorter tube lies in the trachea while the distal end of the longer tube lies in one of the two mainstem bronchi. There are two separate inflation systems for the tubes, with two cuffs, inflation tubes, and pilot balloons, and they are color-coded for identification with the bronchial cuff and pilot balloon being blue. The lumens of both the tubes are "D-shaped". As the right mainstem bronchus is shorter, the right-sided DLT has a slot in the cuff for ventilation of the right upper lobe. There is a radiopaque line running along the length of the tube. The DLT has two curves, a proximal and a distal.

Sizes: The French gauge is used to classify tube size and is based on the external circumference of the tube. Tubes are available in sizes of 26, 28, 35, 37, 39, and 41 F, the ID of each lumen being respectively 4.0, 4.5, 5.0, 5.5, 6.0, and 6.5 mm.

Types: There are several different types of double lumen tubes. Some of them include Carlens, Robertshaw, White, Broncho-Cath **(Fig. 24)**, Sher-I-Bronch, and Silbroncho DLTs. The Carlens tube has a carinal hook and is intended for left bronchial placement. The White DLT is intended for right bronchial placement, and it also has a carinal hook. Robertshaw right and left DLTs are available. They differ in the angle of the bronchial portion, which is 20° in right-sided DLT and 40° in left-sided DLT. The bronchial cuff of the right-sided DLT also has an opening in its lateral aspect for right upper lobe ventilation.

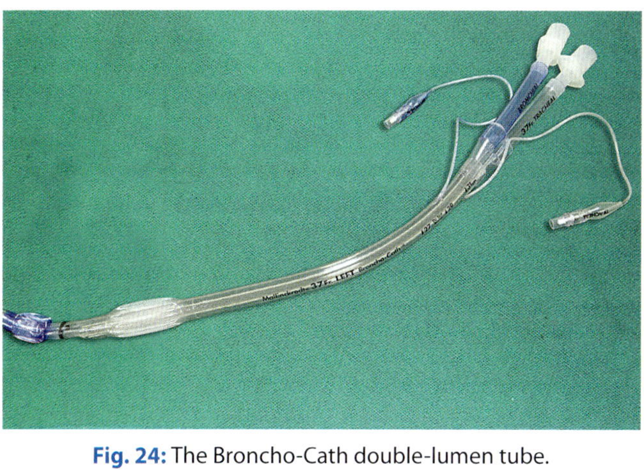

Fig. 24: The Broncho-Cath double-lumen tube.

The Sher-I-Bronch right-sided DLT has two bronchial cuffs, proximal and distal to the right upper lobe ventilation slot. The Silbroncho DLT is made of silicone, and the bronchial segment distal to the tracheal cuff is reinforced with wire to prevent kinking.

Technique of insertion: After direct laryngoscopy, the DLT with the stylet is first inserted with the concavity of the proximal curve facing anteriorly till the bronchial tip is advanced through the larynx, after which the stylet is removed and the DLT is rotated through 90° so that the bronchial lumen points toward the appropriate side. First, the tracheal cuff is inflated and then the bronchial cuff is inflated gradually, the total volume not exceeding 3 mL. Position is checked by auscultation, clamping each lumen separately, and auscultation again. Fiberoptic bronchoscopy is the most appropriate method of confirming correct placement. A 3.6–4.2 mm fiberoptic bronchoscope (FOB) can be used with all adult DLTs.

Tubes with Bronchial Blockers

The Univent tube is a single-lumen tube with a small separate lumen on its concave surface containing a hollow bronchial blocker that can extend about 8–10 cm beyond the tip of the tube. It is available from size 6.0 mm ID to 9.0 mm ID. After intubation, the bronchial blocker can be advanced into either lung. The lumen of the blocker allows ventilation and suction of the lung.

Bronchial Blockers

These are devices that are used to block a selective bronchus with collapse of the lung that is distal to the block. They are placed through conventional single lumen ETTs. The placement of bronchial blocker is less traumatic compared to a DLT.

Arndt Blocker

It is available in three sizes, 5, 7, and 9 F, that are respectively 50, 65, and 78 cm long. There is a small flexible adjustable wire loop at the distal end of the catheter that serves as a guide loop through an FOB to aid in placement of the blocker. It has a narrow lumen to allow oxygen insufflation and suctioning. It has a high-volume low-pressure, elliptical or spherical balloon, minimizing potential trauma to the bronchus. There are distance markings to indicate how far the blocker has been advanced. The ID of the lumen is 1.4 mm.

Cohen Flexitip Blocker

It is available as a 9 F catheter with a length of 65 cm and a central lumen of 1.6-mm diameter. It has a unique deflecting tip to direct the blocker into the bronchus, which is controlled by a wheel-twisting device located in the proximal portion of the unit. It has a spherical, low-pressure, high-volume balloon, with side holes in the distal end for lung deflation. It also has a torque grip to allow blocker rotation.

Fuji Uniblocker

It is available in two sizes, 5 F and 9 F, with respective lengths of 30 and 51 cm. It has a high-volume balloon that is made of silicon and the recommended cuff volume is 3 and 8 mL, respectively for the 5 F and 9 F catheters. It has a torque control to direct the malleable shaft. The ID of the central channel is 2.0 mm.

EZ-Blocker

This blocker comes with a bifurcated "V-shaped" distal end with two color-coded cuffs, one in each limb of the "V". The cuffs are low volume, made of polyurethane, providing optimal seal. The unique bifurcated distal end allows for placement of the cuffs in the right or left bronchus. The shaft is radiopaque. It is available in a single size of 7 F. The central lumen is 1.4 mm in diameter.

AIDS FOR INTUBATION

Bougies

These are devices that are inserted into the trachea and serve as a guide over which the tracheal tube can be advanced into the trachea. They are also called as ETT introducers. Their use for intubation was first described by Sir Robert Reynolds Macintosh.

Description

The original product was the Eschmann tracheal tube introducer, erroneously called the gum elastic bougie; erroneous because it is not gum, it is not elastic, and it does not dilate (bougie is a device used for dilatation). The Eschmann tracheal tube introducer is a 5 mm (15 F) flexible device, 60 cm in length which has a coude tip ("J" or curved tip) of 40° at the distal 2.5 cm and has markings every 10 cm. It is made of braided Dacron with a resin coating. The angled tip helps in the insertion of the device into the trachea even when the larynx is only partially visualized or hidden from view by the epiglottis. The other advantage is the memory of the material, retaining the shape for 10–20 seconds, thus allowing time for use. The 15 F-sized bougie is used for intubation with tracheal tubes of sizes 6–11 mm and the size 10 F bougie is used for intubation with tracheal tubes of sizes 4–5.5 mm. It can be used multiple times after autoclaving, which however makes it brittle.

Some of the recently introduced endotracheal introducers are made of plastic and some are hollow to facilitate oxygen insufflation during a difficult intubation. The Frova intubating introducer (Cook Medical) is one such device that is hollow, angled at 45° for 2 cm from the tip, may have a stiffening cannula and is supplied with Rapifit adapters with Luer-Lock and 15 mm fittings to allow jet ventilation or oxygenation with a breathing circuit. The distal side ports ensure sufficient airflow and prevent whipping during jet ventilation. There are graduated markings in centimeters to assess depth of insertion and it is radiopaque. It comes in two sizes, 8 F (1.6 mm ID) which is 35 cm long for pediatric use and 14 F (3 mm ID) which is 65 cm long for adult use, that are used for tracheal tubes >3 and 6 mm ID, respectively **(Fig. 25)**.

Uses

Endotracheal tube introducers are used for tracheal intubation by direct or videolaryngoscopy, for tracheal intubation through a supraglottic device, for cricothyrotomy and for tracheal tube exchange.

Technique of Use

The tracheal tube introducer can be inserted with or without the tracheal tube loaded on it. The lubricated introducer with the tracheal tube loaded on it should be inserted after direct laryngoscopy from the right angle of the mouth and directed without undue force toward the larynx, or under the epiglottis if the larynx cannot be viewed. The angled tip of the introducer should face anteriorly. If it gets stuck at the anterior commissure, it can be rotated through 180° to advance it into the trachea, when a clicking

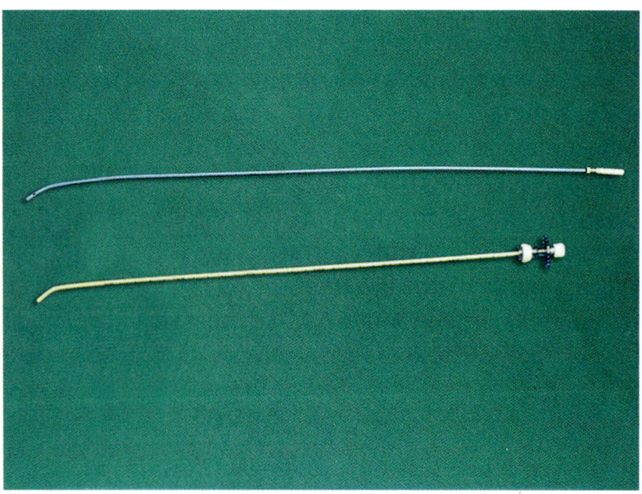

Fig. 25: The adult and pediatric Frova intubating introducers.

sensation will be felt due to the tracheal rings. Intratracheal placement can be confirmed with capnography with a hollow introducer. The tracheal tube is then advanced over the introducer (railroaded) into the trachea. If the tracheal tube gets stuck at the laryngeal inlet, a 90° rotation of the tube will facilitate advancement into the trachea. The bougie is then withdrawn.

Complications

Complications with use of endotracheal introducers include trauma to the oropharyngeal structures, larynx or trachea, insertion into the esophagus, and insertion of the tracheal tube too far leading to endobronchial intubation and accidental slippage of the introducer.

STYLETS

These are devices that are malleable and are inserted into the lumen of the tracheal tubes to change their shape to facilitate intubation. They are made of metal coated with plastic. They should be sufficiently rigid to enable intubation, but also malleable enough for the shape to be changed. If there is no securing device, the stylet should be bent at the machine end of the tracheal tube during use. Stylets should be lubricated before insertion into the tracheal tube. A gently curved shape is used for normal intubations and a hockey stick shape is used for difficult intubations.

Lighted Stylets

This is a stylet with a bright light at the distal end that allows transillumination of the neck tissues to facilitate tracheal intubation and direct visualization of the glottis is not necessary with these devices. It is useful in situations where visibility is poor due to secretions or blood leading to difficulty in using a fiberoptic bronchoscope. The “Trachlight” (Laerdal) is one such device. It has a handle that houses the batteries, a wand and a stiff, retractable stylet within the wand that allows the wand to be shaped into a hockey stick configuration. The length of the wand can be adjusted by sliding it along the handle.

The Trachlight is introduced into the lumen of the tracheal tube and bent to the desired shape. With the patient supine, the jaw is lifted forward and the Trachlight is inserted from the corner of the mouth initially and then brought to the midline after entry into oropharynx. A well-defined circumscribed glow in the neck below the thyroid prominence indicates that the tip of the Trachlight is at the glottis opening. A dull lateral glow indicates that the tip is in the pyriform fossa. A diffuse glow that is not readily detected indicates that the tip is in the esophagus. When it is at the glottis, the stylet is retracted and the tracheal tube is advanced into the trachea and the Trachlight removed from the tracheal tube.

Optical Stylets

The term "optical stylet" was coined by Karl and Berci in the year 1979 to describe a straight rigid endoscope that was used as a tracheal tube stylet for intubation. The straight design limited its use. The fiberoptic stylet laryngoscope, though commercially unavailable now, was the first semi-malleable stylet with fiberoptic technology that was used to aid intubation, and its configuration is used in many modern optical stylets.

An optical stylet is a metal stylet that uses a fiberoptic or video-viewing element in its distal end. There is a distal objective lens at the tip of the optical stylet and a proximal eyepiece for viewing the glottis, and in some devices, this is connected to an external monitor for magnified view. Although most optical stylets use glass fibers to transmit the image to the eyepiece, some use plastic image guides. The size of the ETT that can be used depends on the stylet diameter.

Shikani Optical Stylet

The Shikani optical stylet (Claris Medical) is a semirigid device that is available in adult and pediatric versions. It is a fiberoptic stylet that is malleable in the distal end and comes with a port for oxygen insufflation. The adult version can accommodate tracheal tubes from size 5.5 to 9 mm and the pediatric version can accommodate tracheal tubes from size 2.5 to 5 mm.

The optical stylet is inserted into the lumen of the tracheal tube. It can be used with or without direct laryngoscopy. Visualization of the vocal cords is through the eyepiece or the monitor and the stylet with the loaded tracheal tube is guided toward the larynx. As the tracheal rings are visualized, the tube is advanced further and the stylet is withdrawn.

Bonfils Optical Stylet (Bonfils Retromolar Fiberscope)

Bonfils retromolar fiberoptic stylet (Karl Storz) is a rigid fiberoptic stylet with a 40° anterior curve built into its distal end, a 35,000-pixel light bundle and useable shaft length of 35 cm. It has a moveable proximal eyepiece that can also be connected to a monitor screen. There is an adapter at the proximal end of the shaft of the stylet for attaching the tracheal tube. The adult stylet has a 5-mm external diameter and can accommodate a 6.5-mm ID or larger tracheal tube. The Brambrink pediatric intubation endoscope has an external diameter of 2 mm and a working sheath length of 22 cm and can be used in children as it can accommodate tracheal tubes of ID 2.5–6 mm. Bonfils originally described a retromolar approach to intubation in children with the Pierre Robin syndrome and this is the technique for the use of the Bonfils retromolar scope. The tracheal tube is loaded on the fiberoptic stylet till the stylet is just above the bevel and the stylet tube assembly is inserted from the

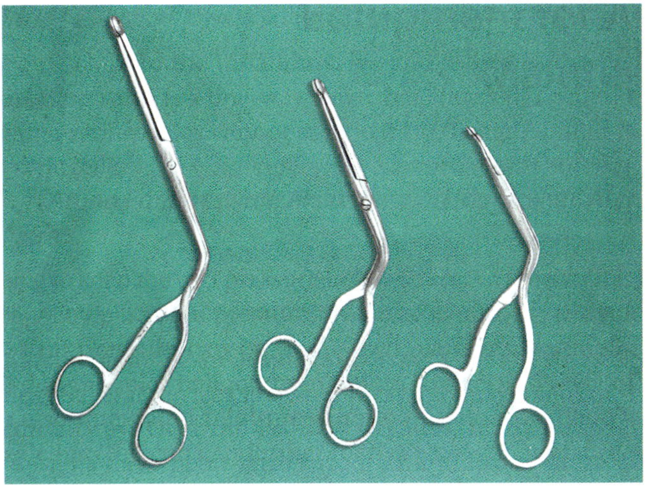

Fig. 26: Magill forceps of three different sizes, adult, child, and infant.

corner of the mouth, behind the molars with a jaw thrust to create a working space and advanced beneath the epiglottis till the tube tip is at the glottis. Then, the tube is advanced off the stylet into the trachea.

MAGILL'S FORCEPS

Named after Sir Ivan Magill, these are stainless steel, angled forceps with a blunt, ridged, and rounded tip. There is an oblique angle between the handle and the blades, so that when the forceps are grasped, the handle is to the right of the blades. This maintains the line of sight and prevents the airway from being obscured from view by the forceps. It is available in three sizes: adult, child, and infant **(Fig. 26)**. It is used to grasp and direct an ETT into the larynx, especially during nasotracheal intubation, to direct a nasogastric tube into the esophagus, to insert a throat pack, and to remove foreign bodies from the upper airway or esophagus.

DEVICES FOR DIFFICULT AIRWAY MANAGEMENT

FIBEROPTIC BRONCHOSCOPIC INTUBATION

History

The first FOB was designed by Ikeda in 1966.

Physics

Fiberoptic scopes work on the principle of total internal reflection of light. When light travels from one medium to another, it is transmitted, absorbed, or internally reflected. Thin, stretched, and glass fibers can be grouped so that light is totally internally reflected along the length of the fiber. So, when light from an object enters at one end of this glass fiber and exits at the other end, a sharp image of the object is retained at the other end.

Parts of a Fiberoptic Bronchoscope

The parts of a fiberoptic bronchoscope include the handle, insertion tube, universal cord, and power source **(Fig. 27)**.

Handle (Body)

This is the proximal portion of the fiberscope that is held in the palm of either hand **(Fig. 28)**. It has a conical connection where it meets the insertion cord

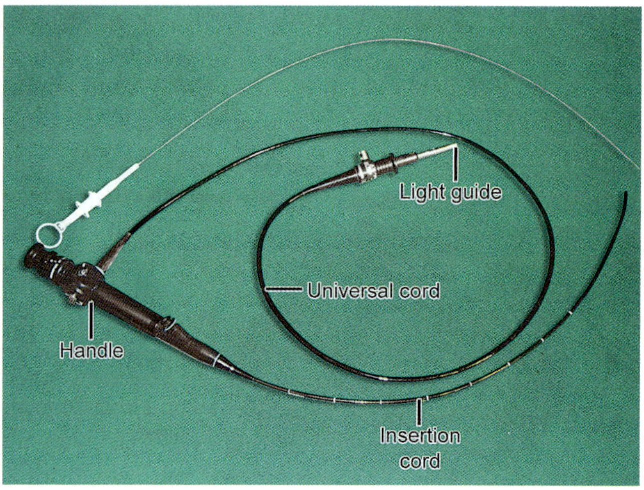

Fig. 27: The flexible fiberoptic bronchoscope.

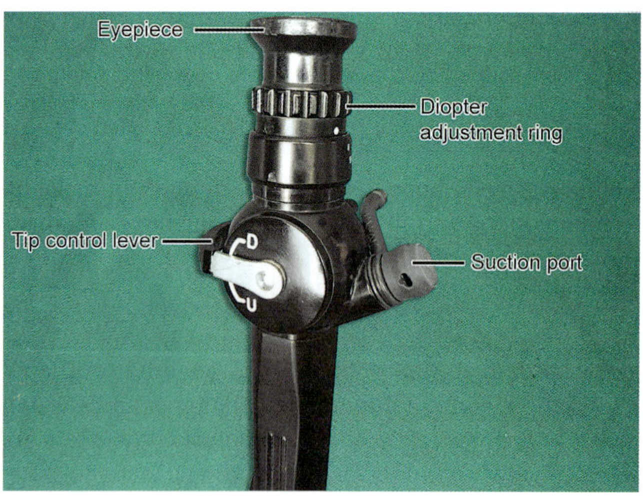

Fig. 28: Parts of the handle (body) of the flexible fiberoptic bronchoscope.

to facilitate loading of a tracheal tube. The blue ring on the body signifies that the whole of the fiberscope can safely be immersed in a disinfectant. It contains:

- Eyepiece
- Diopter adjustment ring
- Lever to control the bending tip of the insertion tube
- Suction button or valve
- Access port to the suction channel

Insertion Cord

It is the portion of the FOB that is inserted into the patient and over which the ETT is passed during fiberoptic intubation. It contains:

- Two light transmission bundles
- One image transmission bundle
- Working channel
- Tip-bending control wires

The outside diameter of the insertion cord is what determines the size of the smallest ETT that can be used. The size of the smallest ETT that can be loaded over the FOB is usually 1 mm greater than the diameter of the insertion cord. There are white indicators every 5 cm from 15 to 40 cm on the insertion cord.

The transmitting bundles contain 10,000 glass fibers, each 8–10 μm in diameter. Each fiber is covered with a thin 1μ film of glass with a different refractive index when compared to the core glass. This process of cladding is done to reduce leakage of light out of the fibers. There are two different types of glass fiber bundles in the flexible fiberscope. One bundle transmits the light from the light source to the object to illuminate it. In this, the fibers are not arranged in any specific manner and this is called the incoherent or light transmission bundle. The other bundle transmits the image from the object to the eyepiece. In this bundle, the fibers are arranged in a specific manner so that the arrangement of fibers in the distal end is identical to the arrangement at the proximal end. This is called the coherent or the image transmission bundle.

Light from an external light source travels via two light transmission (incoherent) fiberoptic bundles to the distal end of the fiberscope and illuminates the object. The light from the object is reflected onto the objective lens at the tip of the fiberscope. The objective lens focuses the light onto the image transmission (coherent) bundle, through which it is internally reflected. The image, which is a composite of lots of small spots of light, each with uniform intensity and color from each fiber, is reconstructed in the eyepiece at the proximal end of the fiberscope. The image can then be focused onto the viewer's retina by a diopter ring so that it is sharp. When viewed in the eyepiece, a pointer is seen which is an "orientation mark". This mark helps in orientating the operator to the anterior direction of the tip.

The insertion cord has a working channel that extends from the handle of the FOB to the distal tip of the scope. This channel has several functions. It can be used to suction secretions or blood during intubation, insufflate oxygen that can help to blow away secretions besides improving the oxygen reserve of the patient, spray local anesthetics, to pass various biopsy and brush instruments and also for insertion of guidewires for anterograde and retrograde fiberoptic intubation techniques.

The distal tip of the insertion cord of the fiberscope can be manipulated by the movement of the bending lever located at the back of the handle. Two wires originating from the bending lever and ending at the tip of the FOB provide the mechanism. The tip can only be moved in one plane of motion (anteflexion and retroflexion). The thumb of the operator is usually used to maneuver the bending lever.

All the components of the insertion cord are held together by a stainless steel spiral wrap and braid and then further covered by a waterproof material.

Universal Cord

This connects the FOB to the light source. It ends in a light guide that is inserted into the power source.

Power Source

This provides adequate illumination for viewing. An intense cold light is generated from a separate power source and is focused on the proximal end of the light guide cable. In portable FOBs, the light source is incorporated into the body of the scope.

Steps in Planning and Execution

- Airway evaluation
- Backup plan
- Explanation and consent
- Premedication
- Monitoring
- Oxygenation
- Judicious sedation
- Upper airway local anesthesia
- Good endoscopy technique
- Choice of tube and technique of railroading

Types of Fiberoptic Bronchoscopic Intubation

- Awake oral
- Awake nasal

- Anesthetized oral
- Anesthetized nasal
- Awake intubation

Good preoperative counseling, good communication with the patient during the procedure, an excellent local anesthetic technique, and adequate sedation are essential for maintaining patient's comfort during awake fiberoptic intubation. Young patients and uncooperative adults may not be suitable for this technique.

Advantages of Awake Intubation

- Preservation of patient's natural airway
- Maintenance of upper airway tone results in adequate space in the oropharynx.
- Protection from aspiration
- Nonsupine positions possible in patients with difficulty in breathing
- Vocal cords can be abducted for entry of FOB into the trachea by asking the patient to take a deep breath.

Disadvantages of Awake Intubation

- Topical anesthesia can be unpleasant as lignocaine has a bitter taste and injections can cause discomfort.
- Transtracheal injection can cause coughing.
- Insertion of the tracheal tube through the nose can cause patient's discomfort.

Awake Oral

With the patient's head in the neutral position, a conduit oropharyngeal airway is inserted into the mouth. After insertion of a lubricated tracheal tube into the airway for a few centimeters, the FOB is inserted through the tracheal tube. As the scope is advanced, the uvula can be seen, after which it is advanced further anteriorly to visualize the epiglottis and the vocal cords. By fine manipulation, the FOB is advanced through the vocal cords into the trachea till the carina. Then, while one operator holds the FOB, the assistant advances the tracheal tube over the FOB till the ETT is at the mid-tracheal level, about 4 cm above the carina.

Awake Nasal

This is easier than oral intubation, as there is no need to bend the FOB acutely. The FOB with the appropriate-sized tracheal tube loaded over it is inserted through the most patent nostril. The septum and inferior turbinate are identified. The FOB is advanced till it comes out of the posterior nares, when the soft palate and uvula will be visible. It is then advanced between the soft palate and the posterior pharyngeal wall and in most patients at this point, the epiglottis, and vocal cords will become visible. The FOB is then advanced into the trachea and the tracheal tube railroaded over it, till in place in the trachea.

Anesthetized Fiberoptic Intubation

Anesthetized fiberoptic intubation can be done with the patient breathing spontaneously through a face mask, nasopharyngeal airway or a supraglottic device. It can also be done after neuromuscular blockade and positive pressure ventilation. As the patient receives oxygen and anesthetic gases with a specially designed face mask, the FOB can be inserted through the sealable diaphragm in the mask or the angle connector. If oxygenation and anesthesia are maintained through a nasopharyngeal airway, FOB can be inserted through the other nostril or the mouth.

Points to Remember for a Successful Fiberoptic Intubation

- Preoperative counseling of the patient, proper planning, good topical anesthesia, and adequate sedation are very important for a successful awake fiberoptic intubation.
- Whether awake or anesthetized, the procedure has to be done with continuous monitoring and with continuous administration of oxygen to the patient.
- The ETT and fiberoptic scope should be immersed in warm water prior to use. The insertion cord of the FOB is warmed to prevent fogging. The ETT is warmed to make it soft and more pliable.
- The size of the ETT in relation to the size of the FOB is important to minimize "play". A tracheal tube of ID 1 mm greater than the OD of the FOB is ideal.
- An awake fiberoptic intubation is easier than an anesthetized intubation. This is because the loss of muscle tone with onset of general anesthesia decreases the air space available to negotiate the scope.
- Nasal fiberoptic intubation is easier than oral fiberoptic intubation. This is because of the acute angle between the oral cavity and the laryngeal inlet while using the oral approach.
- Visualization of the glottis by the FOB can be facilitated by head extension, jaw thrust, and pulling the tongue forward. These maneuvers open up the oropharyngeal space by pulling the tongue, soft palate, and epiglottis away from the posterior pharyngeal wall. They are especially useful in anesthetized FOB intubation, when the upper airway can just be a narrow fissure or slit.
- The bevel-down orientation improves the success of oral fiberoptic intubation as it allows the tracheal tube to slip past the arytenoid.

- The bevel-up orientation improves the success of nasal fiberoptic intubation, as it avoids the epiglottis.
- If there is difficulty in passing the tracheal tube at the laryngeal inlet (aryepiglottic arrest), rotation of the tracheal tube by 90° facilitates advancement.
- An ILMA tube with its soft and silicone tip is the ideal tube for fiberoptic intubation and passes easily and smoothly over the FOB into the trachea.
- Flexible FOB intubation is not a panacea because of the following:
  - It is time-consuming and may not be an appropriate technique for rapidly securing the airway.
  - Vision can be obscured by blood and secretions.
  - An air space is required, which may be absent with masses, tumors, and edema of the oropharyngeal tissues.
  - If the glottis is displaced from the midline, it may not be possible to direct the FOB into the glottis and trachea.

Choice of Fiberoptic Bronchoscopes

There are different manufacturers of flexible fiberoptic intubating bronchoscopes and there are variations among the different scopes with regard to the length and diameter of the insertion cord, the diameter of the working channel, the degree of tip bending and the field of view. The Olympus fiberoptic scopes are available from 2.2 to 5.3 mm external diameter of the insertion cord, with a length of 60 cm, with a suction channel in all except the 2.2 mm neonatal fiberscope. Pentax fiberscopes are available in sizes 2.8–5.1 mm OD of the insertion cord, which are also 60 cm long, with a suction channel. Karl Storz fiberoptic scopes available from 2.8 to 5.2 mm sizes OD of the insertion cord, are 50–65 cm long, with a suction channel.

Flexible Intubating Video Endoscope (Karl Storz)

This is a new flexible intubating scope that can be used in a similar manner to a fiberoptic scope but does not use glass fibers and, hence, does not work on the principle of total internal reflection of light. It incorporates a video chip in the distal end of the insertion cord and high-power LEDs for illumination **(Fig. 29)**. The proximal end is connected to a high-resolution 7-inch monitor for magnified viewing of the image, which can also be used for the C-MAC video-laryngoscope. The insertion cord has an external diameter of 5.5 mm and a length of 65 cm with a 2.3-mm working channel. Though expensive, the advantage of this scope is that there is no risk of breakage of glass fibers, which can occur with the fiberoptic scopes if the insertion cord is bent and there is no separate monitor needed for magnified viewing.

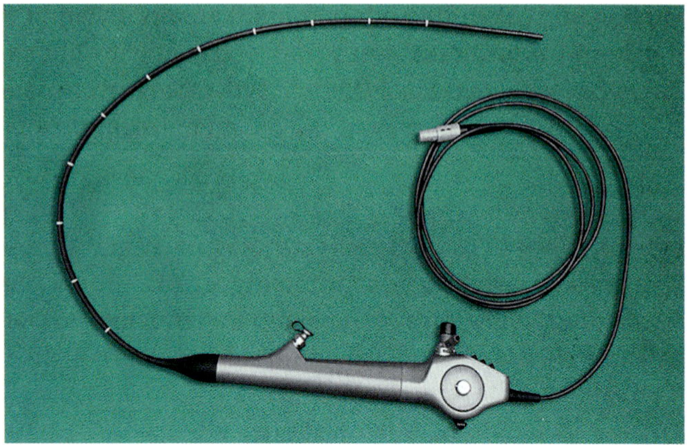

Fig. 29: Flexible intubating videoendoscope.

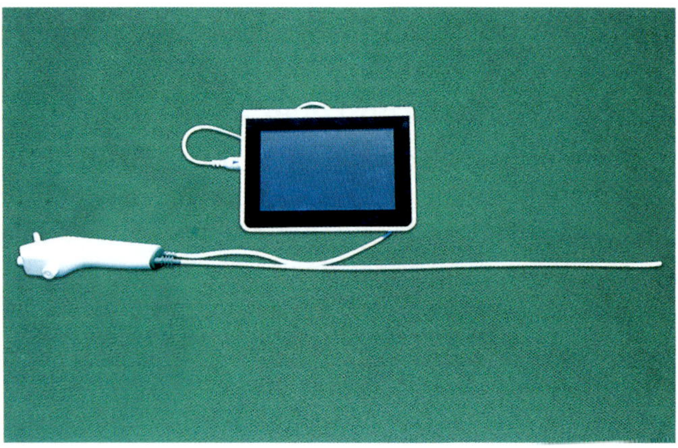

Fig. 30: The Ambu aScope.

Ambu aScope

This is a single use and disposable flexible videoscope that has a video camera at the distal tip and two LEDs **(Fig. 30)**. It is compatible with a rechargeable lightweight 8.5-inch color TFT LCD monitor, Ambu aView. It is sterile straight from the pack and does not require any reprocessing. It is easy to transport and avoids cross-contamination that can occur with reusable fiberscopes. It is available in two versions: The Ambu aScope3 5.0/2.2 and the Ambu aScope3 Slim3.8/1.2. The Ambu aScope3 has an insertion cord with an OD of 5 mm and a 2.2-mm inner channel, on which a tracheal tube of size >6 mm ID can be loaded. The insertion cord has a length of 60 cm and the tip can be moved 150° up and 130° down. There is a tube connector at the proximal end to allow for fixation of the tracheal tube. The operation time is limited by the manufacturer to a maximum of 30 minutes from the time the scope is switched on. The Ambu aScope3 Slim is a slimmer version with the OD of the insertion cord being 3.8 mm, allowing intubation with tracheal tubes of ID 5 mm or greater.

Adjuncts to Fiberoptic Intubation

Conduit Oropharyngeal Airways

These have an open or split design for removal of the fiberoptic scope from the airway after insertion of the tracheal tube. Ovassapian fiberoptic intubating airway has a lingual surface that is flat and gradually widens distally. The flexible curved guides between the vertical sidewalls on the buccal portion of the airway permit removal of the airway from around the tracheal tube. The proximal tubular portion functions as the bite block while the distal half is open posteriorly to provide maneuverability to the fiberscope. The other airways used as conduits for fiberoptic intubation include Williams airway intubator, Berman intubating/pharyngeal airway, and the Patil-Syracuse endoscopic airway.

Masks for Ventilation/Intubation

An endoscopic mask allows mask ventilation and oxygenation during insertion of the fiberoptic bronchoscope. The body of the mask has a hole which is covered with a flexible membrane, which in turn has a small sealable hole for passing the fiberscope. After intubation, the mask is removed over the tracheal tube. Such sealable diaphragms are also available in the angle piece.

Aintree Intubation Catheter (Cook Medical)

This is used for fiberoptic intubation through a supraglottic device. The radiopaque catheter is 56 cm long with an ID of 4.7 mm (19 F) and can be used over fiberoptic scopes of OD 4.5 mm or smaller. Once the catheter is in the trachea, the FOB and the supraglottic device (SGD) are removed and 6.5 mm or larger tracheal tubes can be railroaded over this catheter into the trachea. It has centimeter markings to facilitate accurate placement, a blunt tip and distal side ports to prevent whipping during jet ventilation. It is provided with a removable Rapi-Fit adapter with 15 mm and Luer Lock connectors for attachment to a ventilator device. It can also be used for ETT exchange.

SUPRAGLOTTIC DEVICES

The terminology of supraglottic airways refers to all devices that serve as a conduit for maintaining a patent airway and allow delivery of gases in and out via an airway tube that lies above the level of the glottis. The classical

LMA introduced in the year 1988 by Dr Archie Brain is the first supraglottic airway device (SAD) that has changed airway management primarily from endotracheal intubation to placement of these devices in elective surgical procedures and as a rescue device in difficult airway scenarios.

Classification

The supraglottic airways have been classified by Miller based on the site of sealing, directional effect on sealing, and presence or absence of esophageal sealing properties. They have been further subdivided into single-use and reusable devices.

The classification is as follows:

- Cuffed perilaryngeal sealers without directional sealing: LMA classic, LMA unique, ILMA, and LMA flexible.
- Cuffed perilaryngeal sealers with directional sealing: Proseal LMA and supreme LMA.
- Cuffed pharyngeal sealers with esophageal cuffs: Laryngeal tube (LT), laryngeal tube suction (LTS), and gastrolaryngeal tube.
- Cuffed pharyngeal sealers without esophageal cuffs: Cobra perilaryngeal airway.
- Cuffless preshaped sealers with esophageal sealing: i-gel and Baska mask.
- Cuffless preshaped sealers without esophageal sealing: Streamlined liner of the pharynx airway (SLIPA).

An ideal SAD provides unobstructed access to the airway, reliable ventilation during spontaneous breathing, and positive pressure ventilation with least risk of aspiration, and also prevents pressure-related injuries to the soft tissues and cranial nerves in the periglottic area. But, each device varies with regard to efficacy and safety aspects listed above.

CUFFED PERILARYNGEAL SEALERS

Classic Laryngeal Mask Airway

The LMA classic is the first supraglottic device marketed for clinical use and has been extensively studied and has good evidence supporting the safety of use compared to all the other devices. It is a reusable device made of silicone.

Design

It has an airway tube that is curved and is connected to an elliptical mask at an angle of 30°. The proximal end of the airway tube has a standard 15 mm connector and the distal end terminates into the bowl of the mask. There are two silicone strands at the point of entry of airway tube into the mask called the aperture bars which prevent epiglottic obstruction of the airway lumen. A longitudinal black line is present throughout the posterior aspect of the shaft of the airway tube serving as a marker of misplacement or rotation of the LMA. The mask contains an inflatable cuff, pilot tube, and a pilot balloon **(Fig. 31)**. The disposable version is similar to classic LMA and is made of PVC and is comparatively less compliant.

Sizes

The classic LMA is available in eight sizes from neonates to large adults **(Fig. 32)**. Available sizes and recommended volume of air for cuff inflation are given below **(Table 2)**.

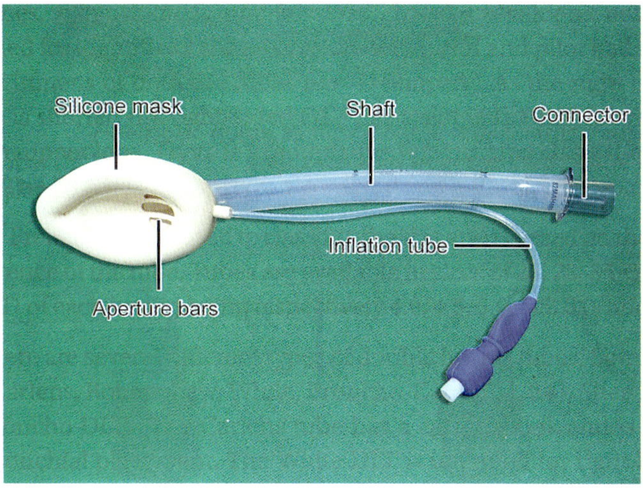

Fig. 31: Parts of the laryngeal mask airway (LMA) Classic.

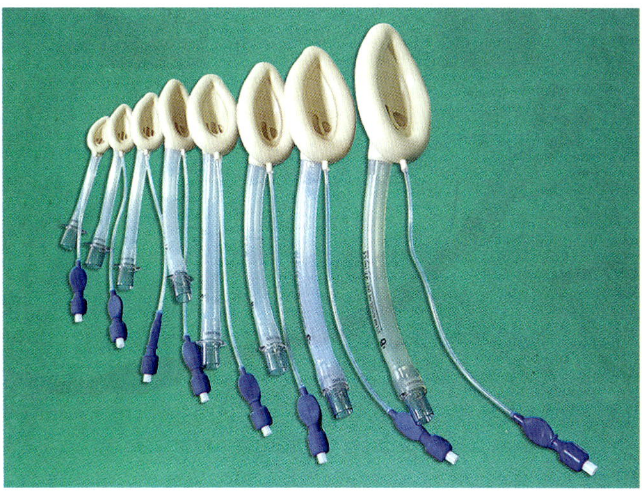

Fig. 32: All available classic laryngeal mask airway (LMA) sizes from 1 to 6.

TABLE 2: Showing different sizes of LMA classic with cuff inflation volume, the ID in mm of the ETT that can be passed through each, and the OD of the flexible fiberoptic bronchoscope to be used with each.

Patient's weight (kg)	*LMA Classic size*	*Cuff volume (mL)*	*ETT size to fit into LMA (ID)*	*Largest flexible endoscope (ID)*
Up to 5	1	4	3.5	2.7
5–10	1.5	7	4.0	3.0
10–20	2	10	4.5	3.5
20–30	2.5	14	5.0	4.0
30–50	3	20	6.0 cuffed	5.0
50–70	4	30	6.0 cuffed	5.0
70–100	5	40	7.0 cuffed	5.5
>100	6	50	7.0 cuffed	

(ETT: endotracheal tube; ID: internal diameter; LMA: laryngeal mask airway; OD: outer diameter)

Insertion Technique

The insertion of the LMA mimics the deglutition process and should be inserted after adequate suppression of pharyngeal reflexes by analgesics and anesthetic drugs. The size of the LMA is chosen appropriately based on the weight and the mask is deflated completely till it is spoon-shaped without any wrinkles. The water-soluble lubricant is applied on the posterior surface of the cuff prior to insertion. The sniffing position is ideal for insertion of the LMA. The LMA is grasped with the thumb and index finger like a pen at the junction of the mask and shaft.

The tip of the mask is pressed against the hard palate and advanced posteriorly and cranially maintaining the contact with the palate throughout and is advanced into the hypopharynx until a resistance is felt. Then the cuff is inflated without holding the LMA by hand so that it accommodates itself around the perilaryngeal structures.

The other methods of insertion include thumb insertion technique, 180 rotation technique, and laryngoscopy-guided placement.

Ideal placement and confirmation of LMA: When the LMA is placed ideally the tip of the LMA rests on the upper esophageal sphincter, the proximal part of the mask is at the base of the tongue and the sides face the pyriform fossa. Positive pressure ventilation with <20 cmH_2O resulting in adequate chest expansion without audible leak and a square pattern of capnography waveform ensures correct placement. Bite block is mandatory with use of classical LMA to prevent obstruction and postobstruction pulmonary edema.

Benefits

The airway can be quickly secured and maintained by blind insertion of the device without the need for laryngoscope or any other accessory. The insertion rate is successful 75–96% in adults. Insertion of an LMA is less invasive than endotracheal intubation with no hemodynamic response. Tolerating an LMA requires less dose of anesthetics without the need for neuromuscular as compared to an ETT. The emergence is smooth, and recovery is faster with minimal coughing, straining, and breath-holding. The risk of bronchospasm is less in those with hyper-reactive airways as it is less invasive.

Uses

It is the first choice of airway in failed mask ventilation or failed intubation.

Used as a primary airway device for elective surgeries and in remote location anesthesia for diagnostic procedures.

It aids fiberoptic intubation with the LMA as a conduit by railroading Aintree intubation catheter into the trachea. The ETT is placed after removal of LMA by passing the ETT through the Aintree catheter.

Contraindications

- Mouth opening <1.5 cm
- Patients at risk of aspiration
- Morbidly obese patients
- Patients with poor lung compliance requiring peak inspiratory pressures of >20 cmH_2O.
- Oropharyngeal obstructive pathology and lesions in the glottis and subglottic regions.

Problems

Dislodgment: The incidence of dislodgment and suboptimal position is more in children especially with use of size 1 and 1.5 resulting in airway obstruction and ineffective ventilation.

Aspiration: The risk of aspiration exists and the storage capacity of the bowl or mask is minimal in case of regurgitation from stomach. The position of LMA varies according to the head and neck position and is not ideal for surgeries in nonsupine positions.

Trauma: An overinflated cuff can press on the soft tissues leading to sore throat and cranial nerve palsies.

Intubation difficulty: Blind intubation is impossible through the classic LMA as it allows passage of smaller size ETT and there is considerable distance between the aperture bars and vocal cords. Removal of LMA is difficult after

ETT placement. Hence, fiberscope-guided Aintree intubation of the trachea is preferred with use of classic LMA. The sealing pressures are lower in the range of 16–20 cmH_2O and are not the ideal choice for positive pressure ventilation.

Laryngeal Mask Airway Flexible

This LMA was designed to prevent kinking and airway obstruction during use in surgical procedures of oral cavity, head, and neck.

Design

Laryngeal mask airway flexible has a wire-reinforced airway tube **(Fig. 33)** which prevents occlusion. The airway tube is narrower and longer than the classic LMA **(Figs. 34A and B)**. The additional length of the airway tube enables the breathing circuit to be connected away from the surgical field and the reduced size helps in providing more space for surgeries in the oral cavity. The flexibility of the airway tube allows bending to any angle and repositioning during surgical procedures without losing the cuff seal. The black line present on the posterior surface of the shaft to diagnose rotation is not present along the entire length of the shaft, unlike a classic LMA.

Sizes

They are available in six sizes starting from size 2 to 6. They are available as reusable and disposable types **(Table 3)**.

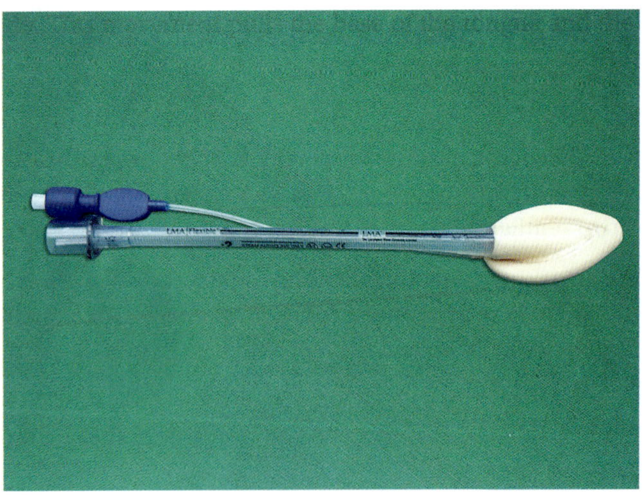

Fig. 33: Laryngeal mask airway (LMA) flexible with a reinforced airway tube that is longer and of smaller diameter.

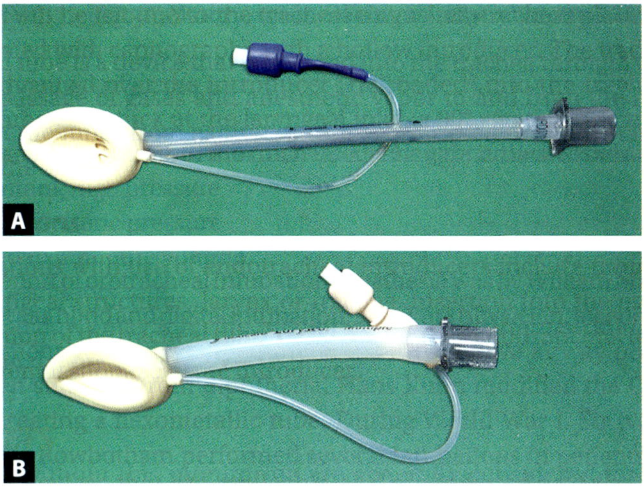

Figs. 34A and B: (A) Flexible laryngeal mask airway (LMA) size 2 showing narrower and longer airway tube when compared to the same size Classic LMA and (B) Classic LMA size 2.

TABLE 3: Showing the available sizes of flexible laryngeal mask airway (LMA) and their cuff inflation volumes.

LMA flexible size	Patient's weight in kg	Maximum cuff inflation volume
2	10–20	10 mL
2.5	20–30	14 mL
3	30–50	20 mL
4	50–70	30 mL
5	70–100	40 mL
6	>100	50 mL

Insertion

The flexible LMA insertion is difficult and may require use of introducer to aid placement. A Stylet or a smaller-size ETT can be inserted into the shaft for added stability during insertion.

Indications

Used in surgical procedures on the head, neck, and for intraoral surgeries like adenotonsillectomy, cleft lip, and palate.

Problems

- *Dislodgment:* It can dislodge easily due to improper application of mouth gag and inappropriate size selection.

- *Airway obstruction:* Airway obstruction due to biting of the shaft and disruption of wires.
- *MRI compatibility:* It is not MRI compatible and the image quality is interfered by the spiral rings.
- *Increased resistance:* Spontaneous ventilation increases the resistance to breathing owing to increased length and smaller diameter of the tube.
- Malrotation and misplacement cannot be diagnosed easily based on the indicators in the airway shaft.

Laryngeal Mask Airway Fastrach

The Fastrach LMA was designed to facilitate ETT placement blindly in order to overcome the limitations faced during intubation with classic LMA. It was introduced in the year 1995.

Design

It consists of three parts that include ILMA, ILMA ETT, and the stabilizing rod **(Fig. 35)**.

It has a rigid and anatomically curved wider and shorter airway tube that ensures passage of the ETT cuff beyond the vocal cords during blind insertion. The ID of the airway tube is 13 mm, which allows size 8 ETT to be placed without any difficulty. The rigid stainless-steel handle facilitates insertion, removal, and adjustment of the device position to enhance effective sealing and optimize alignment with the glottis **(Fig. 36)**.

The epiglottic elevating bar in the aperture of the mask elevates the epiglottis during passage of ETT and the ramp in the floor of the mask guides

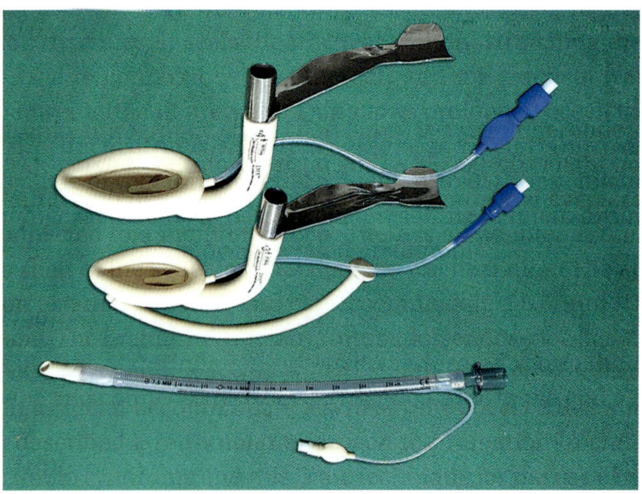

Fig. 35: Intubating laryngeal mask airway (ILMA) sizes 3 and 4 with the stabilizing rod and ILMA endotracheal tube.

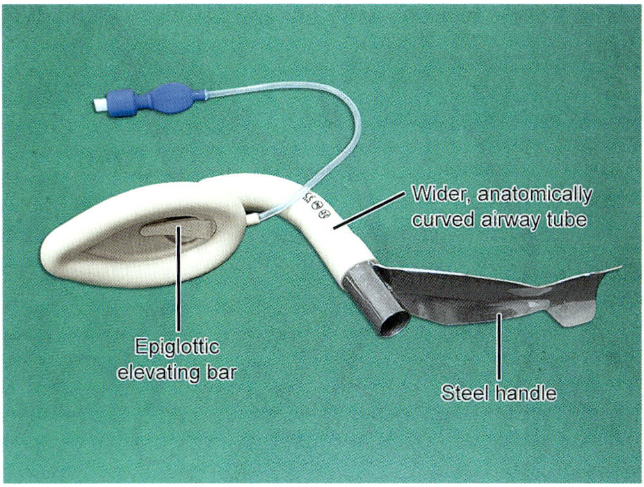

Fig. 36: Parts of an intubating laryngeal mask airway.

the ETT anteriorly into the glottis. The ILMA ETT is silicone-based, soft, straight, and reinforced tube with a high-pressure and low-volume cuff. The tube is tapered at the tip for atraumatic blind insertion through the ILMA. The black longitudinal line of ILMA tube should face the nose of the patient for proper alignment of the bevel against the glottis opening. A transverse black line is present in the ILMA ETT which denotes the point of exit of tube from the ILMA.

Sizes

It is available in three sizes. Size 3 is used in patients weighing 30–50 kg, size 4 in patients weighing 50–70 kg and size 5 in patients weighing 70–100 kg.

Technique of Fastrach-Guided Intubation

The successful placement of ETT through Fastrach is dependent on choosing the correct size ILMA, position of the patient, additional maneuvers to align the aperture of the mask against the glottis, and the type of ETT used for intubation. The correct size is chosen by placing the ILMA next to the patient's head in such a way that the cranial surface of the shaft lies at the level of incisors. Appropriate size ILMA will have the epiglottic elevating bar at the level of thyroid notch. Then the selected LMA is lubricated with water-soluble jelly on the posterior surface.

The head is positioned in neutral position for ILMA insertion.

The ILMA is inserted after opening the mouth by placing the handle parallel to the chest and pressing the tip of mask against the palate and advanced further along the anatomical curvature till the airway tube lies against the chin of the patient. Then, the cuff is inflated to recommended volumes without exceeding 60 cmH_2O and checked for ventilation. If the ventilation is inadequate, the ILMA is withdrawn 6 cm upward without deflation and then inserted again. This movement solves the epiglottic downfolding-related airway obstruction.

Chandy's Maneuver

The device is rotated in a sagittal plane using the handle till the bag ventilation is easiest with adequate tidal volume. This maneuver aligns the airway aperture of the LMA with the glottic inlet.

The second step involves passage of ETT tube till the transverse marking followed by lifting the Fastrach LMA away from the posterior pharyngeal wall using the handle to aid the passage of ETT inside the glottis without impinging on the vestibule or arytenoids.

The ETT connector is removed and attached to stabilizing rod. Then, the ILMA cuff is deflated and taken out while applying counter pressure to the tube.

If regular tubes are used, they should be prewarmed and introduced with a reverse swing to decrease the angle of exit from the ILMA for correct placement in the trachea.

Indications for Fastrach Intubation

- It is a rescue device for unanticipated difficult intubation anywhere in the hospital.
- Indicated as a primary method of intubation in anticipated difficult airway and can be inserted under awake local anesthesia.
- Used to intubate patients with suspected and diagnosed cervical spine injuries. They cause less movement of the cervical spine and do not worsen the injury in unstable cervical spine patients.

Problems

Improper mask selection and malalignment leads to esophageal intubation and impingement on the valleculla. Injuries to the soft tissues and teeth occur if the ILMA is not removed and used as a primary airway for prolonged time. It does not protect from pulmonary aspiration.

CTrach Laryngeal Mask Airway

Design

It is similar to Fastrach and has two fiberoptic channels and a viewing monitor. The fiberoptic channels are present at the epiglottic elevating bar and they transmit the image to the viewing screen. The screen is a detachable unit and is connected by magnetic latch to the CTrach. It is available in 3, 4, and 5 sizes and can be used up to 20 times.

Insertion

The CTrach is lubricated and inserted similar to Fastrach without the viewing monitor. The airway is secured, ventilation is checked, and then the viewer is attached and activated to see the real-time image of the larynx. The glottic image is optimized by readjusting the LMA position till a satisfactory optimal view is obtained which is followed by endotracheal intubation.

Benefits

The real-time image allows manipulating the LMA for proper alignment of the larynx and hence there is a higher rate of success in ETT placement.

Laryngeal Tube, Laryngeal Tube Suction, and Gastrolaryngeal Tube

Design

The airway tube of LT is slim, curved, and short with a blind distal end. It has a proximal large pharyngeal cuff that isolates the laryngopharynx from the oro- and nasopharynx and a distal small cuff that seals the upper esophagus, thereby separating the laryngopharynx from the gastric lumen. Ventilation occurs via the two lumens between the cuffs and the lateral eyes present in the LT. The cuffs are inflated via a single pilot tube and balloon, and the cuff pressure has to be limited to 60 cmH_2O. The connectors are color-coded according to the size.

Size

The laryngeal tube is available for use in seven sizes for all age groups starting from neonates to adults. The appropriate size is chosen based on the weight of the patient for sizes 0–2 and height of the patient for sizes 3–5.

Benefits

The slim profile allows easier placement of the LT in patients with restricted mouth opening, decreased pharyngeal space (oropharyngeal edema as in PIH, enlarged tonsils) where even LMA insertion is difficult.

The oropharyngeal leak pressure is in the range of 22–32 cmH_2O.

Laryngeal tubes are efficacious during both spontaneous and controlled ventilation. It is an approved airway equipment for usage during emergency cardiopulmonary resuscitation.

It allows fiberscope to be passed nasally for placement of ETT with the LT in place without deflation of the cuffs. The smaller airway diameter of the LT limits the size of the ETT placement. In addition, there is difficult negotiation of fiberscope through the small ventilating orifice and is not the ideal SAD serving as a conduit for intubation.

Problems

- Tongue edema due to pressure effects from the pharyngeal cuff can lead to upper airway obstruction after removal of the LT.
- The risk of aspiration is not eliminated with an esophageal cuff.
- Airway obstruction due to nonalignment of the ventilating small orifices can occur with rotation of the airway tube in situ along the longitudinal axis.

Laryngeal Tube Suction

The laryngeal tube suction (LTSII) is a modified version of the LT with a drainage tube extending beyond the airway tube facilitating suctioning and passage of gastric tube. The distal cuff of LTSII is asymmetrical, ovoid in shape sealing the esophagus effectively, and also prevents axial rotation of the airway tubes.

Gastrolaryngeal tube is a modified version of laryngeal tubes that allows passage of gastroendoscope via a separate lumen of 16 mm diameter. It allows passage of gastroscope of external diameter 13.8 mm that provides access to the alimentary tract for performing diagnostic and therapeutic procedures with uninterrupted ventilation. The gastrolaryngeal tube is available only in one size for use in adults who are taller than 155 cm.

Cobra Perilaryngeal Airway

Design

It is a modification of the Guedel's airway that seals the airway at the base of the tongue. It is made of PVC and consists of an airway tube, circumferential cuff proximal to the ventilation orifice, and a distal end that is flattened like the head of a cobra surrounding the ventilation orifice. The head has soft grills on the anterior aspect of the head deflecting the epiglottis away from the ventilation orifice and allows passage of fiberscope and ETT easily **(Fig. 37)**. The ramp present in the head guides easy passage of ETT. The airway pressure should be limited to 20 cmH_2O and the cuff pressure should be limited to 25 cmH_2O.

Insertion

The Cobra is inserted straight between the tongue and the hard palate in the sniffing position without pressing against the hard palate and is advanced caudally until there is resistance. Ideal placement results in the head lying in front of the laryngeal inlet and the cuff at the base of the tongue. The tip of the Cobra does not seal the esophageal inlet like other supraglottic airways and has decreased margin of safety in case of regurgitation and aspiration.

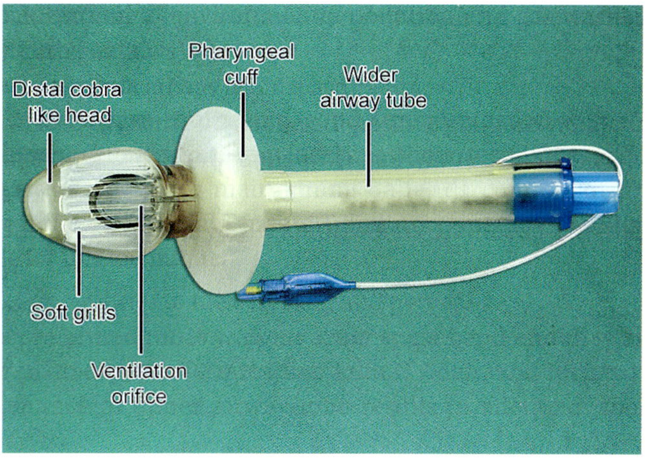

Fig. 37: Parts of the Cobra PLA (Cobra Perilaryngeal Airway).

Size

It is available in eight sizes and can be used in all age groups.

Benefits

The wider and shorter airway tube enables larger size of fiberscope and ETT placement. The incidence of sore throat is less. The sealing pressure is higher than the classic LMA. It has been used as a device to maintain airway during tracheostomy.

Problems

It has less esophageal sealing and does not prevent aspiration.

Ambu Laryngeal Masks

Design

Ambu laryngeal masks are designed with airway tubes with a preformed curvature resembling the anatomy of the upper airway. The airway tube and cuff are molded as a single unit and the internal ribs present inside the tube provide flexibility and integrity with varied position of the head. The cuff is elliptical in shape with no aperture bars and hence allows easy passage of the fiberscope. The tip of the cuff is reinforced to prevent folding at insertion of the device. The pilot balloon is color-coded to identify the size of the Ambu LMA.

Sizes and Types

Ambu laryngeal masks are available in eight sizes from 1 to 6. They are available as single-use devices (Ambu Aura once), reusable (Ambu Aura 40), and flexible (Ambu Aura flexible) type. Ambu AuraGain has an integrated gastric channel for placement of gastric tubes **(Fig. 38)**. Ambu Aura-i resembles the ILMA with a shorter rigid tube and a plastic handle with an integral bite block serving as a rescue device for ETT placement.

The success of placement, alignment to glottis, and sealing pressures are comparable to classic LMA except for time of insertion that has been shown to be relatively shorter than the LMA classic.

Benefits

The insertion is easier and quick due to the preformed anatomical curvature compared to classic LMA.

Proseal Laryngeal Mask Airway

- It is a second-generation supraglottic device that has additional features of safety for preventing aspiration and to provide high-sealing pressures.
- It is a modification of the classical LMA that provides:
    - Reliable separation of the gastrointestinal tract from the respiratory tract.
    - Effective sealing of the glottis to ensure positive pressure ventilation without gastric insufflation.
    - Enables detection of malpositioning of the supraglottic device easily. These features improve the safety of Proseal LMA in clinical practice.

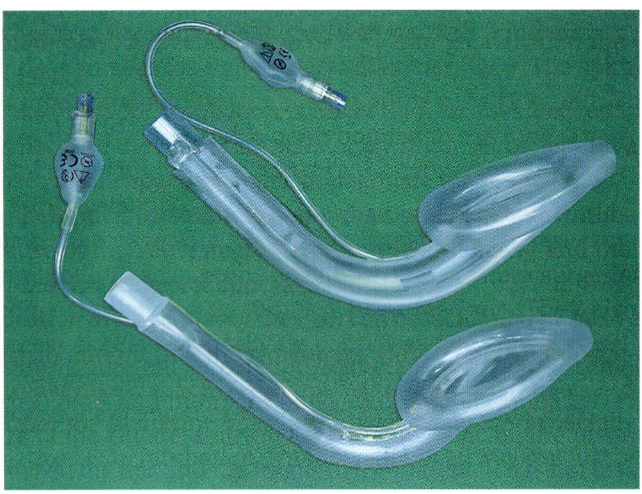

Fig. 38: Two different types of Ambu laryngeal mask. Top panel: Ambu laryngeal mask airway (LMA) with gastric channel (Ambu Aura gain) and bottom panel: Ambu LMA without the gastric channel.

Design

The Proseal LMA is a silicone-based and latex-free supraglottic device consisting of four components: (1) mask, (2) inflation line, (3) drain tube, and (4) and airway tube.

The mask is larger and deeper without grills and also has a dorsal cuff that increases the effectiveness of sealing. The airway tube is wire reinforced, smaller in diameter, and has a drain tube running laterally that terminates at the distal tip of the cuff.

An integral bite block prevents tube damage and iatrogenic airway obstruction **(Figs. 39A and B)**. The red plug acts as a vent for egress of gases and prevents overexpansion of the cuff during autoclaving. The cuff deflator

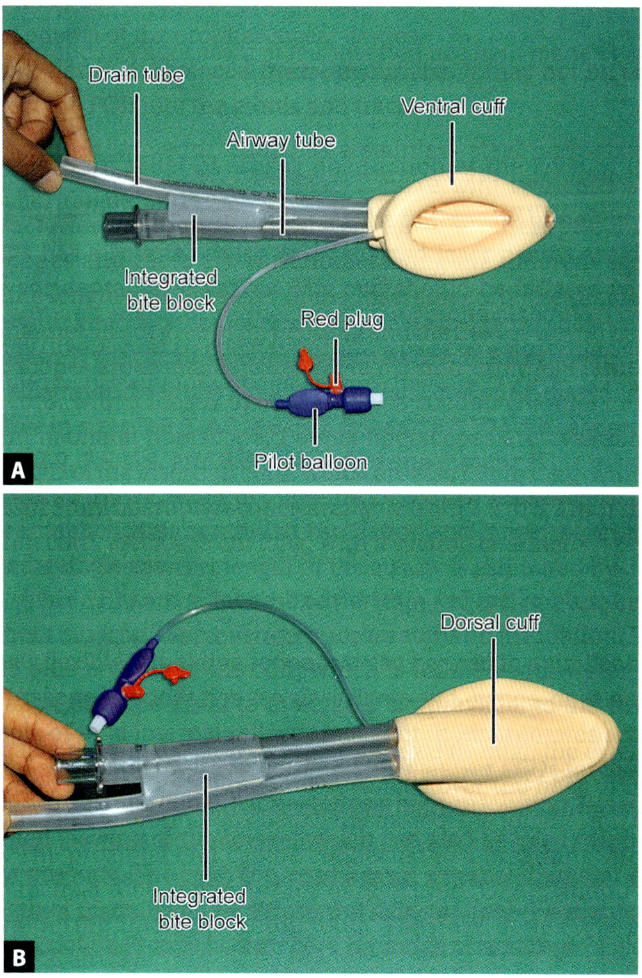

Figs. 39A and B: Parts of a laryngeal mask airway (LMA) Proseal. (A) Ventral aspect; and (B) Dorsal aspect.

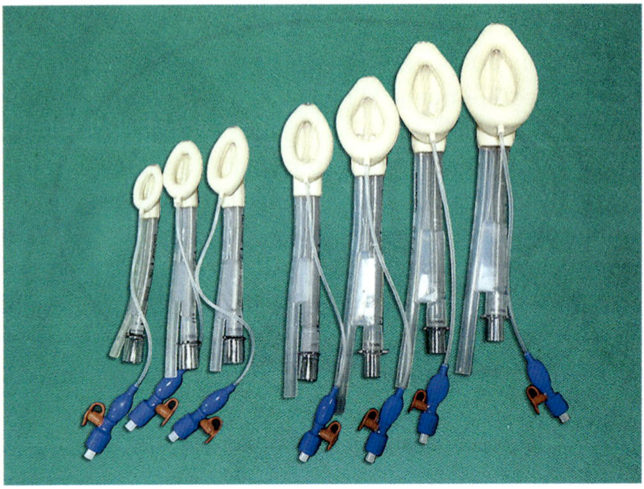

Fig. 40: Different sizes of a laryngeal mask airway (LMA) Proseal from size 1 to 5.

aids complete deflation of the mask ensuring a wedge-shaped mask for preventing traumatic insertion and distal folding over the cuff. The Proseal LMA is available in seven sizes **(Fig. 40)** and the pediatric sizes lack the dorsal cuff.

Technique of Insertion

It can be inserted using the standard index finger insertion, thumb insertion, and a metal introducer tip mounted to the notch between the airway tube and the drain tube. The use of introducer is advisable during pediatric Proseal LMA insertion. An alternative technique involves placement of the gum elastic bougie under direct visual guidance into the esophagus followed by railroading the Proseal LMA, so that the distal tip lies against the esophageal sphincter. The tip of the mask should be pressed against the hard palate and the inserting fingers should press the airway tube cranially to avoid contact with the structures anteriorly.

The tip of the Proseal LMA rests against the upper esophageal sphincter, the upper borders at the base of tongue, the sides of the mask face the pyriform fossa, and the airway tube orifice lies in front of the glottis.

An ideally placed device ensures unobstructed ventilation without any audible leak at cuff pressure of <60 cmH_2O. The passage of orogastric tube through the drain tube into the stomach signifies ideal position of the tip of Proseal LMA. The bite block lies midway between the incisors. The average sealing pressures for Proseal LMA is in the range of 23–32 cmH_2O.

Malpositioning of the LMA can be identified by the following tests:

- When the tip of the Proseal LMA (PLMA) is folded backward, ventilation is obstructed, inflation pressures may be high, and there is absence of gas leak from the drain tube. The gastric tube cannot be passed, and the gel placed on the drain tube does not move with positive pressure ventilation.

- Highly placed PLMA tip in the supraglottis can be identified by the bite block protruding beyond the incisors. The positive pressure ventilation is ineffective, and there usually is audible leak around the PLMA and the drain tube. This leak is corrected by pressing the LMA further downward.
- Glottis placement of the tip results in ejection of the gel placed on the proximal end of the drain tube with obstruction to ventilation and gas leak from the drain tube. Pressing the mask further downward worsens airway obstruction in this type of misplacement.
- Overinflation of the cuff and rise in cuff pressure beyond 60 cmH_2O can displace the LMA drain tube anteriorly resulting in ineffective sealing promoting aspiration.

Indications

- Ideal supraglottic device for positive pressure ventilation in elective surgeries, especially laparoscopic procedures, open abdominal surgeries, nonsupine surgical positions—prone and lateral position and for obese patients undergoing peripheral surgical procedures. The higher leak pressures enable positive pressure ventilation with peak inspiratory pressures up to 30 cmH_2O and the drain tube vents out the gastric fluid and air effectively preventing gastric insufflations and aspiration.
- Used as a rescue device for ventilation in situations of difficult and failed intubation. It is the preferred rescue airway device in pregnancy and failed intubation following rapid sequence induction.

Problems

The risk of aspiration is not eliminated completely in spite of the presence of the drain tube as the position of the LMA is dynamic with changes in cuff pressure and dislodgment can occur even after optimal placement.

The narrower airway tube allows intubation via a fiberscope successful with use of Aintree intubation catheter-guided railroading of the ETT.

Airway obstruction due to mechanical closure of the vocal cords in lighter planes of anesthesia can occur despite ideal placement of the LMA.

Laryngeal Mask Airway Supreme

This device is a modified version incorporating the benefits of LMA unique, Proseal LMA, and Fastrach LMA.

Design

It is a disposable device with an oval-shaped cuff possessing higher leak pressures similar to Proseal LMA, reinforced drain tube tip and anatomically preformed shaft that aids easier insertion. The shaft has two lumens with a central lumen for access to the alimentary tract and an oval-shaped airway lumen. The fixation tab protrudes 2 cm beyond the upper lip ensuring optimal depth of insertion of cuff inside and for easy fixation. The elliptical shape of the cuff is an added advantage that permits the use of this device with reduced interdental space. The fins present on either side of the drain tube prevent epiglottic obstruction of the airways **(Fig. 41)**.

Sizes

Laryngeal mask airway supreme is available in all sizes from 1 to 5.

Merits

- Easier and successful insertion at the first attempt due to the preformed shaft and shape of the cuff.
- Sealing pressures are similar to Proseal LMA.
- The reinforced tip resists folding of the cuff.

i-gel Airway

Design

It is a cuffless single-use device with a mask that resembles the perilaryngeal structures, which creates a cuffless seal with use of appropriate size and correct placement of the airway. It is made of medical grade thermoplastic elastomer gel. The i-gel has a noncompressible proximal shaft that encloses both the airway and drain tube. The drain tube of i-gel is narrower and allows passage of a smaller size Ryle's tube compared to other second-generation

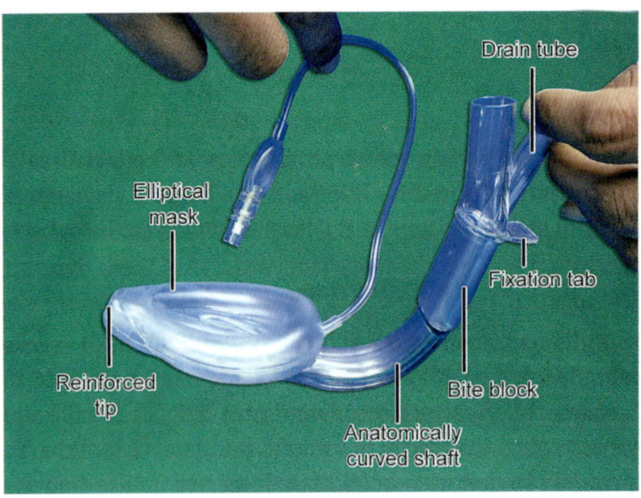

Fig. 41: Parts of the laryngeal mask airway (LMA) supreme.

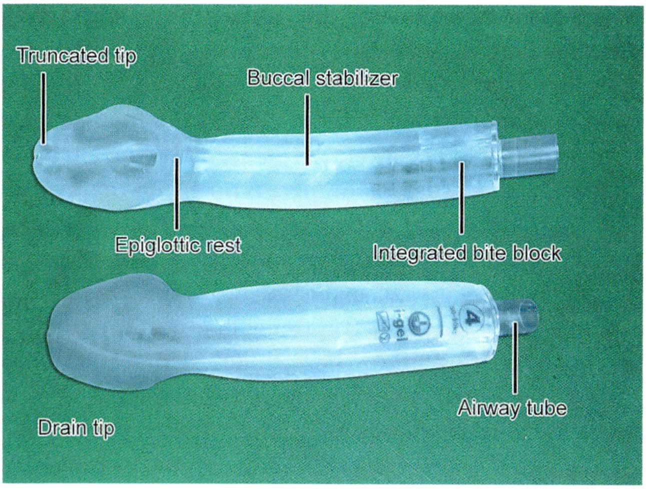

Fig. 42: Parts of the i-gel.

SADs **(Fig. 42)**. The airway tube is shorter and wider with no grills at the end. The epiglottic ridge present at the proximal end of the mask stabilizes the i-gel in position resisting outward movement of the mask. The stem of i-gel is wider, with a curvature mimicking the oropharynx preventing axial rotation. The distal tip of i-gel is truncated reducing the esophageal sealing properties. It is available in 7 sizes pediatric to adult and the size 1 lacks the gastric drain channel.

The sealing pressures are in the range of 20–30 cmH_2O enabling positive pressure ventilation.

The cuffless nature promotes quick insertion and there is minimal displacement and rotation of the device. The shorter and wider airway tube allows easier fiberoptic endoscopy-guided intubation and also allows passage of bigger size ETT compared to LMA.

Demerits

The incidence of failed ventilation with successful placement of the device is high (5%) compared to other devices possibly due to the cuffless nature of the device.

Soft-tissue injuries and cranial nerve palsies can occur due to pressure effects from the rigid parts of i-gel in prolonged surgeries and in nonsupine positions. The esophageal seal is relatively low compared to other devices.

NEWER SUPRAGLOTTIC AIRWAY DEVICES

The Self-sealing Baska Mask

The "Baska Mask" is a sophisticated SAD that has gained attention for its innovative design and functionality, particularly in the field of anesthesia.

Unlike traditional laryngeal masks, the Baska Mask features a self-sealing and noninflatable cuff, which is one of its most significant advancements. This cuff automatically adapts to the patient's pharyngeal and laryngeal anatomy, providing a secure seal without the need for manual inflation. This self-sealing mechanism offers several benefits, including a reduction in the risk of trauma to the airway tissues, as there is no need to apply high pressure to inflate the cuff. This feature is particularly advantageous in patients with fragile or sensitive airway tissues, where traditional inflatable cuffs might cause damage or increase the risk of postoperative sore throat.

The Baska Mask's design also incorporates dual gastric drainage channels, which are a critical safety feature. These channels allow for the continuous drainage of gastric contents, significantly reducing the risk of aspiration—a serious complication in anesthesia. Aspiration of gastric contents can lead to chemical pneumonitis, which can be life-threatening. By providing a means to manage this risk proactively, the Baska Mask enhances patient's safety during procedures where the risk of regurgitation is elevated, such as in emergency surgeries or in patients with a full stomach.

Another notable feature of the Baska Mask is its construction from a soft, pliable material that conforms to the patient's airway. This adaptability not only improves the seal but also makes the mask more comfortable for the patient. The pliable material is less likely to cause pressure necrosis or other forms of tissue damage, which can be a concern with harder, and less adaptable materials used in other airway devices. The design also simplifies the insertion process, making it easier for clinicians to achieve an effective airway seal quickly, even in challenging situations.

In addition to these features, the Baska Mask has a built-in bite block, which helps to prevent the patient from occluding the airway by biting down, a common issue with other supraglottic devices. This bite block is integral to the mask's structure, reducing the need for additional accessories and thereby simplifying the setup process.

However, despite its many advantages, the Baska Mask is not without limitations. For instance, while the self-sealing cuff is highly effective in most cases, it may not provide an adequate seal in patients with abnormal airway anatomy, such as those with large oropharyngeal masses or significant anatomical distortions. Additionally, the mask's effectiveness can be limited in cases where high airway pressures are required, such as in patients with severe pulmonary disease or those undergoing procedures that necessitate high ventilation pressures. In these cases, a more traditional airway management approach, such as endotracheal intubation, may be necessary.

Another limitation is the learning curve associated with the Baska Mask. Although it is designed to be user-friendly, its novel features require proper training and familiarity to optimize its use. Clinicians accustomed to traditional laryngeal masks may need to adjust their techniques when using the Baska Mask, particularly regarding insertion and management of the self-sealing mechanism.

Overall, the Baska Mask represents a significant advancement in supraglottic airway management. Its self-sealing cuff, dual gastric drainage channels, and patient-friendly design offer substantial benefits, particularly in reducing the risk of airway trauma and aspiration. However, its limitations must be considered, and appropriate patient selection is crucial to ensure the best outcomes. Ongoing education and training are also essential to fully realize the potential of this innovative airway device in clinical practice.

The Laryngeal Mask Airway Protector

The LMA protector is a newer generation SAD that offers enhanced features for airway management in anesthesia. It is designed to provide a secure and effective airway seal while minimizing the risks associated with traditional airway devices. One of its key features is the dual gastric drainage channels, which improve patient's safety by allowing continuous drainage of gastric contents, reducing the risk of aspiration during anesthesia. The LMA protector also features a cuff made from silicone, which is designed to minimize trauma to the airway and enhance patient's comfort. The cuff's construction provides a better seal at lower pressures, reducing the risk of complications such as sore throat or tissue damage postoperatively.

Another advantage of the LMA protector is its compatibility with fiberoptic bronchoscopes, which allows for easy visualization of the airway, aiding in both placement and diagnostic procedures. This makes it particularly useful in cases where airway anatomy may be challenging or when precise placement is critical. However, the LMA protector is not without limitations. It may not be suitable for patients requiring high airway pressures, such as those with severe lung pathology, where traditional intubation may be preferred. Additionally, like other supraglottic devices, its effectiveness may be limited in patients with abnormal airway anatomy.

VIDEOLARYNGOSCOPES

Videolaryngoscopy-guided intubation is one of the recent additional tools that has changed the face of difficult airway management in both elective and emergent scenarios. Direct laryngoscopy has been the standard technique for intubation for >70 years. The innovative method of viewing the larynx indirectly for intubation has been used in rigid scopes like Bonfils. Videolaryngoscopy is the latest tool of advanced airway management integrating the digital technology for image capture, optics for transmission of image and the shape of blade angulation for a better and wider visualization.

Principles of Videolaryngoscopy

The distal end of the blade has a miniature camera—complementary metal oxide semiconductor (CMOS) chip. It captures a wider and improved view of the glottic image that is transmitted electronically/optically/system of prisms to a distal or integrated monitor. The LED present at the distal end of the blade illuminates the glottic area and also prevents fogging. The indirect visualization of the glottic image is possible without alignment of the oral, pharyngeal and laryngeal axes. The problems due to line of sight are circumvented by the indirect method of viewing the glottis. The glottic view is wider and superior with a live image on the screen enabling the assistant to help with external manipulation unlike direct laryngoscopy.

Classification

There are different types of videolaryngoscopes based on the type and shape of the blade and the channel for guiding the endotracheal tube.

- Macintosh type blade: Storz V Mac and Storz C Mac.
- Angulated blades: GlideScope, McGrath 5 Series, and Storz C Mac D blade.
- Anatomically shaped blades with channels for ETT: Pentax Airway scope and Airtraq and King Vision.

The tracheal tube is preloaded into the guide channel of the videolaryngoscope prior to laryngoscopy in these types of videolaryngoscopes.

Angulated Blades

The angulated blades have an exaggerated curvature that helps in looking around the corners of the larynx for an enlarged view and a wider vision. They always require a stylet that is shaped similar to the curvature of the blade for ETT placement and are useful when direct visualization of the glottis is impossible.

GlideScope

The shape of the blade is extremely angulated to 60° upward with a camera located in the midway **(Fig. 43)**. This arrangement provides a suprapanoramic view of the glottis irrespective of its position and without the need for alignment of the oral, pharyngeal, and laryngeal axes. The camera is placed more proximally and so the image is of high quality as it is unaffected by secretions or blood. The heating components (LED) provide effective antifog mechanism. The use of styleted ETT bent to 90° makes intubation successful **(Fig. 44)**. Specialized reusable stylets—GlideRites are available to aid intubation.

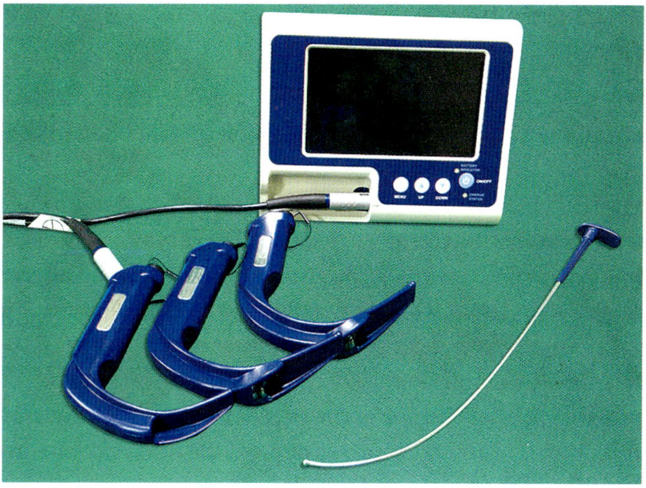

Fig. 43: The GlideScope with three different blade sizes, the viewing monitor, and the GlideRite stylet.

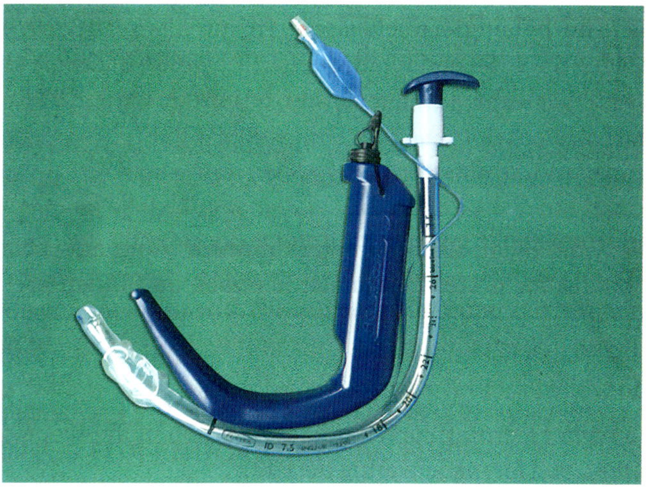

Fig. 44: Endotracheal tube shaped according to the bend of the GlideScope blade.

GlideScope cobalt is a single-use videolaryngoscope with disposable blades, a reusable video baton, and a handle. GlideScope Ranger is a portable version with an antireflective screen that can be used even in the presence of sunlight. GlideScopes are available in four sizes for pediatric usage starting from 0, 1, 2, and 2.5 as single-use blades. The recent version includes slim titanium blades that are available in both Macintosh type and angulated blades. The titanium blades increase the durability, and the slim profile helps in decreasing the height of the blade to aid oral insertion smoothly.

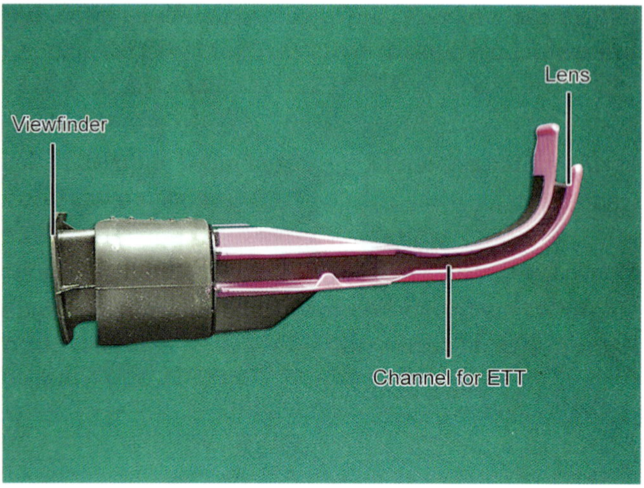

Fig. 46: Parts of the Airtraq videolaryngoscope. Pediatric size 1. (ETT: endotracheal tube)

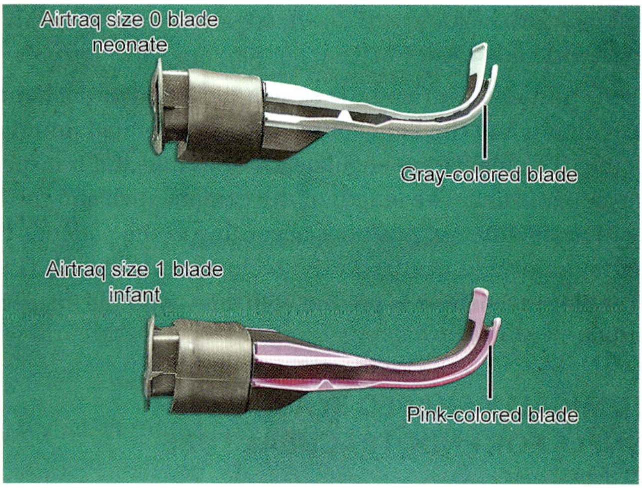

Fig. 47: Two different blade sizes of Airtraq videolaryngoscope. Top picture: The neonatal blade is size 0, is gray-colored, and accepts tracheal tubes of sizes ID 2.5–3.5 mm; and bottom picture: The infant blade is size 1, is pink-colored, and accepts tracheal tubes of sizes ID 4.0–5.5 mm.

color-coded according to the size of the ETT (2.5–8 mm) and is available for all age groups **(Fig. 47)**.

Airtraq Avant has reusable optical components with disposable blades and eye cup. They prevent cross-contamination and allow multiple uses up to 50 times. The disposable blades have lenses at the distal end of the blade and at the eye cup.

Technique

The insertion of the scope is in the midline and then it is advanced while viewing through the viewfinder or an external monitor. Intubation is successful with Airtraq only when the glottic image is visualized in the center of the field. Failure to achieve optimal position is rectified by twisting movements of the scope clockwise and anticlockwise. Failure to intubate after this maneuver is resolved by withdrawing the scope backward followed by upward lifting of the scope to enable ETT placement.

Merits

Studies and case reports have shown improved glottis visualization and ETT placement in anticipated difficult airways, syndromic children, and in patients with limited cervical spine movements. The ETT tube need not be loaded on to a stylet as there is a guiding channel along with the scope.

Demerits

The size of the device is bulky limiting its usage in patients with limited mouth opening. A minimum of 12–13 mm mouth opening is needed for insertion of the pediatric blades and >16 mm mouth opening is needed for insertion of the adult blades. Mucosal injury can arise from repeated movements of the scope for optimal glottic image and because of undue pressure on the soft tissues.

Airway Scope

It is a portable wireless device operated by battery and has a transparent single use P blade with a port for suction. It uses LED with a flexible wire for the charge-coupled device (CCD) unlike other videolaryngoscopes that use CMOS chip for the camera. The viewing monitor and the channel for ETT are an integral part of the scope with a target mark appearing on the monitor for guiding the ETT placement correctly.

MACINTOSH TYPE BLADES

C-MAC Videolaryngoscope

It is the fourth generation of videolaryngoscopes developed by Karl Storz having the unique feature of Macintosh type laryngoscope blades.

Design

The blade is thinner and flat with a maximum of 14 mm thickness that allows insertion of the scope in patients with limited mouth opening (15 mm). The device insertion is easier due to familiarity with the use of Macintosh curved-blade laryngoscope and the thinner profile of the blade.

The smooth beveled margins offer additional advantage of atraumatic insertion. The camera and the LED are placed in the distal one-third of the blade and the image captured by the lens has an aperture angle of 80°. Hence, the tip of the blade is also visualized during advancement serving as a visual guide to position the tip of the blade in the vallecula. The best view of the glottis is seen with this ideal position of the blade.

The image captured is displayed as a high-quality color image on the LCD monitor. It is available in five sizes, as Macintosh blades size—2, 3 and 4, and as Miller blades 0 and 1.

The D blade is angulated **(Figs. 48 and 49)**, elliptically tapered, and rises at the distal end. It is indicated in patients with higher Cormack Lehane scores and with anticipated anteriorly placed glottis.

Merits

It can be used in patients with mouth opening of 1.5 cm. The learning curve with C-MAC videolaryngoscope is faster due to the familiarity with the Macintosh type of laryngoscopic blade.

TruView Picture Capture Device

Design

The TruView laryngoscope has a unique blade shape that is straight in the proximal part with an angulated distal portion that has an optical lens. This provides 46° refraction angle enabling visualization of the anteriorly placed glottis. The image viewed through the eyepiece is displayed on to the monitor

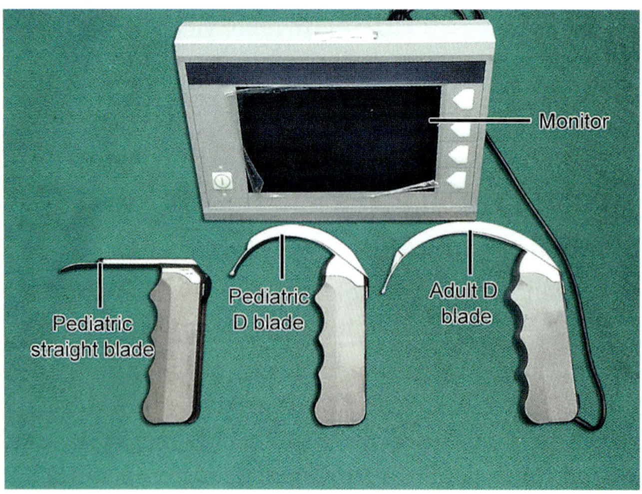

Fig. 48: C-MAC videolaryngoscope with one straight blade and D blade of pediatric and adult sizes.

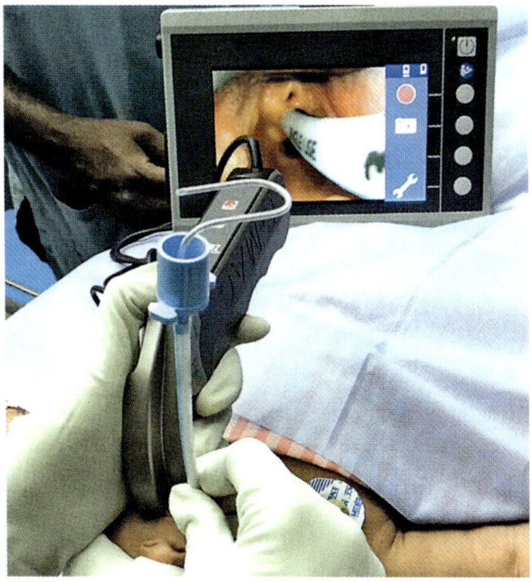

Fig. 49: A child being intubated with a C-MAC pediatric D blade. The glottis is visualized in the center of the upper one-third of the monitor. A styleted tracheal tube bent at the distal end is used for intubation.

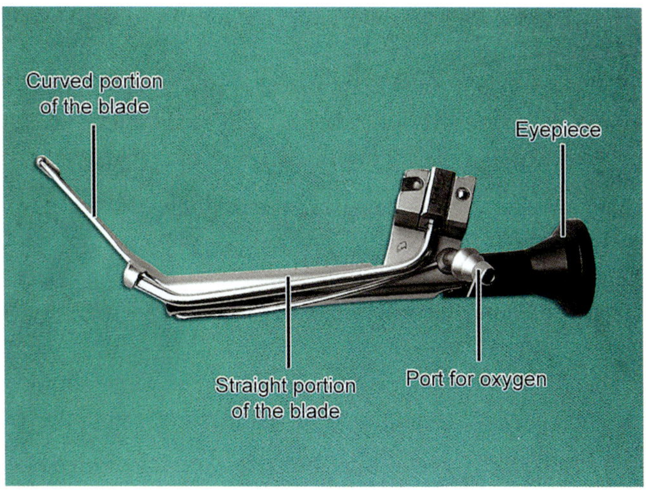

Fig. 50: Parts of TruView laryngoscope.

using magnetic connection of the eyepiece to the camera of the TruView PCD screen **(Fig. 50)**.

The blades are available in five sizes from 0 to 4 and the height of the blade is 8 mm. Size 0 is used in neonates, size 1 in infants, and size 2 in a small child. The blades have ports for insufflating a jet of oxygen that helps to prevent fogging and desaturation during intubation. Studies have shown improved Cormack Lehane scoring with successful intubation with the use of TruView compared to standard conventional Macintosh blades. However, the glottic image is inferior compared to other videolaryngoscopes.

Clinical Uses and Benefits of Videolaryngoscopy

- Used as a primary and alternative intubation device in both anticipated and unanticipated difficult intubation
- Teaching elective intubation in patients with normal airways
- Assessment of upper airway caliber, patency, and ease of visualizing the glottis prior to extubation in a difficult airway, and after major reconstructive surgeries in the head and neck.
- Placement of airway exchange catheters under direct vision before extubation
- Retrieval of foreign bodies
- Assessment of nerve palsies after thyroid surgeries
- Less force is required for optimal glottic image than a conventional laryngoscope with possibly less hemodynamic response to intubation.
- Less cervical spine movements compared to conventional direct laryngoscopy.

Pitfalls with Videolaryngoscopy

- Different techniques of scopy and intubation with each model and brand of videolaryngoscope
- No single scope has all the ideal features.

Pearls for Successful Use of Videolaryngoscopes

- Insertion of the scope should be from the midline, avoiding any sweeping movements of the tongue.
- The image should be optimized to the center and to the upper one-third of the screen in order to have space for manipulating the endotracheal tube.
- In channeled versions of videolaryngoscopes, the scope should be moved backward and forward to get the best view in the center of the field and for placing the ETT tube successfully.
- Stylet bent to the shape of the blade further aids success.
- There are no studies with absolute evidence recommending a particular type of videolaryngoscope at present. But, they do have a definitive role in difficult airway management.

RECENT ADVANCES IN LARYNGOSCOPES—THE VIE SCOPE

The Vie Scope is an innovative intubation device that has been developed to address challenges commonly encountered in airway management, particularly in emergency and difficult airway scenarios. Its design is a departure from traditional laryngoscopes, offering a unique approach to visualizing the vocal cords and facilitating endotracheal intubation. The Vie Scope consists of a straight, clear, and rigid tube with an integrated light source that illuminates the airway, providing a direct line of sight from the mouth to the vocal cords. This straight-to-cuff visualization technique simplifies the process of identifying the glottis, which can be particularly challenging in patients with difficult airway anatomy or in high-pressure situations such as trauma or cardiac arrest.

One of the key advantages of the Vie Scope is its ability to reduce the need for extensive manipulation of the patient's head and neck. Traditional laryngoscopy often requires significant extension of the neck and elevation of the jaw to align the oral, pharyngeal, and laryngeal axes to achieve a clear view of the vocal cords. In contrast, the Vie Scope's straight design allows for a more neutral head position, which is particularly beneficial in trauma patients who may have cervical spine injuries or in situations where spinal precautions are necessary. This feature not only enhances patient's safety but also makes the Vie Scope a valuable tool in prehospital settings where conditions are less controlled and time is of the essence.

The Vie Scope's simplicity is another major advantage. Its clear and straight tube design provides an unobstructed view of the airway without the need for complex adjustments or manipulations. This can significantly reduce the time to successful intubation, which is critical in emergency settings where every second counts. The integrated light source further enhances visibility, ensuring that the vocal cords are clearly illuminated, even in low-light environments. This makes the Vie Scope particularly useful in prehospital settings, such as in ambulances or on the battlefield, where lighting conditions may be suboptimal.

Moreover, the Vie Scope is designed to be compatible with standard ETTs, making it versatile and easy to integrate into existing airway management protocols. This compatibility means that practitioners do not need to learn new techniques or use specialized equipment, which can streamline the adoption of the device in clinical practice. Additionally, the Vie Scope's rigid structure helps to maintain the patency of the airway, reducing the risk of soft-tissue collapse during intubation, which can be a challenge with flexible laryngoscopes.

Despite its numerous advantages, the Vie Scope is not without limitations. One of the primary challenges is the learning curve associated with its use. While the device is designed to be intuitive, practitioners who are accustomed to traditional laryngoscopy techniques may need time and training to become proficient with the Vie Scope. This is particularly important because the device's effectiveness relies on the operator's ability to maintain a direct line of sight to the vocal cords while advancing the ETT. Inexperienced users may initially struggle with this technique, potentially leading to longer intubation times or unsuccessful attempts.

Furthermore, as the Vie Scope is a relatively new device, there is still limited long-term data on its efficacy and safety compared to more established intubation tools. While initial studies and anecdotal reports have been promising, more research is needed to fully understand its role in airway management, particularly in diverse patient populations and clinical settings.

Overall, the Vie Scope represents a significant advancement in airway management technology, offering a simple, effective, and potentially life-saving tool for emergency and difficult airway scenarios. Its design minimizes the need for patient's manipulation, enhances visibility, and reduces intubation times, making it a valuable addition to the arsenal of airway management devices. However, proper training and familiarity with the device are essential to maximize its benefits and ensure patient's safety.

RETROGRADE INTUBATION (TRANSLARYNGEAL-GUIDED INTUBATION)

History

Retrograde intubation was first described in 1960 by Butler and Cirillo. Through the patient's tracheostomy, a red rubber catheter was passed cephalad and retrieved from the oral cavity, through which an ETT was guided into the trachea.

The presently practiced technique was first described by Dr Ralph Waters, a British anesthesiologist in 1963 for treating cancrum oris patients, in whom he passed a Tuohy needle through the cricothyroid membrane, the epidural catheter through the Tuohy needle and retrieved it through the nares using a hook, and used this as a guide to advance the ETT into the trachea.

Indications

- Failed attempts at laryngoscopy, LMA, or fiberoptic intubation.
- Emergency airway establishment in conditions where blood, secretions, or anatomic derangements obscure glottis visualization
- Elective airway access in patients with:
    - Limited mouth opening
    - Oral and oropharyngeal masses
    - Maxillary and mandibular fracture
    - Limited cervical spine movement
- Contraindications
- Unfavorable anatomy (huge thyroid and mentosternal burns contractures)

Coagulopathy

- Local infection
- Disease or disruption of the larynx and trachea

Technique

Classical Technique

The classical technique employs a 17 G Tuohy needle and an epidural catheter. The larynx is stabilized with the left-hand thumb and middle fingers. The skin and subcutaneous tissue over the puncture site is incised with scalpel blade to facilitate entry of the blunt Tuohy needle.

The Tuohy needle with the attached syringe is used to puncture the cricothyroid membrane at an angle of 45° cephalad. Placement of the needle in the lumen of airway is confirmed by aspirating air. Then, an epidural catheter is advanced through the Tuohy needle into the trachea, which will exit through the nasal or oral cavity. Asking the awake patient to protrude the tongue or pulling the tongue anteriorly in case of anesthetized patients will prevent coiling of the catheter in the oropharynx. A hemostat is then applied to the catheter at the neck to prevent further displacement of the catheter. The catheter can be retrieved from the oropharynx using a nerve hook. It is then threaded through the distal end of the ETT or through the Murphy's eye and is then advanced into the trachea. Using the Murphy's eye allows an extra 1 cm of tube to pass through the vocal cords.

Guidewire Technique

This technique involves the introduction of a guidewire instead of the epidural catheter through the cricothyroid or cricotracheal needle and retrieving it from the nose or the oropharynx and using it as a guide to advance the ETT into the trachea.

The retrograde intubation kit **(Fig. 51)** from Cook Medical comes with an introducer needle, a polytetrafluoroethylene (PTFE) catheter introducer needle, 0.038-inch wire guide with two positioning marks, 20 cm from the end, a radiopaque guiding catheter and 2 Rapi-Fit adapters (with 15 mm

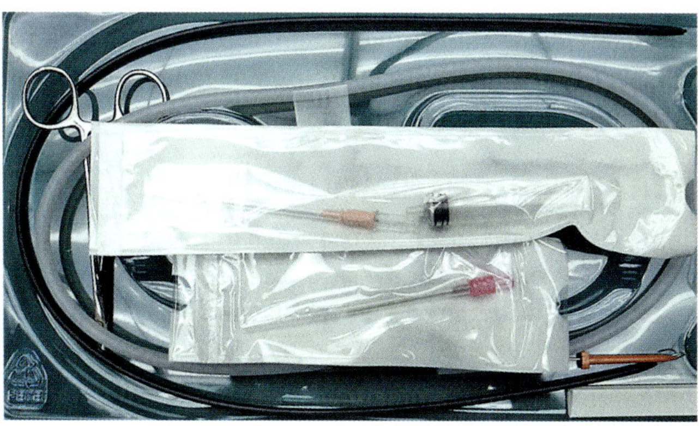

Fig. 51: Cook retrograde intubation kit.

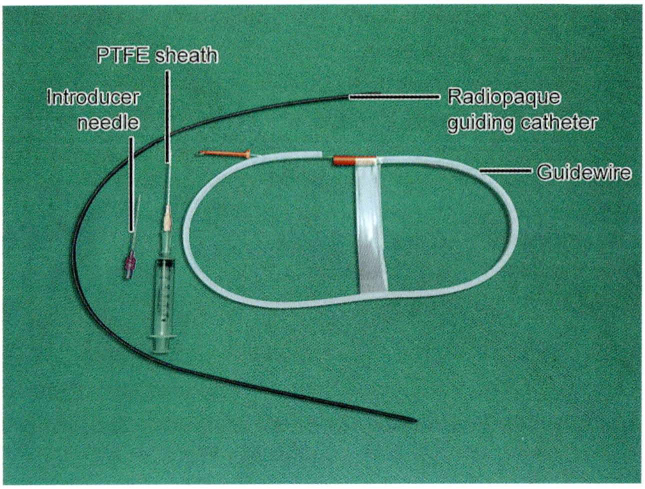

Fig. 52: Parts of the Cook retrograde intubation kit.
(PTFE: polytetrafluoroethylene)

connector and Luer Lock connector) and a hemostat **(Fig. 52)**. The set comes in three sizes of 6 F, 11 F, and 14 F for use with ETTs of ID 2.5 mm or larger, 4.0 mm or larger and 5.0 mm or larger, respectively. After the guidewire is retrieved from the nose or mouth, the guiding catheter is advanced over the guidewire. Then the ETT is passed over the guidewire/guiding catheter assembly and advanced into the trachea. The guidewire/guiding catheter assembly is then removed and the ETT is left in place. The use of a guiding catheter minimizes the play between the ETT and the guidewire.

Fiberoptic Technique

This technique involves the use of a fiberoptic bronchoscope. Once the guidewire is retrieved from the nose or mouth, it is advanced into the suction channel of the FOB to guide the FOB into the trachea. Once the FOB abuts the cricothyroid membrane, the guidewire can either be removed or made relaxed so that the FOB can be further advanced into the trachea and then the guidewire removed. The FOB acts an antegrade guide catheter over which the tracheal tube can then be advanced into the trachea.

TRANSTRACHEAL VENTILATION

This technique involves the insertion of a small diameter cannula or a needle through the cricothyroid membrane into the trachea and ventilation using a high-pressure oxygen source or a jet ventilator. This is used in the "cannot ventilate cannot intubate" situations to buy some time before definitive airway access can be achieved, because it is quicker to perform compared to a cricothyrotomy or tracheostomy and does not require special devices or kits. This technique works on the principle of air entrainment and mass movement of gas. Egress of the inhaled gas is through the normal upper airway. So, maintenance of upper airway patency is important with this technique to avoid barotraumas. As the needle or catheter can easily get displaced, this technique is only used as a temporizing measure and has to be replaced as quickly as possible by a more definitive airway.

Indications

- *Emergency:* Cannot ventilate, cannot intubate situation, where mask ventilation is inadequate to maintain oxygen saturation and supraglottic device placement and/or ventilation through the SGD has failed.
- *Elective:*
  - Laryngeal surgeries
  - Provides ventilation under GA during fiberoptic intubation or tracheostomy in difficult airway.

Equipment

Commercial and preassembled systems are available for transtracheal catheter ventilation. It is important to note that low-pressure systems like the manual self-inflating device and anesthesia-breathing circuits are ineffective for transtracheal catheter ventilation, if the transtracheal catheter is <3 mm inner diameter. The devices' needs for transtracheal catheter ventilation are: (1) source of oxygen; (2) connecting tubing from oxygen source; (3) connection between conveyance tubing and cannula; and (4) cannula.

The oxygen source can be from a central source supplied through wall outlets, oxygen flowmeters or the fresh gas outlet of the anesthesia machine. The supply pressure has to be regulated between 0 and 50 psi, to avoid barotraumas in children. The tubing connecting the oxygen source to the cannula should be of low compliance. A Luer Lock connection is recommended between this tubing and the cannula **(Fig. 53)**. A kink-resistant cannula is preferable.

Several self-assembled devices are used in operating rooms for transtracheal catheter ventilation. A 14 G cannula can be connected through a three-way to oxygen tubing (available with masks) which can then be connected to an oxygen flowmeter. The three-way stopcock can be intermittently occluded to provide ventilation.

A 14 G cannula can also be connected to a 2-mL syringe with piston removed, which in turn can be connected to the 15 mm connector of a size 7 ETT. This can then be connected to the breathing circuit. However, an intravenous cannula is difficult to fix in the neck and invariably kinks and

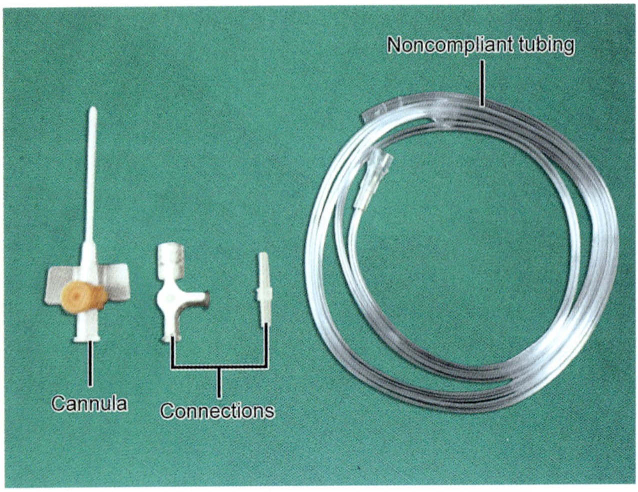

Fig. 53: A self-assembled transtracheal ventilation kit using an intravenous cannula, three-way stopcock, and tubing of low compliance.

the breathing circuit is incapable of providing adequate oxygenation and ventilation through such a narrow cannula.

Jet ventilation through the transtracheal cannula can be done by connecting it to a Manujet "injector". It has a 4-m long pressure hose for connection to a central source or oxygen cylinder, a pressure regulator, which can adjust the pressure between 0 and 50 psi with a locking mechanism to increase safety, a trigger that can be activated manually, a color-coded pressure gauge and a 100-cm long connecting tube with a Luer Lock. The Manujet III is a complete kit with Manujet injector and Ravussin jet ventilation catheters in three sizes, 13 G (adult), 14 G (child), and 16 G (infant). The catheter is made of teflon, is anatomically curved, has a flange, and also has three small lateral holes to keep the catheter away from the tracheal wall to prevent "whipping" during jet ventilation. In addition to the Luer Lock connection for jet ventilation, it also has a 15-mm connection to allow oxygenation using a resuscitator.

Complications

- Air trapping and hypercarbia
- Barotrauma, pneumothorax, and subcutaneous emphysema
- Hematoma

CRICOTHYROTOMY

This is an infraglottic technique of accessing the airway between the inferior border of the thyroid cartilage and the superior border of the cricoid cartilage. This area is the most easily accessible portion of the respiratory system below the glottis.

Relevant Anatomy

Cricothyroid membrane is located between the thyroid cartilage superiorly and the cricoid cartilage inferiorly. It is 10 mm long and 22 mm wide and is avascular in the middle portion of the lower one-third of the membrane, with the superior thyroid vessels crossing over the upper part.

Classification

Cricothyrotomy can be classified into three different types:

1. *Direct needle puncture cricothyrotomy:* This refers to the placement of a needle or a catheter over a needle through the cricothyroid membrane.
2. *Percutaneous dilational cricothyrotomy:* This refers to the placement of an airway catheter or airway tube into the trachea through the cricothyroid membrane, by initially passing a needle, then a guidewire through the needle, then a dilator over the guidewire and finally the airway tube over the dilator.
3. *Surgical cricothyrotomy:* This refers to the use of scalpel and other surgical instruments through the cricothyroid membrane to access the trachea, followed by insertion of a tracheal tube or a tracheostomy tube.

Direct Needle Puncture Cricothyrotomy

In this technique, a large bore metal needle, straight or curved, with a sharp or blunt tip is inserted through the cricothyroid membrane for ventilation.

Rusch Quicktrach cricothyrotomy kit is a preassembled unit containing a stainless-steel needle inside a conical cannula with a fixation flange and a 15-mm connector. It is attached to a 10-mL syringe, a padded neck strap, and a connecting tube. There is also a removable safety stopper on the cannula to reduce the chances of perforation of the posterior wall of the trachea during insertion. The needle tip is conical to ensure the smallest necessary stoma. It is available in two sizes, adult (2 mm) and pediatric (4 mm).

Percutaneous Dilational Cricothyrotomy

This is done using the Seldinger's technique that the anesthesiologists are familiar with as we use it routinely for central venous cannulation. It involves in sequence, puncturing the cricothyroid membrane with a needle or needle in a cannula, passing a guidewire through this, and then a dilator and an airway tube through the guidewire. Several kits are available commercially for this purpose like the Melker's circothyrotomy kit (Cook Medical) and the Portex Mini-Trach II (Smith Medical). The airway tubes are of sufficient diameter to allow ventilation and oxygenation, as compared to a needle cricothyrotomy or transtracheal jet ventilation (TTJV). They can be directly connected to the breathing circuit without need for any special devices or modification of available devices.

Melker's Cricothyrotomy Kit

Melker's cricothyrotomy kit **(Fig. 54)** comes in three sizes of uncuffed airway catheter and one size of cuffed airway catheter. The components of the kit include a tetrafluoroethylene (TFE) catheter needle, curved radiopaque dilator, guidewire with flexible tip, percutaneous entry needle, disposable scalpel, syringe, and tape **(Fig. 55)**. The uncuffed airway catheters come in three sizes with ID of 3.5, 4, and 6 mm with airway catheter lengths of 3.8, 4.2, and 7.5 cm respectively. The cuffed airway catheter has an ID of 5 mm and is 9 cm long.

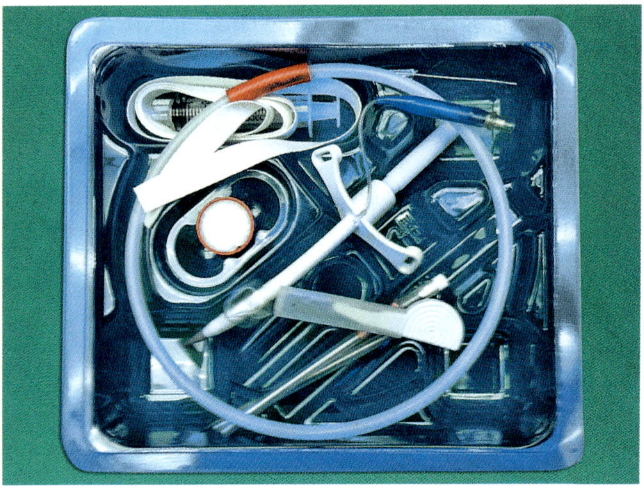

Fig. 54: Melker's cricothyrotomy kit.

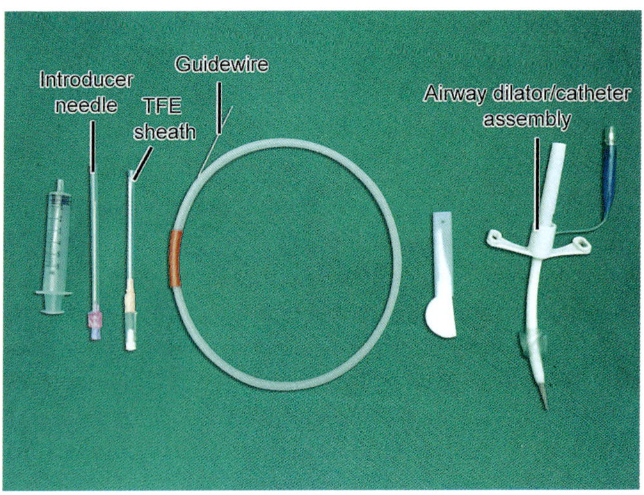

Fig. 55: Parts of the Melker's cricothyrotomy kit. (TFE: tetrafluoroethylene)

Technique

The cricothyroid membrane is first identified in the mid-line of the neck between the thyroid and cricoid cartilage. Using the scalpel, a vertical incision is made in the mid-line while stabilizing the cartilage. The 18 G TFE catheter introducer needle is advanced through the incision into the airway at an angle of 45° to the frontal plane, in a caudal direction. Aspiration of air confirms tracheal placement of the needle, after which the needle is withdrawn while the catheter is left in situ. The guidewire is then inserted into the trachea through this catheter. The guidewire is left in place while the catheter is removed. The tapered end of the airway dilator is inserted into the connector end of the airway catheter till the handle stops against the connector. This airway dilator-catheter assembly **(Fig. 56)** is then inserted over the guidewire till the proximal end of the guidewire is visible at the handle end of the dilator, to avoid loss of guidewire into the airway. The airway dilator-catheter assembly is then advanced over the guidewire into the trachea and then the guidewire and dilator are removed simultaneously, leaving the airway catheter behind in the trachea. In cuffed catheters, the cuff is inflated with 8–10 mL of air using a syringe and the catheter is held in place with the tape. The 15-mm connector of the airway catheter can then be connected to the ventilator device.

Incision of the skin and the cricothyroid membrane prevents catheter kinking and allows easier passage of the airway dilator. A vertical skin incision is better than a horizontal incision as a superior or inferior extension of the incision is feasible to identify the cricothyroid membrane. In the Pertrach percutaneous cricothyrotomy device, the guidewire and dilator is a single unit. So, the introducer needle has to be split for advancing the

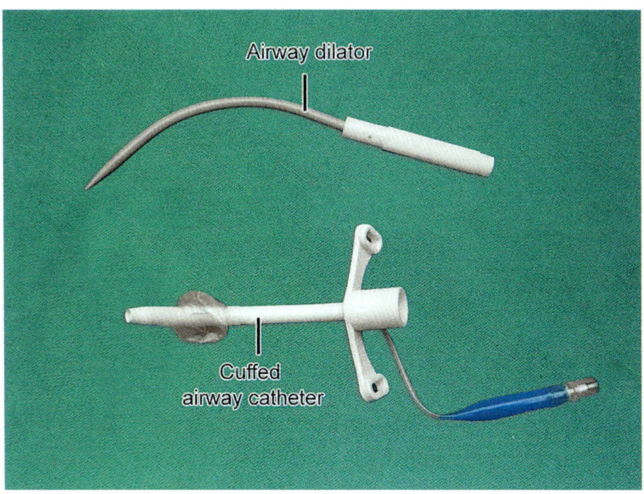

Fig. 56: Melker's cricothyrotomy airway dilator and cuffed airway catheter.

guidewire dilator assembly. The Nu-trake is another percutaneous dilational cricothyrotomy kit.

The Portex cricothyrotomy kit (Smith Medical) incorporates a Veress needle design to confirm tracheal entry, thus limiting the risk of damage to the posterior tracheal wall. The airway tube has an ID of 6 mm and has a Portex Soft Seal cuff. The device is preassembled and comes in compactly packed "trauma bags" for emergency use.

Surgical Cricothyrotomy

This involves surgical instruments to access the cricothyroid space. After midline vertical skin incision with its center over the cricothyroid membrane and palpating the cricothyroid membrane with the index finger, a horizontal incision is made over the cricothyroid membrane. Then, a tracheal hook is inserted and gentle traction is applied on the inferior margin of the thyroid cartilage. Next, to enlarge the cricothyroid space, a Trousseau dilator is inserted into the airway through the incision and moved vertically. The tracheal hook is removed, and the tracheostomy tube is inserted along between the blades of the dilator with the obturator in place at an angle of 90° to the patient. The Trousseau dilator is then gently removed as the tube is advanced. The cuff of the tracheostomy tube is then inflated, the obturator removed, an inner cannula if present inserted and the tube's position is confirmed and it is taped to the neck.

A rapid four-step technique (RFST) has been introduced for surgical cricothyrotomy. The steps include:

1. Cricothyroid membrane identification
2. Incision through skin and cricothyroid membrane
3. Traction on the membrane with a tracheal hook
4. Tracheal intubation

Indications

Cannot ventilate and cannot intubate situation, when two attempts at supraglottic airway insertion have failed.

Contraindications

- Age under 12 years
- Tracheal transection or laryngeal fracture
- Intrathoracic airway obstruction
- Relative contraindications:
  - Difficulty in identifying anatomic structures due to hematoma, abscess, and other swellings
  - Trauma, previous radiation therapy, surgical scars, etc.

Complications

- Trauma to vessels causing bleeding, pneumothorax and subcutaneous emphysema, and vocal cord injury
- Displacement of airway catheter with loss of airway
- Tracheal stenosis
- Infection

TRACHEOSTOMY TUBES

Most modern tracheostomy tubes are made of silicone, polyvinylchloride, polyurethane, as they are lighter and more pliable, compared to tubes made of metal. PVC tubes are thick-walled, while polyurethane tubes have a thinner wall and hence a larger lumen. As the length from the tracheostomy stoma to the carina is short, tracheal tubes are nonbeveled, shorter, and have the cuff closer to the tip as compared to an ETT to avoid endobronchial intubation. They can be arc-shaped or angled more acutely. Tracheostomy tubes are provided with an introducer or obturator that has a smooth, rounded, and beveled tip. This obturator is inserted into the outer cannula during insertion. Tracheostomy tubes are of different types:

Cuffed or Cuffless

Cuffless tracheostomy tubes are used in patients who are not at risk of aspiration and who do not require positive pressure ventilation. Since there is no cuff, the air can also pass into the upper trachea and larynx, and allows speaking and coughing. They are used on a long-term basis.

Cuffed tracheostomy tubes are used in patients who require positive pressure ventilation and when there is a risk of aspiration. The cuff is located in the distal end of the outer cannula and has an inflation system similar to an endotracheal tube.

Single or Dual Cannula

Dual cannula tracheostomy tubes have an outer and an inner cannula. The outer cannula passes into the trachea and the size of the tracheostomy tube is stated as the ID of the outer cannula. These dual cannula tubes also have a removable inner tube, which is taken out to clean secretions, without the necessity of removing the entire tracheostomy tube itself. As the presence of the inner cannula decreases the diameter and increases resistance, these cannot be used in patients with limited respiratory reserve.

Single cannula tracheostomy tubes have only the outer cannula and do not have the inner cannula. Resistance to breathing is lesser with these tubes, as they are of a larger diameter.

Fenestrated or Nonfenestrated

Fenestration is a hole in the back of the outer cannula that lies below the larynx when the tracheostomy tube is in place. Fenestration allows the movement of air through the upper airway to enable vocalization.

Tracheostomy tubes are also available with longer stems, foam cuffs, inbuilt distal pressure monitoring, and suction catheters and speaking valves.

PERCUTANEOUS DILATIONAL TRACHEOSTOMY

This is a minimally invasive technique that can be done by the bedside of the patient without surgical visualization of the trachea. It involves the insertion of a tracheostomy tube through the subcricoid area, by initial puncture of the skin all the way through to the trachea, followed by dilatation of the trachea to allow the passage of the tracheostomy tube.

Technique

There are several techniques of percutaneous dilational tracheostomy. Some include:

Ciaglia Multiple Dilation Technique (Named after Dr Pasquale Pat Ciaglia Who Developed It—1985)

In this technique, after initial puncture of the skin and the trachea with a needle, a guidewire is passed into the trachea. Then, a set of seven dilators from 12 to 36 F can be inserted as required in a multistep process for progressively increasing the opening in the tracheal wall. In the final step, the tracheostomy tube fitted over the last dilator is inserted into the trachea between the first and second tracheal rings, or between the second and third tracheal rings.

Ciaglia Blue Rhino Single Dilation Technique (1999)

In this technique, instead of using multiple dilators, a single and sharply tapered curved dilator is used to dilate the trachea in one step. The kit **(Fig. 57)** consists of a Ciaglia Blue Rhino percutaneous dilator with preloaded guiding catheter, 15 G introducer needle, 15 G fluorinated ethylene propylene polymer (FEPP) sheath needle, a J-tipped guidewire with positioning marks, 14 F dilator, and tracheostomy tube loading dilators **(Fig. 58)**. After insertion of the guidewire into the trachea, a 14 F shortintroducer dilator is advanced over the guidewire for initial dilation and then removed. After activating the EZ Pass hydrophilic coating by immersing the distal end of the Ciaglia Blue Rhino in sterile water or saline, the Ciaglia Blue Rhino advanced dilator with the guiding catheter is introduced as a single unit over the guidewire. It is then advanced and pulled back several times to dilate the tracheal access

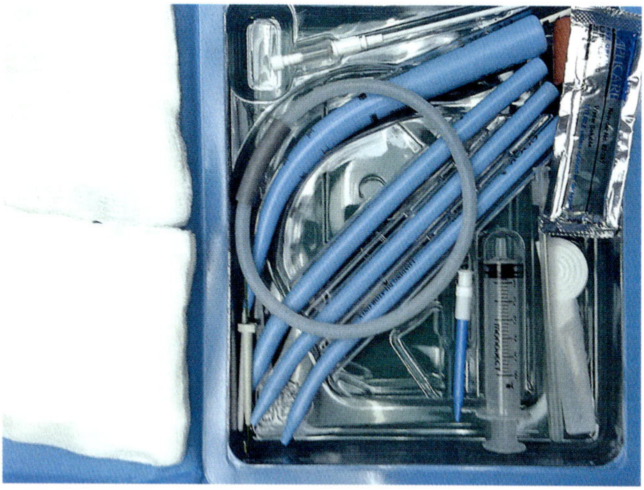

Fig. 57: The Ciaglia Blue Rhino percutaneous tracheostomy kit.

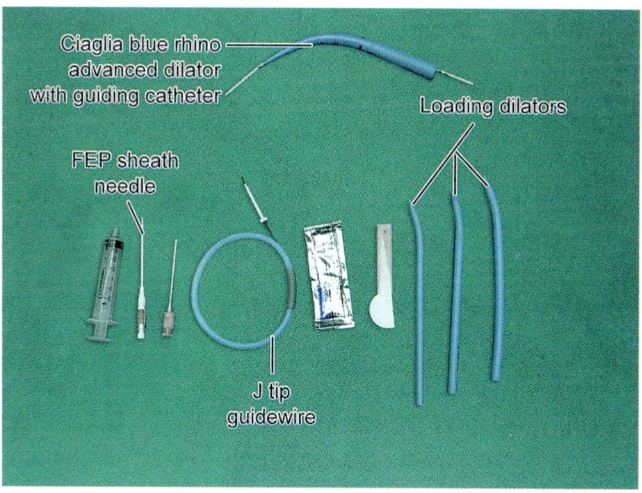

Fig. 58: Parts of the Ciaglia Blue Rhino tracheostomy kit.
(FEP: fluorinated ethylene propylene)

site effectively. The Ciaglia Blue Rhino advanced dilator is removed, leaving the guidewire and guiding catheter assembly in position. The tracheostomy tube loaded on the dilator is then advanced into the tracheal through this assembly. The dilator, guiding catheter, and guidewire are removed, leaving the tracheostomy tube in place.

Rapitrach Technique

Introduced by Schachner, this involves insertion of a guidewire into the trachea followed by a metal tracheotome whose jaws are opened inside the trachea to dilate it, and then a tracheostomy tube is inserted between the jaws of the instrument. Due to the risk of damage to the trachea and the tube, this method has largely been abandoned.

Griggs Technique (1990)

This involves the use of guidewire dilating forceps (GWDF). It is a one-stage dilating technique using a modified Howard Kelly forceps to dilate the soft tissue and the trachea. The guidewire is passed through the hole in the tip of the forceps after which it is advanced into the tracheal lumen and then the forceps are opened to enlarge the tracheal lumen. It is quicker to perform but the incidence of complications could be higher.

Fanconi (Translaryngeal Tracheostomy)

This is done under endoscopic guidance. In this technique, a needle is inserted through the trachea is directed cranially instead of caudally and a guidewire passed through it is retrieved from the mouth. A special device cone cannula (flexible plastic cone with a metal tip that is joined to an armored tracheal cannula) comes with the kit and acts as both the dilator and the tracheostomy tube. This is attached to the guidewire at the level of the mouth and pushed through the oropharynx, larynx, and trachea. The metal tip comes out of the skin and is cut off, and the cannula is rotated downward. The tracheal stoma is thus created from inside to outside and the incidence of bleeding is lesser.

PercuTwist Technique or Rotational Dilatational Tracheostomy (2002)

This technique involves the use of a special screw type dilator with threads to dilate the soft tissue and the trachea, after which it is removed, and the tracheostomy tube is advanced over the guidewire into the trachea.

Ciaglia Blue Dolphin Balloon-assisted Tracheostomy (2005)

This technique combines balloon dilatation and tracheal tube insertion in one step. The kit includes the Dolphin tracheostomy introducer, Cook inflation device, 18 G introducer Echo Tip needle, 18 G FEP sheath needle, guidewire with positioning marks and a 14 F dilator. After insertion of guidewire and initial dilation with the short 14 F dilator, the balloon catheter/dilator/tracheostomy tube assembly is inserted over the guidewire and the balloon is inflated with saline at 11 atm for 15 seconds. After deflation of the balloon, the whole assembly is advanced into the trachea till the tracheostomy tube is in place and then the rest of the assembly is removed. The incidence of posterior tracheal wall injuries is believed to be lesser due to the radial rather than coaxial forces being generated.

Indications

Adult intubated patients in the ICU for pulmonary toilet or weaning off mechanical ventilation.

Contraindications

- Anatomically unsuitable (e.g., neck masses, fixed flexion deformity, obesity, and burns)
- Coagulopathy
- Children
- Positive end-expiratory pressure (PEEP) requirement >20 cmH_2O
- Advantages compared to surgical tracheostomy
- Operative time is shorter.
- Incidence of complications is lesser.
- Better cosmesis
- It can be done by the bedside.
- Decreased incidence of wound infection

Complications

- Bleeding
- Injury to posterior tracheal wall
- Loss of airway during the procedure
- Subcutaneous and mediastinal emphysema
- Pneumothorax
- Infection
- Vocal cord injury
- Laryngeal damage

ADJUNCT FOR GUIDED EXTUBATION

Airway Exchange Catheter

Exchange of tracheal tubes or extubation in a patient with a difficult airway may result in loss of the airway due to difficulty in reintubation. If the tracheal tube is removed over a catheter or bougie, this can serve as a guide for railroading another tracheal tube.

The airway exchange catheter (Cook Medical) is used for this purpose. It is supplied in four different sizes: (1) 8 F (1.6 mm ID), (2) 11 F (2.33 mm ID), (3) 14 F (3.0 mm ID), and (4) 19 F (3.4 mm ID) for placement of ETTs of size 3, 4, 5, or 7 mm or greater ID, respectively. It is 83 cm in length, except the pediatric 8 F catheter that is 45 cm long. It has a soft and blunt atraumatic tip with distal side ports to prevent whipping during jet ventilation. It is radiopaque and comes with removable Rapi-Fit adapter **(Fig. 59)** with 15 mm and Luer Lock connectors to allow the use of ventilator devices or capnograph during the tracheal tube exchange.

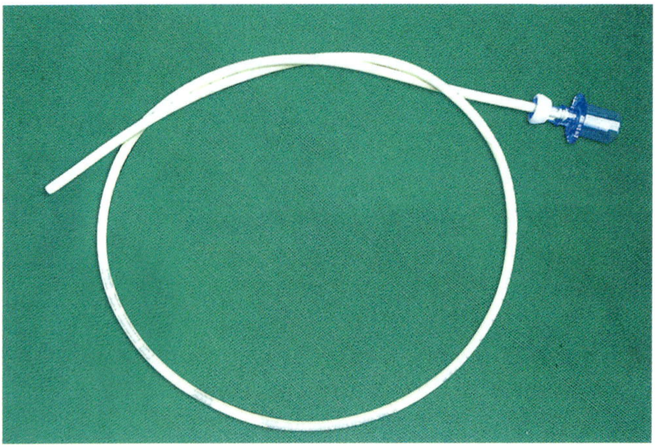

Fig. 59: Cook airway exchange catheter.

Newer airway exchange catheters are available for use with DLTs, which are made of a softer material with the distal 7 cm flexible to avoid trauma. These are available in two sizes, 11 F and 14 F for use with tracheal tubes 4 and 5 mm or larger ID, respectively, and are 100 cm in length.

Airway exchange catheters can be left in situ for several hours, and the patients tolerate it well due to the small diameter as compared to tracheal tubes.

DIFFICULT INTUBATION TROLLEY

A portable and difficult intubation trolley **(Fig. 60)** should be available as a one-stop shop for all airway-related equipment that may be needed during difficult airway management as this avoids unnecessary delays. The common contents of such a trolley include:

- Rigid laryngoscope blades of alternative design and size from those routinely used
- Endotracheal tubes of all assorted sizes
- Fiberoptic bronchoscope
- Videolaryngoscope
- Laryngeal mask airway, ILMA, and other supraglottic devices
- Tracheal tube introducer (Frova) or bougie, Aintree intubation catheter
- Alternate blades (like McCoy)
- Light wand
- Cricothyrotomy kits
- Jet ventilator
- Transtracheal jet ventilation cannula
- Retrograde intubation kits
- Tracheostomy tray and tubes
- Airway exchange catheters

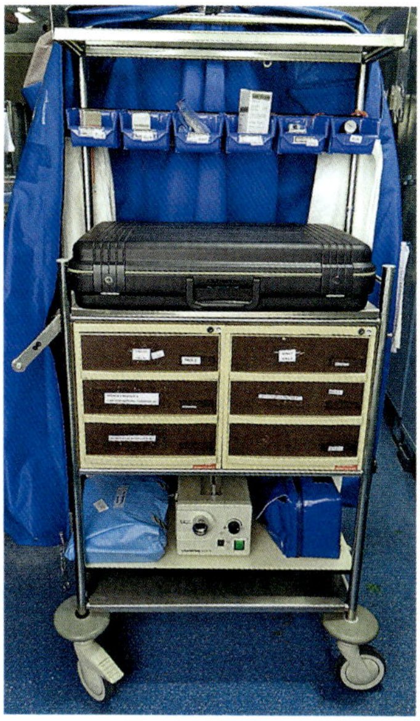

Fig. 60: Difficult intubation trolley.

SUGGESTED READING

1. Cavus E, Dorges V. Videolaryngoscopes. In: Hagberg CA (Ed). Benumof and Hagberg's Airway Management, 3rd edition. Philadelphia: Elsevier Saunders; 2013. pp. 536-48.
2. Cook T. Face masks and supraglottic airways. In: Calder I, Pearce A (Eds). Core topics in airway management, 2nd edition. Cambridge UK: Cambridge University Press; 2011.
3. Cook TM, Howes B. Supraglottic airway devices: recent advances. Continuing education in anaesthesia. Crit Care Pain. 2011;11(2):56-61.
4. Cook TM. Airway management equipment. In: Davey AJ, Diba A (Eds). Ward's Anaesthetic Equipment, 6th edition. China: Elsevier Saunders; 2012. pp. 139-205.
5. Dorsch JA, Dorsch SE. Chapters 16-21: Airway equipment. In: Dorsch JA, Dorsch SE (Eds). Understanding Anesthesia Equipment, 5th edition. Philadelphia: Lippincott Williams and Wilkins; 2008. pp. 444-684.
6. Gil KSL, Diemunsch PA. Fiberoptic and flexible endoscopic aided techniques. In: Hagberg CA (Ed). Benumof and Hagberg's Airway Management, 3rd edition. Philadelphia: Elsevier Saunders; 2013. pp. 365-411.
7. Hernandez MR, Klock PA, Ovassapian A. Evolution of the extraglottic airway: a review of its history, applications, and practical tips for success. Anesth Analg. 2012;114:349-68.
8. Miller DM. A proposed classification and scoring system for supraglottic sealing airways: a brief review. Anesth Analg. 2004;99:1553-9.
9. Niforopoulou P, Pantazopoulos I, Demestiha T, Koudouna E, Xanthos T. Videolaryngoscopes in the adult airway management: a topical review of the literature. Acta Anaesthesiol Scand. 2010;54(9):1050-61.

10. Paolini JB, Donati F, Drolet P. Review article: Video-laryngoscopy: another tool for difficult intubation or a new paradigm in airway management? Can J Anaesth. 2013;60(2):184-91.
11. Popat M. Fiberoptic endoscopy equipment. In: Popat M (Ed). Practical fiberoptic intubation. Oxford: Butterworth Heinemann; 2001.
12. Pott LM, Murray WB. Review of videolaryngoscopy and rigid fiberoptic laryngoscopy. Curr Opin Anaesthesiol. 2008;21(6):750-8.

WEBSITES

1. http://www.theairwaysite.com/pages/page_content/Airway_home.aspx. The definite airway site. Last accessed Nov., 2024.
2. http://aam.ucsf.edu/. The Anesthesia Airway Management (AAM). Last accessed Nov., 2024.
3. http://www.airwayworld.com/. Airway world from founders of difficult airway course. Last accessed Nov., 2024.

CHAPTER 7

Monitoring Technology

Ahalya Kodali, Bhavani Shankar Kodali

INTRODUCTION

In the recent times, newer monitoring equipment has been added to our monitoring armamentarium. These noninvasive technological advances provide substantial insight into the hemodynamic performance of a patient during anesthesia that were hitherto possible only via invasive means. This chapter will highlight the underlying basic operational principles of commonly used monitoring devices that have enhanced safety of a patient under anesthesia. Knowledge of functionality of monitors is essential for proper clinical interpretation of the data provided by these devices. This chapter includes inspired O_2 monitoring, capnography, pulse oximetry, cardiac output (CO), etc.

INSPIRED OXYGEN

Monitoring of fraction of inspired oxygen concentration (FiO_2) is considered crucial to prevent administering hypoxic gas mixture. Anesthesia machines without the facility to monitor FiO_2 should be made obsolete. The oxygen analyzer may be present in the inspiratory limb (fuel cell; **Figs. 1 and 2**), or as a sidestream paramagnetic analyzer sampling gases between patient and breathing system **(Fig. 3)**.

Galvanic Oxygen Analyzer (Fuel Cell)

Two electrodes are contained in potassium hydroxide bath. Oxygen molecules flow through a Teflon semipermeable membrane and pick up electrons from a cathode (gold or silver), combine with water, and travel to the lead anode. An electric current is generated between the two electrodes, which is proportional to partial pressure of oxygen **(Fig. 1)**. The reaction that occurs is:

$$O_2 + 4e^- + 2H_2O \rightarrow 4(OH)^-$$
$$Pb + 2OH^- \rightarrow PbO + H_2O + 2e^-$$

The electrode needs to be calibrated for 21% and 100% to be accurate in the measurement range. The response time is pretty quick, 20 seconds. The accuracy is around ±3%.

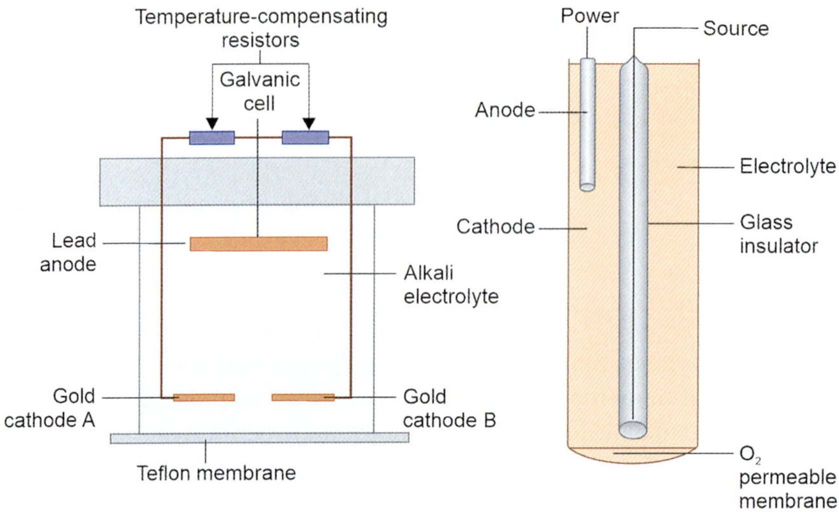

Fig. 1: Schematic representation of galvanic and polarographic oxygen analyzer. The main difference is supply of power.

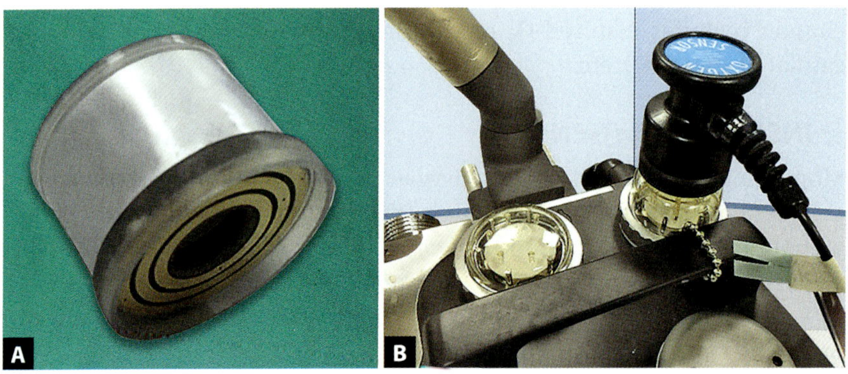

Figs. 2A and B: Oxygen sensor in the inspiratory limb of breathing system.

Polarographic Analyzer (Clark Electrode)

Here, the principle is similar to above but uses 9 V battery. Oxygen flows through a Teflon membrane and the current is generated between a silver cathode and a platinum anode. The current generated, once again, is proportional to the partial pressure of oxygen **(Fig. 1)**. These analyzers need not be replaced more often than 2 years depending on the manufacturer specifications.

Paramagnetic Analyzer

Oxygen is a parametric gas and infrared (IR) technology cannot be used to measure oxygen concentration **(Fig. 3)**. Oxygen, being strongly paramagnetic, is attracted into a magnetic field by the virtue of having unpaired electrons in

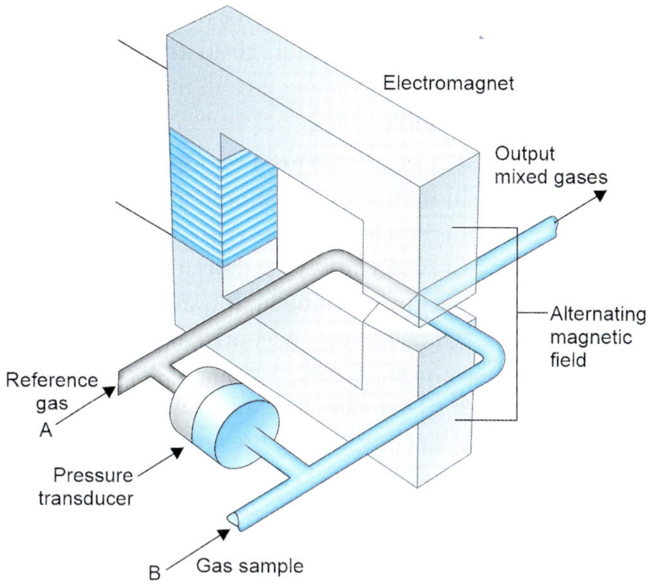

Fig. 3: Paramagnetic analyzer. (A) Reference gas and (B) sample gas resulting in paramagnetic rotation.

their outer electron ring. Other gases in the anesthetic mixture are weakly paramagnetic. The system uses a switched electromagnetic field and pressure transducer. The electromagnetic field is generated at approximately 110 Hz. A differential pressure is generated between the reference sample (air) on one side and the sample to be measured on the other side. The transducer is capable of detecting pressure fluctuations of approximately 20–50 μbar, which are converted to direct current (DC) voltage proportional to oxygen concentration.

CAPNOGRAPHY

Capnography is a continuous monitoring of instantaneous CO_2 concentration and graphic display (waveform) in respired gas. This CO_2 waveform is also called a *capnogram*, and a device that generates the CO_2 waveform is called a *capnograph*. Use of capnography monitoring can reliably and quantitatively provide vital respiratory information in intubated patients. Alterations in CO, distribution of pulmonary blood flow, and metabolic activity can also be reflected by the change of CO_2 concentration in expired gases. The American Society of Anesthesiologists (ASA) mandates the use of capnography in all patients undergoing anesthesia. Many intensive care units utilize capnography as an adjunct to assure patient safety and the adequacy of ventilation. It is strongly recommended by many societies to use capnography to monitor ventilation during sedation. Furthermore, the

American Heart Association is strongly in favor of monitoring the quality of chest compression during cardiopulmonary resuscitation.

Principles of Capnography

Whereas a variety of techniques can be used for CO_2 measurement, such as mass spectrometry, Raman scattering, and photoacoustic measurement, by far the most widely used method is the *infrared absorption spectrometry*. The principle of this technique is based on the fact that CO_2 is a polyatomic gas that absorbs IR radiation of a specific wavelength. CO_2 shows strong absorption in the far IR light at 4.3 μm, which lies way beyond the visible wavelength (0.4–0.8 μm). The basic elements of an IR spectrometry include an IR light source, a sample chamber, and an IR detector. The absorption of the IR light is also governed by the *Beer-Lambert law*; that is, the absorption is proportional to the concentration of the absorbing gas in the sample chamber **(Fig. 4)**.

Types of Capnographs

Depending upon the location of the CO_2 sensor, capnographs can be divided into two types: Sidestream (aspiration) and mainstream (flow-through) capnographs **(Fig. 5)**. In sidestream capnograph, the gas sample is continuously aspirated by a fine tube from the breathing circuit (usually located at the T-piece), it then passes to a measuring unit containing a CO_2 sensor. The CO_2 concentration is determined by comparing the IR light absorption in the sample cell with a chamber free of CO_2. A unique advantage of sidestream capnograph is that it allows monitoring of spontaneously breathing nonintubated patients as sampling of the expired gas can be obtained from face mask or nasal cannula. In mainstream capnograph, a cuvette containing a CO_2 sensor with IR source and detector is inserted between the breathing circuit and the endotracheal tube (ETT), and therefore, the CO_2 measurement takes place within the breathing circuit. Compared to sidestream capnography, the advantages of the mainstream capnography

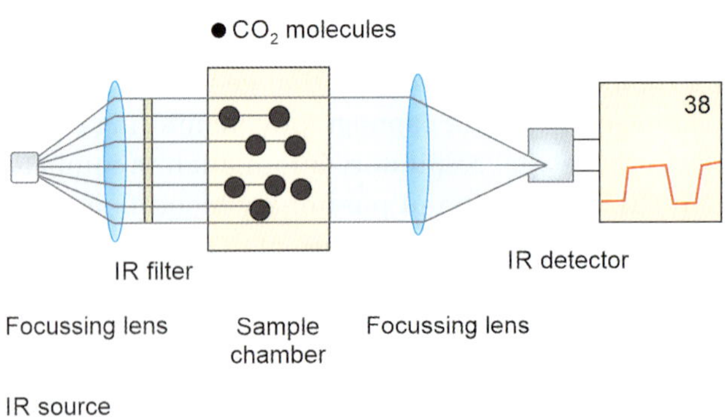

Fig. 4: Infrared (IR) spectrometry.

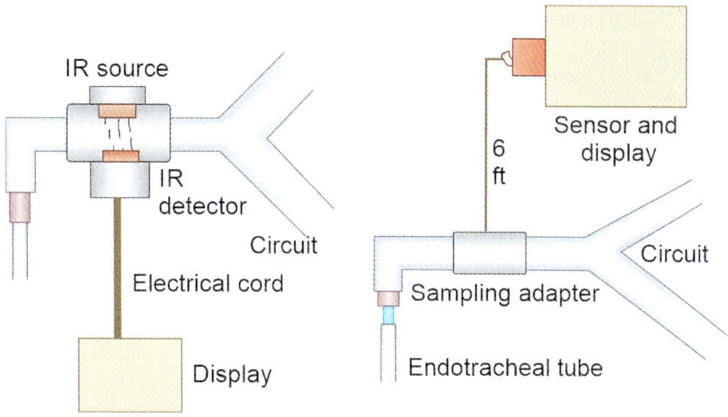

Fig. 5: Sidestream (aspiration) and mainstream (flow-through) capnographs. (IR: Infrared)

include a faster response time, no gas being subtracted from the breathing circuit, and no need for sampling pumps. The disadvantages include the relatively heavy measuring adapter with electrical cord (causing ETT kink), added dead space, and the expense for the repair of damage. Needless to say that the newer generation of mainstream sensors is remarkably lighter and smaller.

Calibration

Capnographs must be calibrated periodically, at different intervals based on manufacturer's models, but usually at least daily. Modern instruments use a self-calibration process and maintain a satisfactory degree of accuracy, which is usually about ±0.1% in the range of 0–10% CO_2 (0–76 mm Hg). They are fairly accurate even in the extended range up to 100 mm Hg, which is useful in rare cases of hypoventilation or malignant hyperthermia.

Normal Capnogram

A capnogram can be displayed as CO_2 versus time (time capnogram), or versus volume (volume capnogram). The time capnogram, however, is the method most commonly used in anesthesia and other clinical practices, since the volume capnogram needs elaborated equipment for plotting the trace. Thus, all capnograms mentioned in this chapter are referred to as time capnogram unless indicated otherwise **(Fig. 6)**.

A standard nomenclature has been assigned for delineating various phases of capnogram. A capnogram can be considered as two segments (an inspiratory segment and an expiratory segment) and two angles (an alpha and a beta angle). The inspiratory segment is also designated as phase 0. The expiratory segment is further divided into phase I, II, and III, and occasionally phase IV, which represents the terminal rise in CO_2 concentration **(Fig. 6)**. Phase I represents the initial stage of expiration; there is no rise in expired

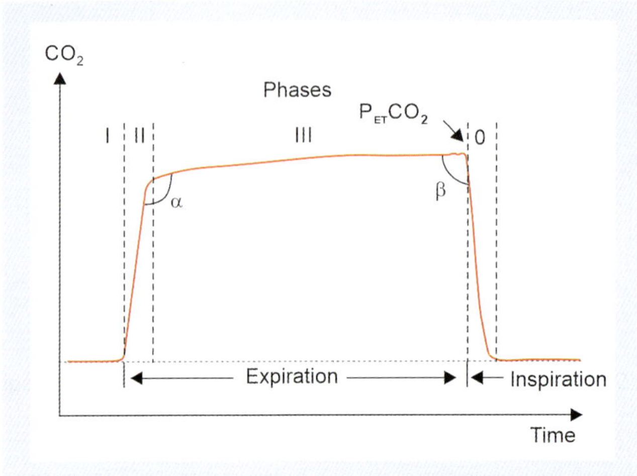

Fig. 6: Nomenclature of capnogram.

CO_2 as anatomical and apparatus dead space gases are exhaled. As expiration continues, there is a sharply rising upstroke (phase II) due to the mixing of dead space gas with CO_2-containing alveolar gas followed by a plateau phase (phase III). The CO_2 concentration at the end of plateau is referred to as end-tidal CO_2 ($EtCO_2$), in terms of end-tidal partial pressure of carbon dioxide ($P_{ET}CO_2$). $P_{ET}CO_2$ is the best reflection of partial pressure of alveolar CO_2 (P_ACO_2), or partial pressure of arterial CO_2 ($PaCO_2$) and, normally, the $PaCO_2$ - $P_{ET}CO_2$ difference is about 5 mm Hg due to the dead space. It is important to note that the expiratory plateau is not an isocapnic trace, but rather it progresses with a very slight and steady increase in the partial pressure of CO_2 (pCO_2) as the alveolar fraction is expelled from the lungs. As the patient begins to inspire, fresh gas is entrained and there is a steep downstroke back to the baseline (phase 0). The angle between phase II and III is called alpha angle, which increases as slope of phase III increases. Normally, it is about 100°–110°. Airway obstruction increases the angle due to increasing the slope. The response time of the capnograph, sweep speed, and the respiratory cycle time also affect the angle. On the other hand, the angle between phase III and phase 0 is called beta angle, which is normally about 90°. During rebreathing, this angle increases. Occasionally, an upward blip or spike known as phase IV can occur toward the end of phase III. This is akin to the phase IV single-breath nitrogen curve. This terminal elevation represents emptying of alveoli with long time constants containing higher CO_2 concentration.

Abnormal Capnograms and Clinical Considerations (Figs. 7A to F)

To analyze the abnormal capnogram, five characteristics should be inspected: Size (height), shape, frequency, rhythm, and baseline. For example, in patients

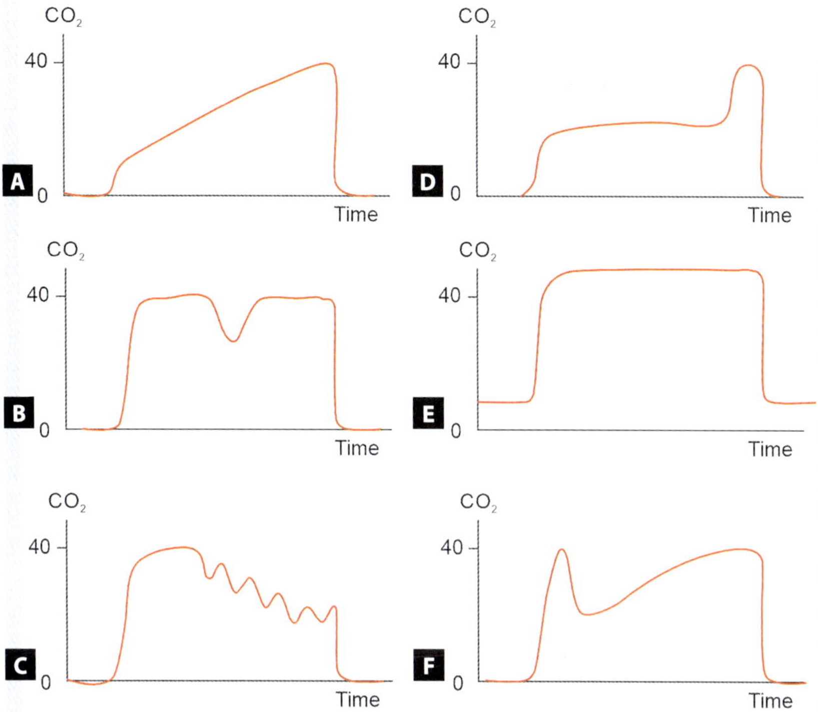

Figs. 7A to F: Examples of several abnormal capnograms. (A) Capnogram of a patient with severe chronic obstructive pulmonary disease (COPD) or other causes leading to the increased airway resistance, such as asthma, endobronchial intubation, or endotracheal tube kinking. No plateau is reached before the next inspiration. The gradient between end-tidal partial pressure of CO_2 ($P_{ET}CO_2$) and arterial CO_2 is increased; (B) Downward wave during plateau phase indicates spontaneous respiratory effort; (C) cardiogenic oscillations appear as small, regular, tooth-like humps at the latter part of the expiratory phase. The rate of the "humps" is identical to the patient's heart rate; (D) a leak in the sampling line during positive-pressure ventilation; (E) failure of inspired CO_2 to return to zero due to an incompetent expiratory valve or exhausted CO_2 absorbent; (F) bifid waveform of expired CO_2 in patient with emphysema undergoing elective surgery after unilateral lung transplantation. The initial upstroke represents gas from the normal (transplanted) lung, which is followed by gas exhaled from the remaining (emphysematous) lung.

with obstructed airway (e.g., emphysema, asthma), the capnogram shows a slow rate of rise of the phase II (upstroke) and the increased slope of phase III (plateau). In an unrecognized esophageal intubation, the capnograms are flat or may have occasional baseline blips. However, after attempted face mask ventilation (driving some expired gas into the esophagus and stomach), or in patients who have recently consumed carbonate beverages, some CO_2 waves can be observed due to gastric CO_2 returning to the breathing system. But such

CO_2 tracing only has a peak effect with a progressively decreasing amplitude, and it does not resemble the usual end-tidal plateau. The CO_2 concentration decreases to zero after about five breaths of ventilation. **Figures 7A to F** show a number of capnograms in a variety of clinical scenarios.

The $P_{ET}CO_2$ concentration measured from the capnography provides important clinical information about ventilatory status of the patient. Since the measurement of $P_{ET}CO_2$ is an estimate of $PaCO_2$, the characteristic abnormal CO_2 waveforms and the concentrations can help in the diagnosis of many clinical or technical abnormalities. **Table 1** summarizes the common causes that may be reflected by $P_{ET}CO_2$ changes during anesthesia care. These include alterations in metabolism, circulation, ventilation, airway, or breathing system. Abnormal CO_2 measurements can also occur as a result of malfunction of sampling or measurement of CO_2.

Though it is believed that capnograms predominantly identify respiratory abnormalities, it can forewarn major impending depression of cardiovascular system, such as hypotension associated with massive blood loss, impending circulatory arrest, or pulmonary embolism. For further reading on capnography, refer to http://www.capnography.com.

INHALATIONAL AGENT MEASUREMENT

Since the introduction of Drager's Narko-Test in 1971 that measured agent concentration by the relaxation effect of halothane on a silicone rubber, several technologies have been developed to measure inspired and expired inhalational agent concentration accurately. These include Raman spectroscopic analysis, mass spectroscopy, IR photoacoustic spectrometry,

TABLE 1: Factors that may change $P_{ET}CO_2$ during anesthesia.

Increase in $P_{ET}CO_2$	*Decrease in $P_{ET}CO_2$*
Due to increasing CO_2 production: • Increases in metabolic rate sepsis • Malignant hyperthermia • Shivering/seizure • Hyperthyroidism	*Due to decreasing CO_2 production:* • Decreases in metabolic rate • Hypothermia • Hypothyroidism
Due to decreasing CO_2 elimination: • Hypoventilation • Rebreathing • CO_2 absorber exhaustion	*Due to increasing CO_2 elimination:* Hyperventilation
	Due to decreasing alveolar: *CO_2 delivery* Hypoperfusion pulmonary embolism
Due to artifact: Malfunction of CO_2 measuring system	*Due to artifact:* • Malfunction of CO_2 measuring system • Gas sampling tube leak or loose connection

simple IR spectrometry, and piezoelectric crystal agent analysis. Except IR analysis, none of the other technologies survived due to high cost. For example, Raman spectroscopy uses a laser light, and when it strikes gas molecules such as nitrogen, nitrous oxide, oxygen, or anesthetic agents, most of the scattered energy is reabsorbed and re-emitted at a shifted longer wavelength specific for each agent. Photomultiplier tubes are used to measure the shifted wave spectrum to identify various gases in a gas mixture. In the IR photoacoustic technology, the IR beam expands and contracts the molecules at a specific frequency producing sound and a microphone picks up these sound signals for analysis. The frequency is specific for each agent. The monitors were susceptible to external noises and did not survive in the market. The current technology uses IR light. Anesthetic agents absorb IR light in the wavelength range of 8–13 µm in contrast to 4–5 µm absorbed by carbon dioxide, nitrous oxide, and water vapor. Complex technologies are used to determine anesthetic agent concentration accurately despite overlapping spectrums of anesthetic agent on each other **(Fig. 8)**. Currently, IR technology is used to monitor carbon dioxide, nitrous oxide, and end-tidal inhalational agent in anesthetic practice.

SPIROMETRY AND GAS FLOW SENSORS

In the past, tidal volume and minute ventilation were measured using conventional wright's respirometer **(Fig. 9)**.

It consists of lightweight, extremely low-resistant vanes that move with flowing gases and a needle on the dial provides the reading. A variety of spirometers are available to be used in clinical practice and some of them have digital output displayed on a screen **(Fig. 10)**. Spirometry devices

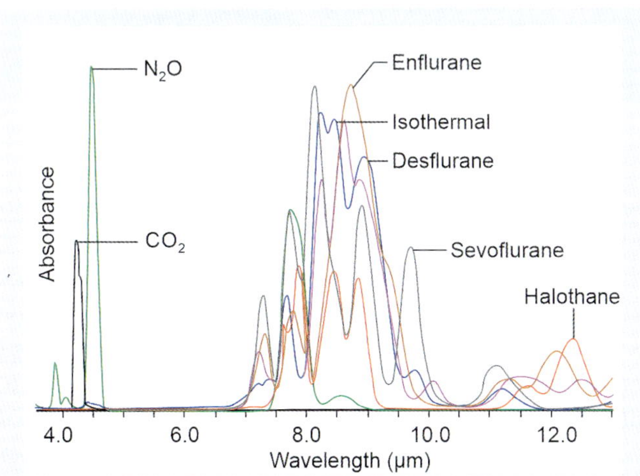

Fig. 8: Different absorption spectra for inhalational agents.

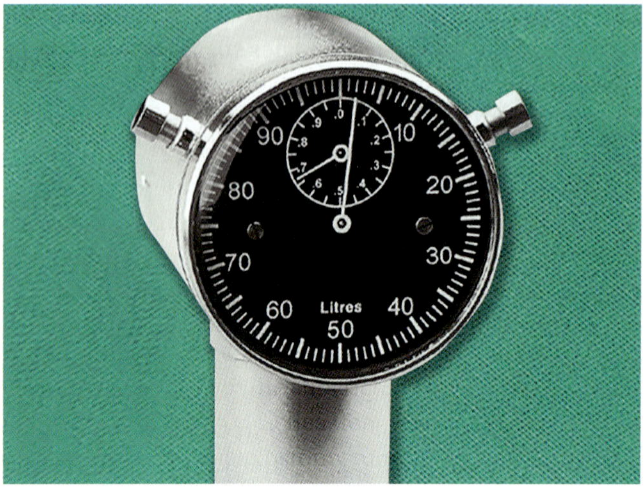

Fig. 9: Wright's respirometer.

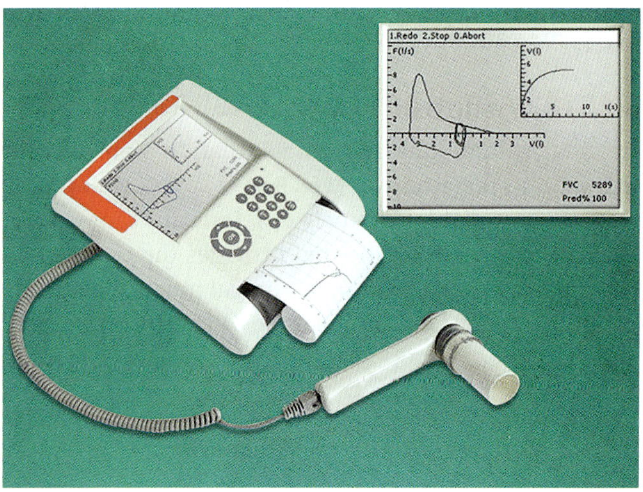

Fig. 10: Digital spirometer.

are still used to measure tidal volume, minute ventilation, and forced vital capacity (FVC).

Modern anesthesia machines use electronic flow meters that are accurate with fast response time. The current technologies include rotating vane spirometers, pneumotachometers, hot wire anemometers, or ultrasound flowmeters. A pneumotachometer uses a restrictor to create a pressure drop. A differential pressure transducer senses the pressure drop. The output signal is calibrated so that accurate flow readings are produced. An orifice is a simple example of a flow restrictor. A disadvantage of fixed orifices is nonlinear relationships between flow and pressure drop. The 7900

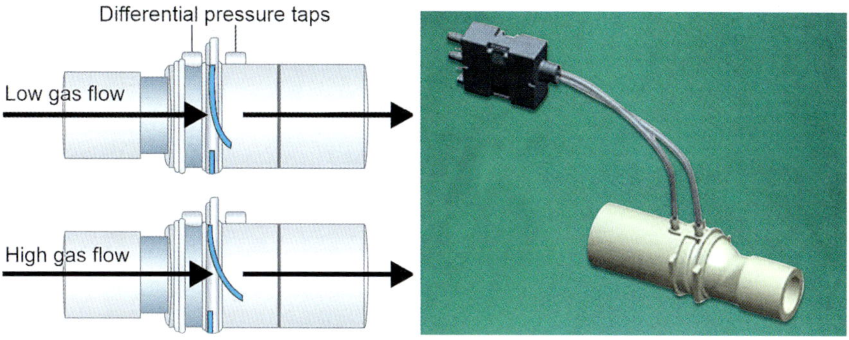

Fig. 11: GE flow sensor.

Smartvent® in the Aisys®, Advance®, and Aestiva® use variable orifice to cater to adult and pediatric gas flows **(Fig. 11)**. Moisture contamination resulting in inaccurate flow readings is a possibility. This is overcome by a modified flow sensor that has a taper and grooves in the housing assembly to divert water away from the vital areas of measurement.

In addition, some anesthesia machines use discrete thermistors to warm the gas flows. Air from anesthesia machines, which is warm and moist, helps provide the patient with a comfortable breathing situation and may reduce sore throats caused by breathing cold, dry air. As such, the temperature of the air delivery system is often monitored and controlled to help ensure that the air stream is maintained at the desired level of warmth. The 192 and 194 Series discrete thermistor sensors are installed directly into the air stream and are designed to monitor and control the temperature of the air. The sensor is coupled to a microcontroller designed to measure the air stream temperature and to send a signal to the controller, which controls and regulates the temperature of the air stream.

Hot wire anemometer technology is used by Drager on their anesthesia machines **(Fig. 12)**. This is an ultrafast system with low inspiratory and expiratory resistance. One flow sensor accommodates different ages of patients, except for the specific needs of neonates in critical care. The principle behind hot wire anemometers is based on a heated element from which heat is extracted by the colder impact airflow. The temperature of the hotwire is kept constant via a regulation switch, and the current (amp draw measured internally) is directly proportional to the air velocity. Turbulent flows can cause errors in the measurement. The anesthesia machines use this technology to measure flow and volumes to generate flow and volume curves.

Flow–Volume Loops/Flow–Time Loops

In addition to assessing pulmonary functions (tests such as tidal volume, minute ventilation, FVC, etc.), one of the vital advantages of spirometry is

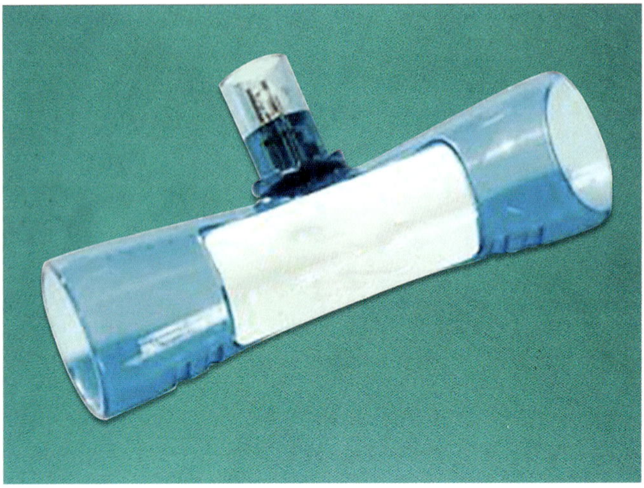

Fig. 12: Drager hot wire anemometer.

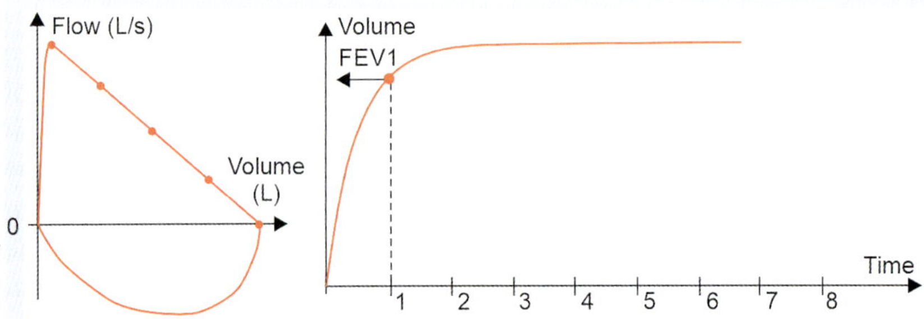

Fig. 13: Normal flow/volume loops (left graph); normal flow/time (right graph).

to assess dynamic respiratory function via flow–volume loops. The flow–volume loops help to differentiate between obstructive lung disease and restrictive lung disease. It can also provide a fair assessment of the location of the obstruction, intrathoracic versus extrathoracic.

Figure 13 shows a normal forced inspiration and expiration. The loop begins on the X-axis at "0", where the flow and volumes are at zero. During the forced inspiration, a curve resembling a semicircle (below the X-axis) depicts the peak inspiratory flow tapering toward zero flow at the end of the inspiration. During forced expiration, the curve rapidly mounts to a peak: Peak expiratory flow. After the peak, the flow rapidly decreases as expiration continues. The descending limb may be straight, or slightly convex, as the flow decreases from peak expiratory flow to the baseline (FVC). The flow–time loop shows the forced expiratory volume in 1 second (FEV1)/FVC ratio to be over 80%.

Obstructive Lung Disease

The forced inspiration is normal but expiration shows a remarkable concave upstroke rather than a straight line or a slightly convex line. The air in the larger airways can be expired normally and therefore peak expiratory flow will be normal. When the air from larger airways is expired, the gases from the lower airways exit slowly due to obstructed lower airways. This will result in lower expiratory flows during expiration, resulting the concave expiratory curve. FVC can be normal but flow-time curve shows decreased FEV1/FVC ratio forced expiration curve values from 25% to 75% portion of the expiratory curve will be lower than normal. FEV1/FVC value <70% is considered to have obstructive lung issues **(Fig. 14)**.

Restrictive Lung Disease

In a restrictive lung disease, the inspiratory and expiratory flow characteristics are normal but overall lung volumes are decreased. Therefore, the curves look normal, but the volumes are low. FVC will be low, but FEV1/FVC will be normal **(Fig. 15)**.

Mixed Lung Disease

Many patients may have a mixed lung disease, both restrictive and obstructive and the flow–volume loop is shown in **Figure 16**.

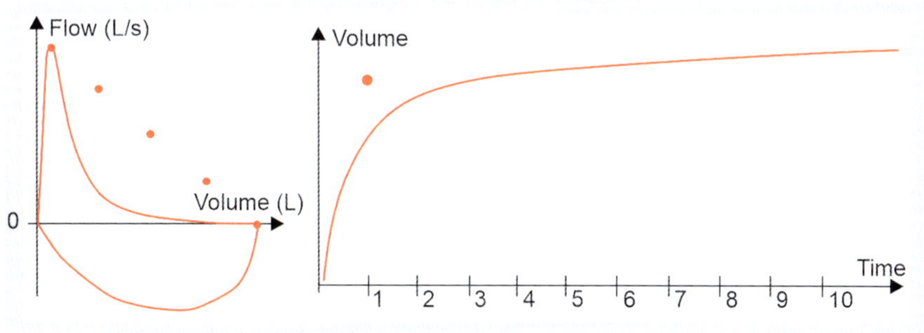

Fig. 14: Obstructive lung disease.

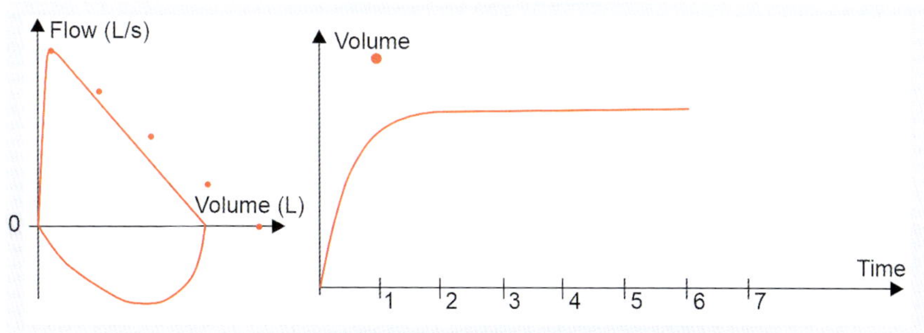

Fig. 15: Restrictive lung disease.

Variable Larger Airway Obstruction

In a variable *extrathoracic* obstruction, the obstruction is pushed outward by the force of the expiration. However, during inspiration, the obstruction is sucked into the trachea resulting in partial airway obstruction during inspiration. This results in flattening of the inspiratory curve in the flow-volume loop. Examples: large extrathoracic goiter, vocal cord paralysis, and laryngeal tumors **(Fig. 17)**.

In a variable *intrathoracic* obstruction, the tumor obstructing the intrathoracic portion is sucked outward during inspiration with normal morphology during inspiration. However, during obstruction, the tumor is pushed into the trachea resulting in the airway obstruction during expiration **(Fig. 18)**.

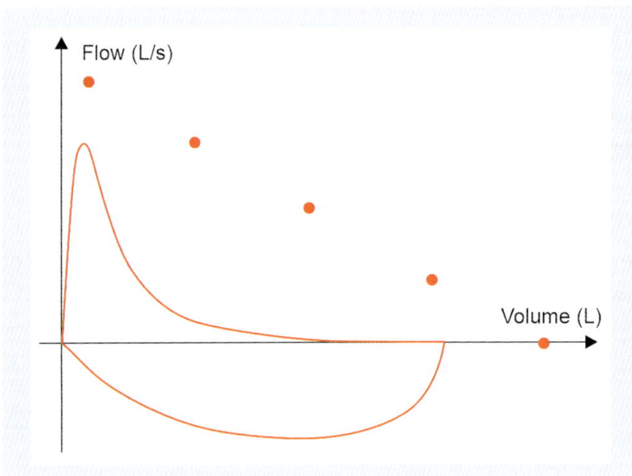

Fig. 16: Mixed lung disease.

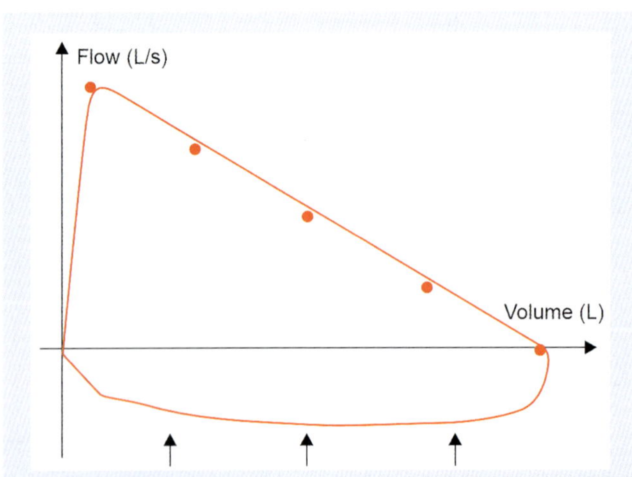

Fig. 17: Variable extrathoracic obstruction.

Fixed Large Airway Obstruction

Fixed large airway obstruction can be intra- or extrathoracic. The airflow is obstructed during inspiration as well as expiration. The resulting flow–volume loops demonstrate flattening of both curves. This flow–volume loop can occur in tracheal stenosis or tumor in the trachea **(Fig. 19)**.

PULSE OXIMETRY

Pulse oximetry (oximeter) is a standard of care for monitoring oxygen during anesthesia. It is a noninvasive method of measuring oxygen saturation of hemoglobin (SpO_2) and pulse rate on a continuous basis to detect hypoxia.

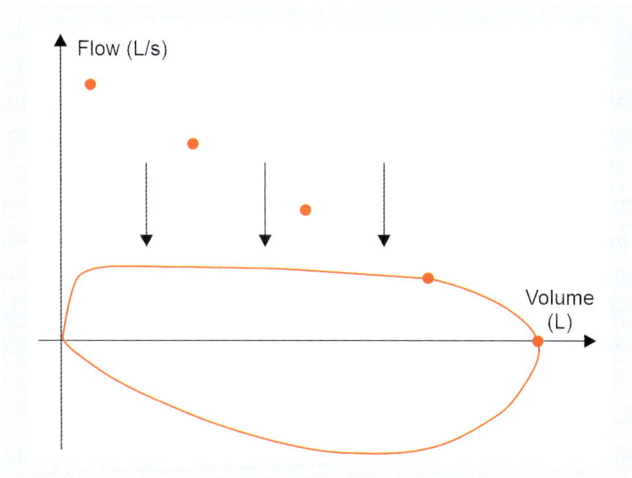

Fig. 18: Variable intrathoracic obstruction.

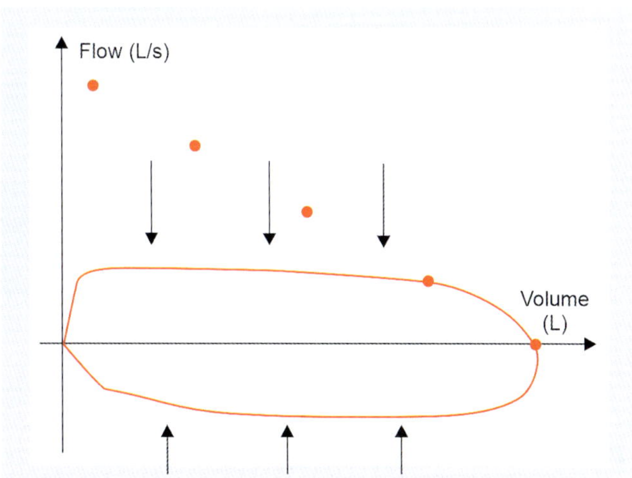

Fig. 19: Fixed large airway obstruction.

Principles of Pulse Oximetry

The general principle of pulse oximetry is based on *Beer-Lambert law* by measuring the transmission of the red (600–750 nm wavelength) and IR (850–1000 nm) lights through the *pulsatile* tissue beds, which subsequently determines the light absorption characteristics of oxygenated and deoxygenated hemoglobin (Hb). According to *Beer-Lambert law*, the intensity of transmitted light decreases exponentially as both the concentration of the substance (due to absorption), and the distance traveled through the substance increase. Oxygenated Hb absorbs more IR light and allows more red light to pass through and thus appears bright red to the naked eye. In contrast, deoxygenated (or reduced) Hb absorbs more red light and allows more IR light to pass through, and thus appears blue or cyanotic **(Fig. 20)**.

Sensing the pulsatile arterial flow is required for pulse oximetry to work. At the measuring site, there are many constant light absorbers that are always present. They are the skin, soft tissue, bone, veins, capillary, and nonpulsatile component of arterial blood. This constitutes the baseline absorption of the light. The pulsatile expansion of the arteriolar bed increases the light path length and further increases light absorbency over the baseline (*Beer-Lambert law, see* earlier). Therefore, the change in light absorption during arterial pulsation is the basis of oximetry determinations. The variation in the absorbability of light during pulsatile flow as compared to baseline is displayed as arterial waveform of (plethysmography).

Pulse Oximetry Sensor

Pulse oximetry sensor consists of a pair of small red (R; 660 nm) and IR (940 nm) light-emitting diodes (LEDs) and a single silicone photodetector

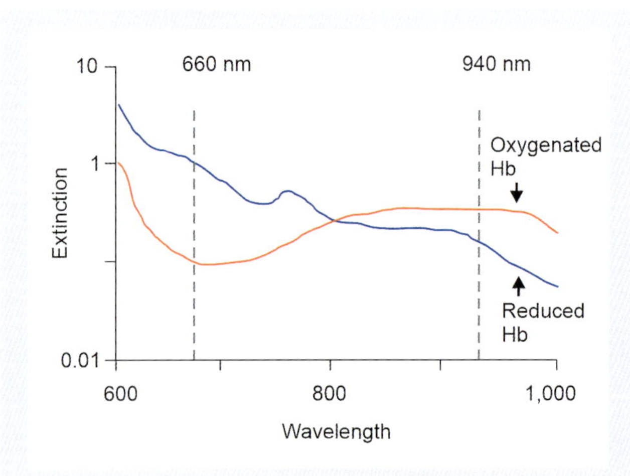

Fig. 20: Absorption of red and infrared light by oxygenated and reduced hemoglobin (Hb).

mounted inside either a rigid spring-loaded clip, a flexible probe, or an adhesive wrap.

Two modes of sending light through the measuring site exist: Transmittance and reflectance. In the transmittance sensor, as shown in **Figure 21**, the LEDs and photodetector are opposite of each other with the measuring site in-between. The light passes through the site. In the reflectance mode, the LEDs and photodetector are mounted side by side on top of the measuring site and the light bounces from the LEDs to the detector across the site. The transmittance mode is the most commonly used type **(Fig. 21)**.

The absorption ratio of R/IR is calculated by a microprocessor and is compared to a "look-up" table (based on experimental studies in healthy human volunteers) that converts the ratio to a SpO_2 value. For example, an R/IR ratio of 0.5 equates to approximately 100% SpO_2, 1.0 to approximately 85% SpO_2, while a ratio of 2.0 equates to 0% SpO_2.

Functional versus Fractional Hemoglobin Saturations

It should be noted that the SpO_2 measured by pulse oximetry differs from the arterial oxygen saturation (SaO_2) measured by a laboratory CO-oximeter. Pulse oximetry measures the *functional Hb* SaO_2, which is defined as hemoglobin capable of carrying oxygen. It is the ratio of oxyhemoglobin (O_2Hb) to O_2Hb plus reduced Hb:

Functional $SaO_2 = O_2Hb/(O_2Hb + \text{reduced Hb})$

Laboratory CO-oximeter measures the *fractional Hb* SaO_2, which is defined as the ratio of O_2Hb to total hemoglobin, which includes nonfunctional Hb such as methemoglobin (MetHb) and carboxyhemoglobin (COHb) (incapable of carrying oxygen):

$$\text{Fractional } SaO_2 = O_2Hb/(O_2Hb + \text{reduced Hb} + \text{MetHb} + \text{COHb})$$

Therefore, the SpO_2 number measured by pulse oximetry (functional SaO_2) should be higher than the SaO_2 reported by the laboratory blood gas. In the usual clinical circumstances, however, the patients' concentrations of MetHb and COHb are so low that the values of both functional and fractional saturations are nearly identical.

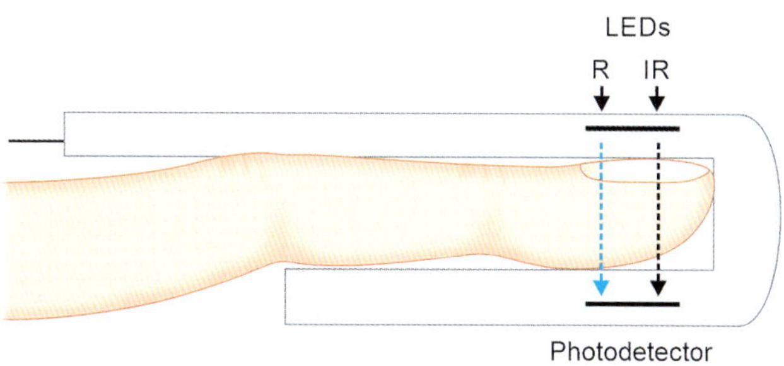

Fig. 21: Transmittance sensor. (IR: infrared; LEDs: light-emitting diodes; R: red)

Calibration and Practical Limitations

Pulse oximetries are calibrated during manufacture and automatically check their internal circuits when they are switched on. They cannot be altered by the users. They are accurate in the range of oxygen saturations from 70% to 100% with a standard error of ±2% but less accurate in the range of 70–50% (±3%).

Limitations of the effectiveness and accuracy of pulse oximetry:

- *Nonfunctional Hb (COHb and MetHb)*: The light absorption of COHb and O_2Hb at 660 nm are identical; that means the COHb is red and it is "detected" by the pulse oximetry as O_2Hb; therefore, in the presence of large amounts of COHb (e.g., CO poisoning or heavy tobacco smokers), the pulse oximetries read the sum of O_2Hb and COHb, which will register a falsely high SpO_2 reading. In this situation, the CO-oximetry is required to measure the COHb level. In contrast, MetHb has identical absorptions at 660 nm and 940 nm wavelengths. This 1:1 absorption ratio is interpreted by the pulse oximetry as 85% of SpO_2 *regardless* of the true saturations.
- A reduction in peripheral pulsatile blood flow due to vasoconstriction, hypovolemia, severe hypotension, hypothermia, shock
- Surgical dyes such as methylene blue, indocyanine green, and indigo carmine transiently decrease the pulse oximetry readings. These dyes absorb light in the region of 660 nm.
- Excessive ambient lights such as high-intensity overhead lights in the operating room (OR) or some IR heat lamps can interfere with the photodetector signal sensing.
- Artifacts due to motion, shivering, radiofrequency diathermy apparatus
- Nail polishes, especially black, blue, and green color

NONINVASIVE ARTERIAL BLOOD PRESSURE MONITORING

Arterial blood pressure is commonly determined noninvasively by direct palpation, auscultation, Doppler probe, or commonly used oscillometry method. Direct palpation reveals systolic pressure but not a diastolic component. Auscultation method uses the concept of classic Korotkoff sound. The sounds appear at systolic reading and disappear or muffle at diastolic reading. The mean pressure is calculated as diastolic pressure +1/3 of pulse pressure (difference between systolic and diastolic pressure).

Automated blood pressure devices use oscillometric method. A transducer in the blood pressure cuff system senses the blood pressure oscillations during the deflation process after an initial inflation of the cuff. The lowest cuff pressure that senses the maximum oscillations is determined as mean arterial pressure (MAP). Depending on the oscillometric device, systolic

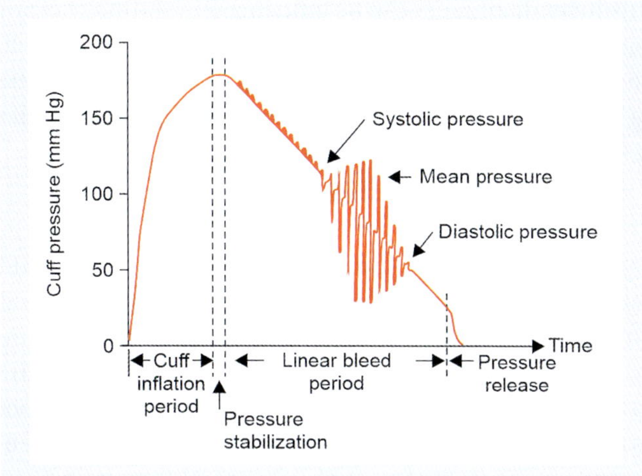

Fig. 22: Observed oscillations in cuff pressure during deflation. The amplitude of oscillations is greatly exaggerated.

and diastolic pressures are determined using an algorithm. The systolic and diastolic pressures are determined where the amplitude of oscillations is a specific ratio of the maximum oscillation amplitude **(Fig. 22)**. A narrow cuff overestimates the blood pressure, whereas a wide cuff can underestimate. Since the transducer measures the oscillations, it is imperative that motion, or shivering, can induce errors in the measurement of blood pressure. Vascular tone changes from any cause can also influence the measurements. More importantly, the MAP may remain the same at more peripherally measured sites, but the pulse pressure may widen with higher systolic and lower diastolic pressures.

INVASIVE ARTERIAL PRESSURE MONITORING

Intraluminal pressure changes are conveyed via a fluid column to a transduce diaphragm that oscillates in response to the pressure waveform. The diaphragm movements are converted to an electrical signal. The transducer enables this function by acting as a part of a capacitor, inductor, or, most commonly, as strain gauge. The strain gauge uses variable resistors, the electrical resistance which changes with changing length. The diaphragm of the transducer moves a small plate connected to four strain gauges. With the movement of the diaphragm, two gauges are compressed and the other two stretched. All four strain gauges form part of a Wheatstone bridge. The movement of the diaphragm is hence converted to intraluminal pressure waveforms seen on the monitor with digital readings. The system is calibrated such that a 50 microvolt change in potential corresponds to a pressure change in 10 mm Hg. Modern equipment does not require external calibration as the units are manufactured to tight standards.

The transducer diaphragm can be influenced by the effect of atmospheric pressure on the transmural pressure of the tubing system as well as by the hydrostatic column of the fluid in the tubing. These effects can be obviated by zeroing the transducer and maintaining the transducer's level at the measuring site.

Zeroing

By exposing the transducer system to ambient atmosphere and zeroing, the unit removes the effect of ambient pressure on the transmural pressure of the tubing system. Zeroing is performed by opening the transducer to atmospheric pressure and electronically setting the effect of atmospheric pressure to zero. Occasionally, this zero baseline can drift and hence periodic checking is recommended. A drift of 5 mm Hg can result in substantial errors in low-pressure measurements, such as central venous pressure (CVP) measurements.

Leveling

Leveling refers to the placement of zeroed transducer at the level of measurement; for example, at the superior border of the right atrium to measure pressure at the level of the heart. This procedure eliminates the hydrostatic pressure of the fluid column in the tubing. A 10 cm change in the height will increase or decrease the pressure by about 7.5 mm Hg. For standardization purposes, the transducer is leveled at the midaxillary line for arterial pressure monitoring. For intracranial procedures, placing the transducer at the level of tragus will reflect the pressure at circle of Willis accurately. As long as the transducer is maintained at the site of the measurement, the insertion point of the cannula into an artery does not matter.

Resonance and Damping (Fig. 23)

An arterial pressure waveform is a sum of several sine waves (Fourier analysis). Transducer systems have their own natural oscillatory frequency, or resonant frequency. If this resonant frequency coincides with one of the frequencies making substantial contribution to the arterial waveform (resonance), distortion of the signal will occur. The natural frequency of arterial pressure monitoring is designed to be around 40 Hz. This is above the frequencies contributing to the arterial waveform and therefore minimizes the effect of resonance. The natural frequency of the monitoring system should be beyond natural frequency of the arterial system. This is very important for arterial measurements, unlike CVP measurements, where there are high-frequency systems contributing to steep waves. Generally, CVP waveforms are of low frequency and do not have steep phases unlike arterial pressure waveforms.

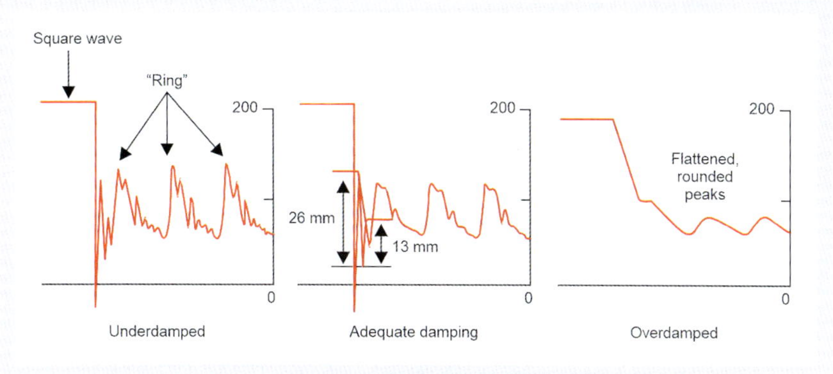

Fig. 23: Effect of damping coefficient on arterial wave morphology. Note the differences in systolic (peak) pressure.

Damping, on the other hand, decreases amplitude of oscillations in an oscillatory system. This diminishes the rate of change in signal. This is generally measured by the damping coefficients. Air bubbles, blood clot, or soft tubing can result in damping effect.

MONITORING CARDIAC OUTPUT

Minimal and Noninvasive Methods

Introduction

Early and aggressive resuscitation has been the cornerstone in limiting organ damage and hemodynamic failure both in the OR and in critical care units (CCU). Studies have listed various hemodynamic markers to determine early progression of systemic collapse. CO measurement is an indirect indication of global tissue perfusion and systemic oxygen delivery. Monitoring CO has been essential in discovering physiologic derangements in the early stages of development. CO is the product of stroke volume (SV) and heart rate (HR) and is a measure of the amount of blood ejected by the ventricles per minute.

Therefore, factors affecting SV and HR such as rhythm, contractility, preload, and afterload also affect CO. Patients with an optimized CO have less postoperative complications and decreased lengths of admission. Similarly, CO optimization in the intensive care unit (ICU) has resulted in improved fluid management protocols, decreased mortality, and shorter lengths of stay. Thermodilution via pulmonary artery catheter (PAC) has been the gold standard in CO measurement. However, the process is invasive, requiring placement through a large vein (subclavian, internal jugular, or femoral) and advancing the catheter until it passes into the pulmonary artery **(Fig. 24)**. A known dose of cold saline is injected via the catheter into the right atrium, and the change in blood temperature is recorded by a thermistor near the

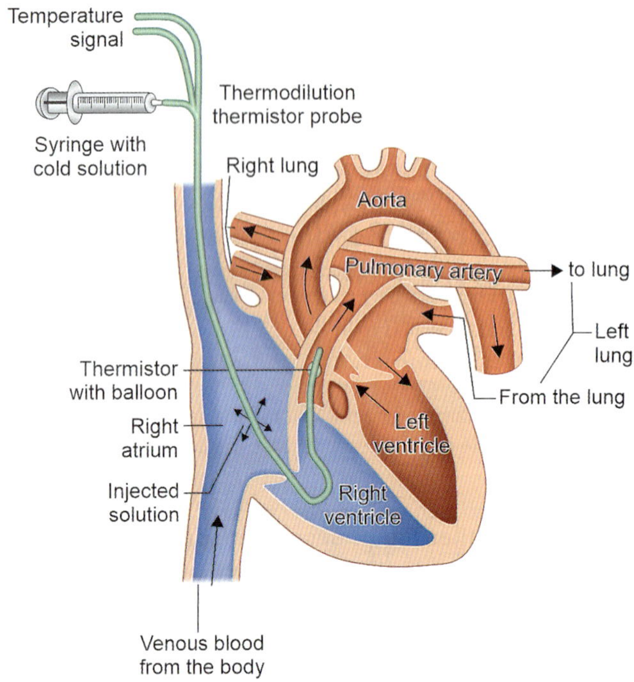

Fig. 24: Thermodilution cardiac output measurement.

end of the PAC. CO is calculated using thermodilution curves and a modified Stewart–Hamilton equation. The amount of indicator injected (n) is related to its mean concentration (c), cardiac output (Q), and the time for which it is detected ($t_2 - t_1$). V is volume of the indicator, T_{core} and $T_{indicator}$ are core temperature and temperature of the indicator, respectively.

$$\dot{Q} = \frac{n}{\int c\,dt} = \frac{k(T_{core} - T_{indicator})\,V_{indicator}}{\int_{t_1}^{t_2} -\Delta T\,dt}$$

Continuous CO can be measured via a modified PAC system where a filament is passed into the right atrium along with the PAC. The filament is heated, and the change in temperature of the blood is measured.

Complications of PAC include pneumothorax, arrhythmia, infection, pulmonary artery rupture, valvular injury, thrombosis, and embolism. In addition, valvular dysfunction, mechanical ventilation, and intracardiac shunts have been associated with inaccurate CO readings. Therefore, newer devices and alternative systems have been developed over the years to provide accurate and reproducible CO measurements comparative to PAC but are less invasive, more cost-effective, and are not easily influenced by disease state.

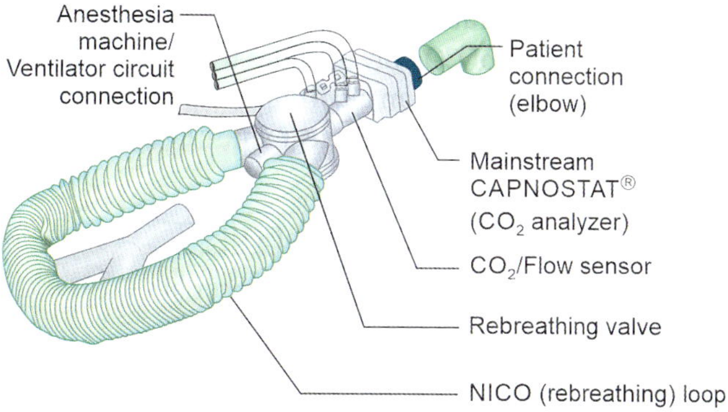

Fig. 25: NICO System: Partial CO_2 rebreathing monitor.

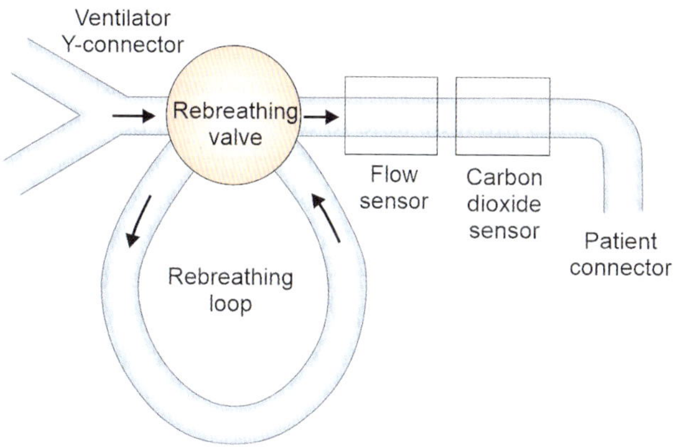

Fig. 26: Diagrammatic representation of NICO.

Minimally Invasive Methods (Via Endotracheal Intubation)

NICO System: Partial CO_2 Rebreathing Monitor

The NICO System (Novametrix Medical Systems, Walling-ford, CT, United States/Respironics, Murraysville, PA, USA) is a setup, which consists of a proprietary rebreathing loop, which is connected to the ventilator circuit along with an IR CO_2 sensor, a differential pressure pneumotachometer, and a rebreathing valve as shown in **Figures 25 and 26**. Patients must be sedated, intubated, and mechanically ventilated in order to utilize this system.

Every 3 minutes, the rebreathing valve is opened and partial rebreathing is initiated for 30–50 seconds. During this time, approximately 150 cc of dead space is introduced into the breathing circuit. CO is calculated by determining the normal and rebreathing CO_2 ratios using a modified Fick's principle and the following rule: The amount of CO_2 entering the lungs via the pulmonary artery is equal to the expired CO_2 plus the amount exiting the lungs via the pulmonary veins and is therefore proportional to CO. Simply put, the $P_{ET}CO_2$ during the nonrebreathing period is compared to that of the subsequent

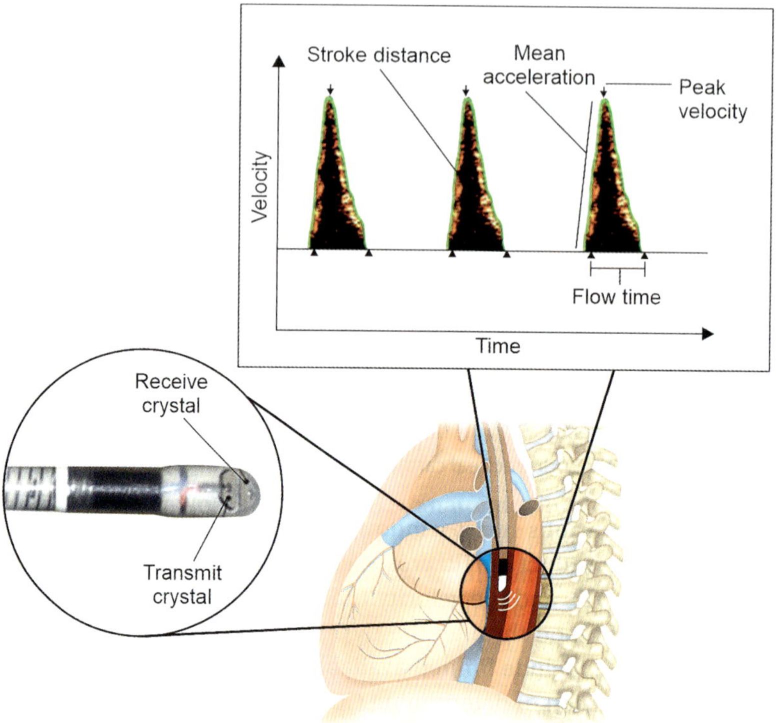

Fig. 28: Esophageal Doppler positioning.

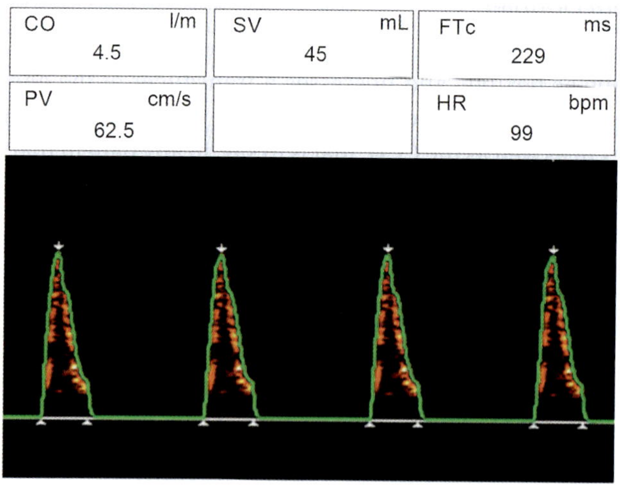

Fig. 29: Rotation of esophageal Doppler probe to obtain. (CO: cardiac output; FTc: flow time corrected; HR: heart rate; PV: peak velocity; SV: stroke volume)
Source: Best waveform, www.deltexmedical.com.

variability and structural changes of the aorta (i.e., coarctation, cross-clamp, or an aneurysm), which can falsely alter the calculation of blood flow. Regardless, studies have determined that the ED can be useful when assessing hemodynamic stability and monitoring fluid therapy.

Minimally Invasive Methods (Via Arterial Line)

Pulse Contour Analysis

The principle of pulse contour analysis is based on the hypothesis that SV is proportional to the area under the curve of the systolic segment of an arterial waveform **(Fig. 30)**. This area, when divided by aortic impedance, measures SV from which CO can be determined using the algorithm in **Figure 31**.

There are four pulse contour systems that are commercially used, and each has a proprietary algorithm to calculate for patient-specific calibration and accurate aortic impedance determination: LiDCO system, PiCCO system, FloTrac system, and the pressure recording analytic method (PRAM). In addition, the algorithms for pulse contour analysis can also provide measures of stroke volume variation (SVV) and pulse pressure variation (PPV).

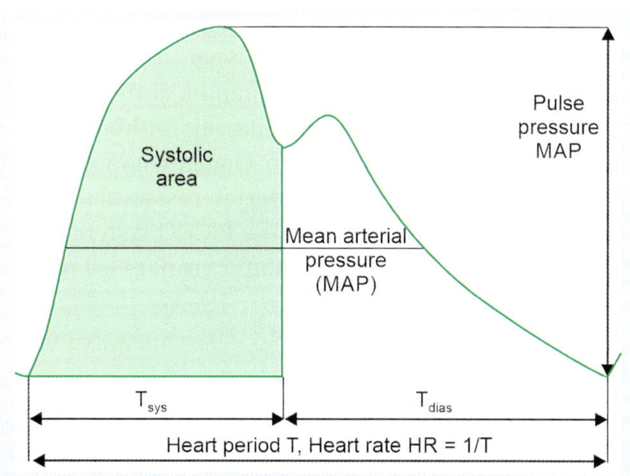

Fig. 30: Pulse contour analysis. (T_{dias}: duration of diastole; T_{sys}: duration of systole)

$$\text{PCCO} = \underbrace{\text{cal}}_{\substack{\text{Patient-specific}\\\text{calibration factor}\\\text{(determined by}\\\text{thermodilution)}}} \bullet \underbrace{\text{HR}}_{\substack{\text{Heart}\\\text{rate}}} \bullet \int_{\text{Systole}} \Big(\underbrace{\frac{P(t)}{\text{SVR}}}_{\substack{\text{Area}\\\text{under}\\\text{pressure}\\\text{curve}}} + \underbrace{C(p)}_{\substack{\text{Aortic}\\\text{compli-}\\\text{ance}}} \bullet \underbrace{\frac{dp}{dt}}_{\substack{\text{Shape of}\\\text{pressure}\\\text{curve}}} \Big)\, dt$$

Fig. 31: Pulse contour cardiac output (PCCO) algorithm.

Remember that SVV is the change in SV during the phases of the respiratory cycle, and that the SVV/PPV ratio can be utilized for trend analysis in fluid management.

PiCCO System

The first pulse contour device created, the PiCCO system (PULSION medical system, Munich, Germany) combines pulse contour analysis with transpulmonary thermodilution to measure not only SV and CO but also several other hemodynamic parameters. It is the most invasive of the pulse contour systems, requiring both a central venous line (femoral or internal jugular) and an arterial line (femoral preferred, but radial, axillary, and brachial can be acceptable). Indicator solution is bolused via the central venous line and blood temperature changes are measured by the thermistor-tipped arterial catheter. These changes determine CO and calibrate the pulse contour analysis to determine SV. In addition, parameters such as intrathoracic blood volume (ITBV), global end-diastolic volume (GEDV), and extravascular lung water (EVLW) can be determined via the PiCCO system. GEDV and ITBV are a measure of cardiac preload, and EVLW is a measure of pulmonary edema. As with the other pulse contour devices, SVV/PPV can also be determined for fluid management. Apart from being significantly more invasive, instances of valvular regurgitation, aortic aneurysm, rapidly changing body temperatures, arrhythmias, air bubbles, and clots can significantly decrease accuracy. In addition, changes in vascular compliance, aortic impedance, and peripheral arterial resistance can influence accuracy. Studies have determined that the PiCCO system correlates very well with PAC, especially during off-pump coronary artery bypass graft surgeries.

LiDCO System: Pulse Power Analysis

The LiDCO system (LiDCO, Cambridge, UK) uses the principle of pulse power analysis, which theorizes that the fluctuations of blood pressure around its mean value can be attributed to the SV. The measurement of SV can be falsely altered by four factors:

1. Nonlinear compliance of the aortic tree
2. Arterial wave reflection which is affected by SVR
3. Dampening of the transducer system
4. Flow of blood in the systolic aorta-filling is pulsatile, but emptying is continuous.

Taking each factor into account, the LiDCO algorithm combines the principles of pulse contour analysis with lithium indicator dilution to monitor SV and SVV. A peripheral or central venous line is required in addition to an arterial line which is attached to a disposable lithium sensitive sensor.

A bolus of lithium chloride is administered via the peripheral line, and the concentration of lithium is measured via the arterial line sensor. This value is a "patient-specific calibration factor", which corrects the SV value determined via pulse contour analysis. The doses of lithium are very minimal and have no physiologic effects on adults. The accuracy of the LiDCO method decreases in patients on lithium therapy in instances of aortic regurgitation, intra-aortic balloon pump (IABP), dampened arterial line, postaortic surgery, severe peripheral arterial vasoconstriction, arrhythmias, and intra- or extracardiac shunts. Initial studies with LiDCO have shown good correlation when compared with PAC, and current studies are determining its reliability in gauging fluid responsiveness and guiding management.

FloTrac System and Vigileo Monitor

The FloTrac/Vigileo system (Edwards Lifesciences, Irvine, CA, USA) can calculate CO via a proprietary sensor attached to the end of a standard arterial line (usually radial). The entire system is based on the principle that there is a linear relationship between pulse pressure and SV. The FloTrac algorithm shown below uses data from the arterial waveform and calibrates the results using standardized patient demographic data to determine SV, SVR, and SVV. SD_{AP} is the standard deviation of 2,000 data points (arterial waves sampled every 20 seconds at 100 Hz) and reflects pulse pressure. The conversion factor, μ, depends on arterial compliance (derived from patient biometric characteristics such as sex, age, height, weight), MAP, and waveform characteristics (degree of wave asymmetry and peakedness, skewness, and kurtosis, respectively). This conversion factor is calculated every minute and thus curtails the need for external calibration required in LiDCO and PiCCO systems.

$$SV = SD_{AP} X \mu$$

The major advantage of this device is that it is truly minimally invasive, requiring only a peripheral arterial line. A major disadvantage is that the accuracy of the readings became unreliable in instances of low SVR as seen in sepsis or liver failure. Although the FloTrac system has evolved into its current third-generation form, this particular limitation has not been thoroughly resolved and shows poor correlation when compared to PAC. In addition, the entire system depends on a continuous and undisturbed arterial waveform and is therefore very operator-dependent.

Pressure Recording Analytic Method

The PRAM-MostCare system (Vytech, Padova, Italy) determines SV by measuring the area under the arterial waveform during the entire cardiac cycle. It uses high resolution, sampling the waveform multiple times at 1,000 Hz, to analyze the pressure wave morphology in real time and separates the systolic and diastolic phases using the dicrotic notch as a marker. The area under the pressure wave (P/t) is established for the systolic and diastolic phases, and two impedance values are calculated through which SV is determined. The advantage to this system is that it is minimally invasive, requiring only an arterial line. The disadvantage is that it has not yet been thoroughly studied and comparative analysis has been variable.

Truly Noninvasive Methods

Thoracic Bioimpedance

The thoracic bioimpedance (TEB) system applies the definition of bioimpedance to the entire thorax. The underlying assumption is that the thorax is a cylinder perfused and filled with blood (the major vessel being the aorta) and when an electric current is passed from one end to the other, the electrical resistance (impedance) can be measured and used to calculate CO. Electrodes are placed, two on either side of the neck and two on either side of the lower thorax. A high-frequency low-amplitude current is passed from the outermost electrodes on either side, and the current is read by the innermost electrodes. Therefore, in **Figure 32**, the current is passed from the black to green electrodes (outer pair) on either side of the thorax and the current is measured in the white and red electrodes (inner pair). The change in voltage between the white and red electrodes is the impedance, and is on tissue fluid volume, as well as pulmonary, venous, and aortic blood. When CO fluctuates aortic blood flow will have a proportional change, and therefore the impedance between electrodes will change.

An algorithm uses the bioimpedance value to calculate CO and SV. Limitations to this system are dependent on the ability to inject and read

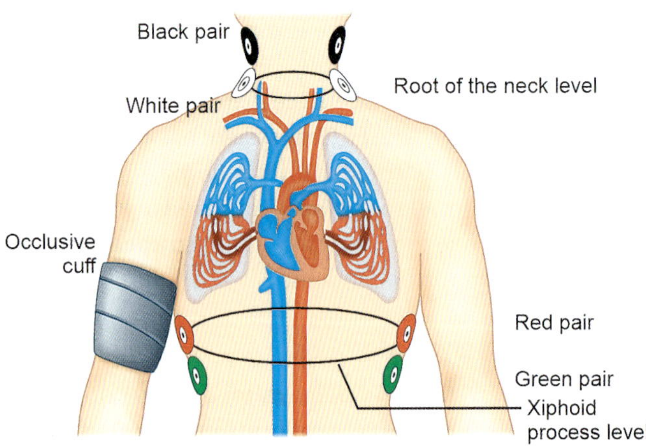

Fig. 32: Thoracic impedance measured between electrodes (black and white pair, and white and green pair).

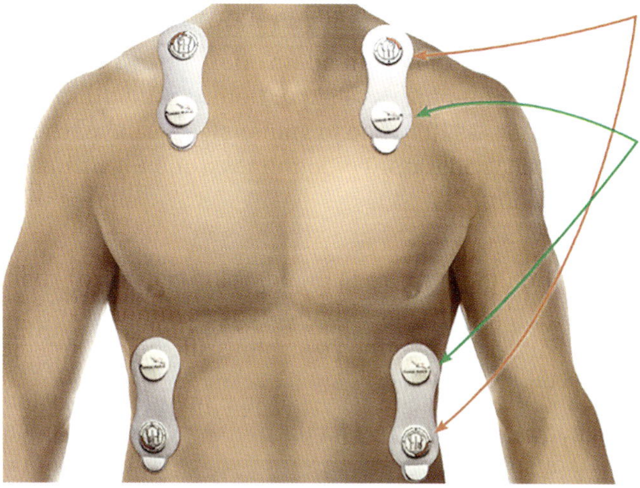

Fig. 33: Thoracic Bioreactance (NICOM) system. Each sticker contains outer and inner electrodes.

an accurate current, and include electrocautery, arrhythmias, patient body habitus and movement, placement of electrodes, and changes in the skin such as temperature and diaphoresis. Studies have shown that there is a poor correlation of the absolute value of CO when compared to invasive methods and have suggested that the benefit of the TEB system is trend analysis and not for a diagnostic purpose.

Thoracic Bioreactance: NICOM System

Thoracic Bioreactance is an evolved version of TEB that is less susceptible to external noise and interference. The NICOM device (Cheetah Medical, Portland, OR, USA) uses four stickers, two placed on the upper thorax and two placed on the lower thorax **(Fig. 33)**. Each sticker contains two electrodes, an outer and an inner. Similar to TEB, a 75 kHz current is passed from one outer electrode to the other (red arrows) and the reading is picked up by the voltage input amplifier on the inner electrodes (green arrows) **(Fig. 33)**. An impedance phase shift is generated from the difference in voltage between the outer and inner electrodes **(Fig. 34)**. The SV and subsequently CO are calculated from this phase shift and the average between the left and right electrodes is displayed on the monitor. Studies have shown that there is a good correlation between CO determined by NICOM versus PAC.

Changes to the blood flow in the thorax (colored arrows) are converted to phase shifts, which are displayed on the NICOM monitor.

The equation used by NICOM to determine SV: C = current; VET = ventricular ejection time; $d\Phi/dt_{max}$ = peak rate of change of the phase shift.

$$SV = C \times VET \times d\Phi/dt_{max}$$

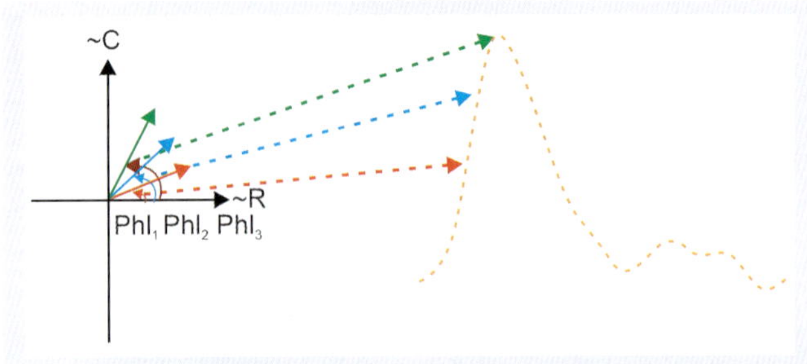

Fig. 34: The impedance shift generated between outer and inner electrodes measures cardiac output.
Source: Lee AJ, Cohn JH, Ranasinghe JS. Cardiac output assessed by invasive and minimally invasive techniques. Anesthesiol Res Pract. 2011;2011:475151.

Summary of Cardiac Output Measurements

Although PAC is the current gold standard, newer methodologies are aiming to be less invasive and easy to use, but still provide the same accurate and reproducible CO measurements. The minimally invasive devices use equipment such as esophageal probes, ETTs, and arterial lines to gather data when calculating CO. This equipment is readily available in the OR and should be used in surgeries where hemodynamic stability is key (i.e., cardiac, vascular, thoracic, liver). The noninvasive methods use electrodes, which are easy to place and transmit data immediately. These methods are useful in cases where hemodynamic instability is unexpected and quick assessment is necessary when required. Finally, some of the newer methods aim to show trends in CO over time rather than absolute measurements and aid in assessing and managing fluid status. As new devices are developed, research is currently underway to determine their accuracy and reproducibility as well as the correlation with PAC.

TEMPERATURE DEVICES

A conventional method of temperature monitoring has been mercury thermometers. Although accurate, they are not used during anesthesia due to the risk of breaking and lack of feasibility to direct the data to an electronic monitor. IR thermometers are a possibility but have not made their way into anesthetic practice, as IR devices are limited to measuring skin and tympanic membrane temperature and are insufficiently accurate for clinical use. The commonly used temperature-monitoring device is based on three electrical techniques: Resistance thermometer, thermistor, and thermocouple.

Resistance Thermometers

A change in temperature causes a change in electrical resistance, which is detected using a Wheatstone bridge circuit. They are accurate and can

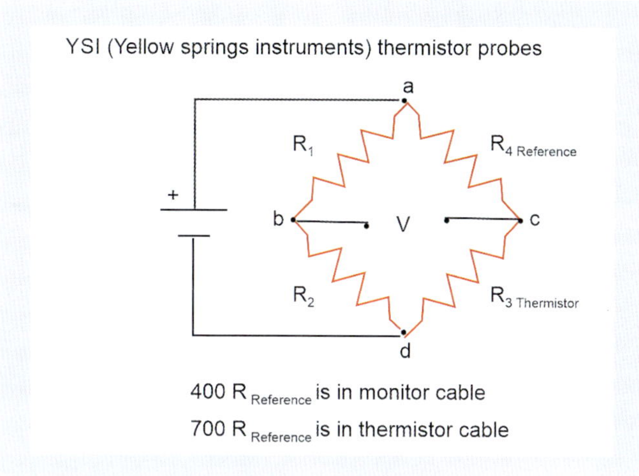

Fig. 35: Thermistor probe.

measure changes in temperature of very small magnitude, up to 0.0001°C. The principle of Wheatstone bridge, first described by Samuel Hunter Christie in 1833, was applied by Sir Charles Wheatstone to measure several variables in 1843. To date, the Wheatstone bridge remains the most sensitive and accurate method of precisely measuring resistance values.

Figure 35 shows a circuit consisting of a power source and four resistors connected in a square. The resistors are connected to each other at junctions that are labeled *a* through *d*. The circuit contains a potentiometer, labeled *V*, which detects the voltage difference between *c* and *b*. If we consider each resistor separately, each resistor has its own current (*i1*, *i2*, *i3*, and *i4*), resistance (R_1, R_2, R_3, and R_4), and voltage (V_1, V_2, V_3, and V_4), which are related to each other through Ohm's law. The law states that the current through a conductor between two points is directly proportional to the potential difference across the two points. The Ohm's law equation I (current) is equal to potential difference which is ΔV by R.

A Wheatstone bridge circuit can be used to compare an unknown resistance R_X with others of a known value, for example, R_1 and R_2, have fixed values, and R_3 could be variable. If we connected a voltmeter between points *C* and *D*, and then varied resistor R_3 until the meters read zero, this would result in the two arms being balanced and the value of R_X to be known as shown.

At zero potential across the bridge, $R_1/R_2 = R_3/R_4$.

Thermistors

Thermistors are semiconductors composed of fused heavy metal oxides including manganese, nickel, zinc, iron, and cobalt. Changes in temperature

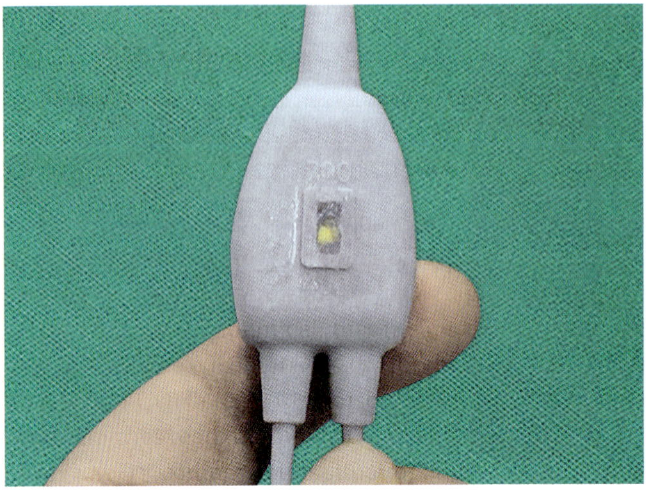

Fig. 36: Thermistor probe: Two-thermistor assembly.

result in changes in resistance of these semiconductors. Although the change is nonlinear, the semiconductors can be manufactured to result in linear changes in resistance within the working range of body temperature. These semiconductors can be small and have rapid response time. The disadvantages are drift, resistance changes over time, and need for frequent calibration.

Thermocouple

The thermocouples work on the Seebeck effect. EstonianGerman physicist Seebeck demonstrated that the electrical potential in the juncture points of two dissimilar metals changes with changes in temperature. If the circuit is completed by a reference junction of whom the temperature is known, the temperature of the measuring junction can be measured. The metals used are copper and constantan (alloy of copper and nickel). The thermocouples are small, accurate, have a rapid response, and are relatively cheap.

Thermistor probes are the ones commonly used in the ORs **(Fig. 36)**.

The 700 series probes were considered to be more accurate. The investment in a more expensive two-thermistor assembly was reasonable when the probes were reusable. Eliminating the reference thermistor from the thermistor assembly and building it into the cable became more reasonable with disposable products. Many cables now have a reference resistor that is either in the circuit or out of the circuit depending on the setting of the small switch. Here we see the switch glued in the "400" position to assure users do not missed it.

SUGGESTED READING

1. Asopa A, Dushane TE, Karthik S. Hemodynamic patient monitoring. In: Vacanti CA, Sikka PK, Urman RD, Deshwitz M, Segal BS (Eds). Essentials of Clinical Anesthesia, 1st edition. Cambridge: Cambridge University Press; 2011. pp. 155-72.
2. Bhavani-Shankar K, Kumar AY, Moseley HS, Ahyee-Hallsworth R. Terminology and current limitations of time capnography. J Clin Monit. 1995;11:175-82.
3. Bhavani-Shankar K, Mosely H, Kumar AY, Delph Y. Capnometry and anaesthesia. Can J Anaesth. 1992;39:617-32.
4. Kodali BS. Capnography outside the operating rooms. Anesthesiology. 2013;118(1):192-201.
5. Lee AJ, Cohn JH, Ranasinghe JS. Cardiac output assessed by invasive and minimally invasive techniques. Anesthesiol Res Pract. 2011;2011:475151.
6. Marik PE. Noninvasive cardiac output monitors: a state-of-the-art review. J Cardiothorac Vasc Anesth. 2013;27(1):121-34.
7. Mehta Y, Arora D. Newer methods of cardiac output monitoring. World J Cardiol. 2014;6(9):1022-9.
8. Xiong Z, Kodali BS. Pulse oximetry and capnography. In: Vacanti CA, Sikka PK, Urman RD, Deshwitz M, Segal BS (Eds). Essentials of Clinical Anesthesia, 1st edition. Cambridge: Cambridge University Press; 2011. pp. 186-90.

WEBSITES

1. Spirometry Interpretation: Flow-Volume Loop. [online] Available from http://www.spirometry.guru/fvc.html [Last accessed October, 2024].
2. http://www.capnography.com. Kodali BS.
3. Cardiac Engineering. (2024). Device development. ECOM monitor images. [online] Available from http://www.cardiacengineering.com/ecom.html [Last accessed October, 2024].

CHAPTER 8

Preuse Check of Anesthesia Equipment

Yasodananda K Areti

"What one intends to use, must be checked before use."

INTRODUCTION

A major contributory cause of anesthesia misadventure has been the use of anesthesia machines and/or breathing systems which have not been adequately checked by an anesthetist before use. Major causes of mortality and morbidity using conventional anesthesia machines (older models) are shown in **Table 1**. The American Society of Anesthesiologists (ASA) closed claim analysis revealed that claims due to anesthesia equipment decreased over the decades and outcomes in claims were less severe due to the advances in new anesthesia workstations. However, despite these advances, critical mishaps continue to occur, and most of them involve provider error with or without equipment failure. 35% of claims were judged as preventable by proper preanesthesia machine check.

There are innumerable number of workstations in different countries and one checklist cannot check all machines. Hence, different bodies in different countries have devised checklists to suit the equipment they use.

In 1993, a preanesthesia checkout recommendation was approved by the Food and Drug Administration (FDA), and widely accepted to be an important component of safe anesthesia practice. Since that time, new anesthesia delivery systems have been developed, and a single checkout procedure is no longer applicable to them all.

TABLE 1: Causes of mishaps in conventional machines. Most importantly, human misuse was three times more common than failure of equipment.

Cause	*Mortality and morbidity*
Breathing circuit: Misconnection or disconnection, leading to hypoventilation or barotrauma	39% (contribute to 70% of death or brain damage)
Vaporizer (awareness or overdose)	21%
Ventilator (high TV or PIP)	17%
High-pressure gas supplies	11%
Other components	15%

(PIP: peak inspiratory pressure; TV: tidal volume)

BOX 1: Preanesthetic recommendation (to be completed daily).

- Verify auxiliary oxygen cylinder and self-inflating manual ventilation device are available and functioning
- Verify patient's suction is adequate to clear the airway
- Turn on anesthesia delivery system and confirm that AC power is available
- Verify availability of required monitors, including alarms
- Verify that pressure is adequate on the spare oxygen cylinder mounted on the anesthesia machine
- Verify that the piped gas pressures are ≥50 psig
- Verify that vaporizers are adequately filled and, if applicable, that the filler ports are tightly closed
- Verify that there are no leaks in the gas supply lines between the flowmeters and the common gas outlet
- Test scavenging system function
- Calibrate, or verify calibration of the oxygen monitor and check the low oxygen alarm
- Verify carbon dioxide absorbent is not exhausted
- Breathing system pressure and leak testing
- Verify that gas flows properly through the breathing circuit during both inspiration and exhalation
- Document completion of checkout procedures
- Confirm ventilator settings and evaluate readiness to deliver anesthesia care. (Anesthesia Time Out). Items 2, 4, 7, and 11–15: to be completed prior to each procedure

Hence, the ASA subcommittee on equipment and facilities in 2008 has recommended a template for developing checkout procedures. An appropriate preanesthetic checkout for the available workstations should be devised **(Box 1)**. Each department must ensure that no one is allowed to operate the machines without understanding or checking them. The provider is responsible for all checkouts along with the technician trained for the purpose.

AUTOMATED CHECKOUT

Clinicians fail to check their equipment thoroughly, often not successful in detecting machine faults, or they do not check their machines at all. Despite extensive instructions, anesthesia residents, at best, could only perform 81% of a checkout procedure. Hence, automated checkout is incorporated in newer machines/workstations. They are unique in having a system checkout routine that is electronic and automated. The operator follows instructions to activate flows of gases, occlude the breathing circuit during the leak check, switch from manual to mechanical ventilation, open and close the pop-off valve, or manually check various functions (suction, or emergency oxygen cylinder supply). The automated checkouts are intended to cover all the steps of the Food and Drug Administration (FDA) checklist. The system checkout is logged, but may be bypassed in an emergency.

Despite these automated procedures, not every fault, obstruction, crossed connection, disconnection, or incompetent valve may be detected as discovered by the user. Additionally, equipment faults may develop during anesthesia that were either not present or not apparent on the preoperative check. It may not be obvious to the clinician as to what the machine is testing. Hence, in addition to automated checkouts, anesthesiologists must develop appropriate manual checklists to suite the apparatus being used. The checklist developed should not be so superficial that its value is doubtful or so detailed that it is impractical to use.

Items that are not evaluated by the automated checkout need to be identified, and supplemental manual checkout procedures included as needed. The Association of Anaesthetists of Great Britain and Ireland (AAGBI) developed a checklist as part of the AAGBI safety guidelines. The checking procedure described in this publication is reproduced in an abbreviated form, as a sheet entitled Checklist for Anesthetic Equipment 2012 **(Tables 2 and 3)**. A similar laminated sheet should be produced by each

TABLE 2: AAGBI safety guidelines (Contd...Table 3).

- Checks at the start of every operating session.
- Do not use this equipment unless you have been trained.
- Check self-inflating bag available.
- Perform manufacturer's (automatic) machine check.

Power supply	• Plugged in • Switched on • Back-up battery changed
Gas supplies and suction	• Gas and vacuum pipelines—"tug test" • Cylinders filled and turned off • Flowmeters working (if applicable) • Hypoxic guard working • Oxygen flush working • Suction clean and working
Breathing system	• Whole system patent and leak free using "two-bag" test • Vaporizers—fitted correctly, filled, leak free, plugged in (if necessary) • Soda lime—color checked • Alternative systems (Bain, T-piece)—checked • Correct gas outlet selected
Ventilator	• Working and configured correctly
Scavenging	• Working and configured correctly
Monitors	• Working and configured correctly • Alarms limits and volumes set
Airway equipment	• Full range required, working, with spares

Contd...

Contd...

Record this "check in the patient's record", do not forget!

- Self-inflating bag
- Common gas outlet
- Difficult airway equipment
- Resuscitation equipment
- TIVA and/or other infusion equipment

(AAGBI: the Association of Anaesthetists of Great Britain and Ireland; TIVA: total intravenous anesthesia)
Source: Permission obtained from the AAGBI.

TABLE 3: The AAGBI safety guideline. It is advisable to develop one similar laminated checklist to suit individual equipment in one different institute. The laminated sheet should be hung to each one machine.

Check before "Each Case"	
Breathing system	• Whole system patent and leak free using "two-bag" test • Vaprorizers—fitted correctly, filled, leak free, plugged in (if necessary) • Alternative systems (Bain, T-piece)—checked • Correct gas outlet selected
Ventilator	Working and configured correctly
Airway equipment	Full range required, working, with spares
Suction	Clean and working

The Two-Bag test:
A two-bag test should be performed after the breathing system, vaporizers and ventilator have been checked individually.

- Attach the patient end of the breathing system (including angie piece and filter) to a test lung or bag.
- Set the fresh gas flow of 5.1/min and ventilate manually. Check the whole breathing system is patent and the unidirectional valves and moving. Check the function of the APL valve by squeezing both bags.
- Turn on the ventilator to ventilate the test lung. Turn off the fresh gas flow, or reduce to a minimum, open and close each vaporizer in turn. There should be no loss of volume in the system.

This checklist is an abbreviated version of the publication by the Association of Anaesthetists of Great Britain and Ireland "Checking Anesthesia Equipment 2012". (Endorsed by the Chief Medical Officers)

(APL: adjustable pressure-limiting; AAGBI: the Association of Anaesthetists of Great Britain and Ireland)
Source: Permission obtained from the AAGBI.

institute for the machines they use. This sheet should be attached to each anesthetic machine and used to assist in the routine checking of anesthetic equipment.

CHECKING VARIOUS COMPONENTS

There are still several machines in use and in the market for developing countries, which do not feature automated checkouts. Once the principle behind various checkouts is understood and learnt, the safety to the patient is improved. This chapter details such checkout details.

Gas Supply

Cylinders

The type of cylinder attached as backup should be noted. One should ensure that pin index is properly seated and no more than one Bodok seal is located on the yoke and one spare is readily available for replacement. Appropriate tools to open and close cylinders must be available readily on the machine. The pressure in the cylinder should be noted (maximum is 137 atmospheres), and if pressure is less than half, the cylinder should be changed or one must ensure that a backup full cylinder is readily available. While attaching the cylinder, it should be supported; the gas outlet should be facing away from the operator. Just before mounting, the spindle valve should be opened and closed off immediately (cracking the cylinder), to blow off any dust particles. Once the pressure is checked, the amount of backup oxygen should be calculated (*see* Chapter 2) and the cylinder should be closed in order to prevent accidental depletion of cylinder contents.

Pipelines

These should be connected to either valve outlet or pendants firmly and securely. The pressure in the pipeline should be read on the gauges present on the machine or displayed on the monitor screen (normal values: 45–60 psi; 3–4 atmospheres; 300–400 kPa). A tug test should be performed to ensure secure connection after connecting the pipeline every time.

Single hose test: This test is performed mainly to ensure that oxygen from pipeline correctly reaches the oxygen flowmeter. All cylinders must be closed, and only oxygen pipeline should be connected. When flow control valves are turned on, flow should be registered only in the oxygen flowmeter. Then nitrous oxide pipeline should be connected. There should be no change in oxygen flowmeter. At this point, the oxygen pipeline should be disconnected. As the oxygen pressure falls, the oxygen flow starts to decrease. At one-point, low oxygen alarm should become audible and nitrous oxide flow quickly falls to zero. Thus, the single hose test identifies that there is no crossing of connections, and also tests the oxygen fail-safe device.

Ensuring Hypoxic Gas Mixture is Not Delivered

Various safety mechanisms are incorporated to ensure that hypoxic gas mixtures are not delivered. These include color coding, diameter index safety system (DISS), pin index system, oxygen fail-safe systems and low oxygen pressure alarm (*see* Chapters 3 and 7).

The most important in this respect is inspired oxygen monitors, using fuel cells in the inspiratory limb of circle system, and paramagnetic analyzers between patient and Y-piece of circle system. The functionality of these should be checked and they should be calibrated periodically (*see* Chapter 7).

- Ensure FiO_2 monitor reads 21% in room air.
- Verify low O_2 alarm is enabled and functioning.
- Reinstall sensor in circuit and flush breathing system with O_2.
- Verify that monitor now reads >90%.

Some machines have LINK-25 system (minimum inspired oxygen >25%) and some machines have proportionating devices (minimum inspired oxygen >30%). Hence, the inspired oxygen concentration should be checked using different flow combinations. In machines with three flowmeters, mechanical or electronic switch prevents the simultaneous administration of air and nitrous oxide (*see* Chapter 3). One must be aware of as to which mechanism is available on the machine that is used.

Vaporizers

The vaporizer that is to be used should have been filled adequately, and mounted appropriately. The leak tests on the machine should be performed with vaporizer in "off" and "on" position. Some machines have only one slot to mount the vaporizer and a slot just to mount alternate vaporizer. One must ensure as to which one is being used and functional. The back bar on most machines can have two vaporizers. But the interlock system should be checked so that only one of the vaporizers can be used at any given time. Vaporizer should be left in "off" position after completing the test.

CIRCLE BREATHING SYSTEM

Circle system is the most commonly used breathing system and one should be familiar with checking all the components and aspects of this system. One must ensure that all the components are assembled and the fresh gas flow (FGF) is connected securely to the FGF outlet of the machine.

Ensure that soda lime is not exhausted by checking the color of soda lime. However, regeneration of surface soda lime after overnight nonuse may mislead one to believe that soda lime is fresh. Rapid change in color may occur after a case is started indicating soda lime exhaustion. Some departments change to fresh soda lime every Monday morning.

Open FGF and the operator may breathe through a facemask to ensure that there is appropriate movement of unidirectional valves, and there is no undue resistance to breathing. This rules out any stuck valves.

Two-Bag Test

This tests the appropriate function of unidirectional valves in the circle system. The ventilator switch should be in manual position. The test lung should be attached to the "Y-piece." A reservoir bag (RB) has to be attached to the manual ventilation arm. The RB should be squeezed to mimic inspiration, alternating with a squeeze of test lung to mimic expiration. One must observe appropriate movement of unidirectional valves and adequate ventilation of the test lung.

Testing the Competence of Unidirectional Valves (Three-Bag Test)

One RB is mounted on the reservoir arm, and "man/auto" switch set to manual mode. The patient circuit is disconnected from unidirectional valve. A test lung or RB is attached to the inspiratory unidirectional valve (IUDV) and another is attached to expiratory unidirectional valve (EUDV). Prime the system with FGF. A squeeze on the manual RB should inflate the test lung on IUDV, but not on the one mounted on EUDV. One should not be able to empty the test lung on IUDV into the manual RB. After completing the test, the bags on UDV should be removed and patient's circuit should be assembled correctly.

Checking the Ventilator

The "man/auto" switch is turned to "auto" mode. The ventilator parameters have to be set for the patient that needs to be anesthetized next. The ventilator is turned "on" and appropriate movement of test lung and unidirectional valves should be observed. Once satisfied, the ventilator is turned off, and the switch should be turned to manual mode ready for use.

Alternate Breathing Systems

Verify backup ventilation equipment is available and functioning. A self-inflating resuscitator should be available and functional **(Fig. 1)**. If one plans to use breathing system other than circle system, the particular system should be assembled and checked with a test lung for proper functioning.

Leaks

Most of the leaks in the workstations are usually detected by the automated checkouts. Different authors use different nomenclature for various parts of machines. The nomenclature used in this book is given in Chapter 3.

High-Pressure System

Once the pressure in the cylinder is checked, the spindle valve should be closed, and one must ensure that the flowmeters are turned off. If there is

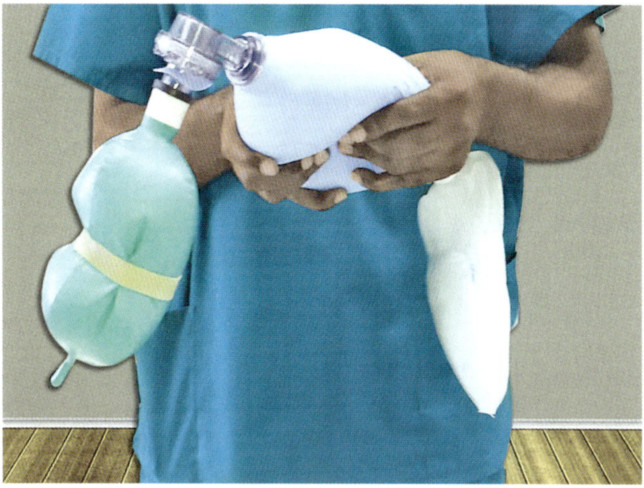

Fig. 1: Checking backup ventilation device (self-inflating resuscitator) using test lung.

no leak, the pressure in the gauge does not come to zero. In machines with mandatory minimal flow, the power should be turned off. Application of soap water at the yolk will identify if the leak is at the level of Bodok's seal.

Intermediate-Pressure System and Low-Pressure System

Positive pressure test: A pressure gauge is attached to the common gas outlet (CGO). Adjust the FGF till the gauge indicates 70 mm Hg. When FGF is turned off, the gauge pressure should not fall. If it starts falling, adjust the FGF till the pressure remains constant. The FGF at this point is equal to the leak. This test should be performed with the vaporizers in "on and off" position to evaluate if the leak is due to vaporizer. If the machine has a back pressure prevention valve at the CGO, this test should not be performed.

Universal negative pressure test: All flowmeters are turned off. An emptied suction bulb is attached to CGO. If there is no leak, the bulb will remain collapse **(Fig. 2)**. In machines with mandatory minimal flow, the power should be turned off.

Breathing Systems

- *Adjustable pressure-limiting (APL) valve* should be tested for correct relief at 30 cmH_2O and also at 50 cmH_2O.
- *Leaks in circle:* APL valve should be closed, and breathing circuit should be checked in manual position for leaks using positive pressure leak test at 30 cmH_2O.
- *Leaks in ventilator:* In order to check any leaks in the ascending bellows ventilator (ascending during expiration), the bellows should be taken to maximum expiratory position, and Y-piece is occluded. If there is a leak

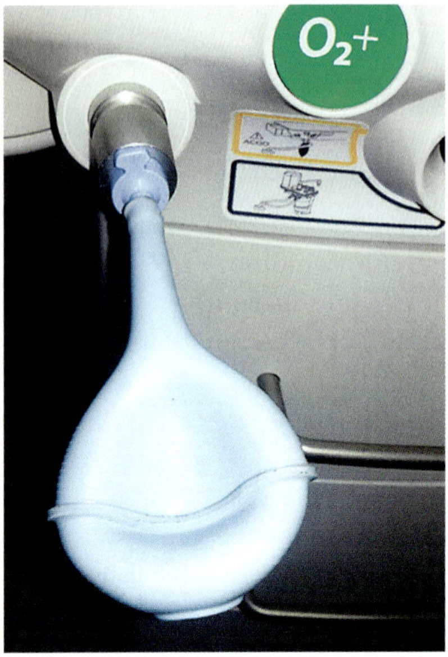

Fig. 2: Universal negative pressure leak test at the common gas outlet.

in the ventilator bellows, the bellows will slowly fall to the lowest position. In descending limb ventilators (descend during expiration), the bellows are taken to the maximum inspiratory position and Y-piece is occluded. If there is a leak, the bellows will suck air and fall to end-expiratory position.

Scavenging System

- Ensure proper connections between the scavenging system and both APL (pop-off) valve and ventilator relief valve.
- Adjust waste gas vacuum (if available).
- Fully open APL valve and occlude Y-piece.
- With minimum O_2 flow, allow scavenger RB to collapse completely and verify that absorber pressure gauge reads about zero.
- With the O_2 flush activated, allow the scavenger RB to distend fully, and then verify that absorber pressure gauge reads <10 cmH_2O.

Suction

Adequate level of vacuum should be available. The negative pressure should be around 100–150 mm Hg. Alternately, vacuum level is checked as shown in **Figure 3**. This will indicate negative pressure around 100 mm Hg.

Monitors

Check all the monitors you are likely to use. Ensure that they are calibrated, and the alarm levels are set properly. The most important monitors with reference to equipment are:

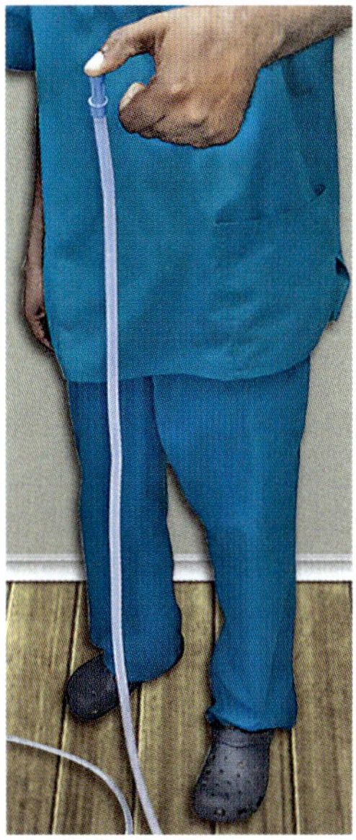

Fig. 3: Checking adequacy of suction.

- Inspired oxygen
- Pulse oximetry
- Capnography
- Airway pressures
- Minute volume
- Anesthesia agent

Airway Management

All the equipment planned for airway management should be checked and kept ready. Alternate equipment and drugs to manage difficult airway should be available and checked. A difficult airway trolley and protocol should be developed and kept in readiness in the suite (*see* Chapter 6).

Equipment for Total Intravenous Anesthesia

If total intravenous anesthesia (TIVA) is planned, appropriate equipment and drugs should be checked (drugs, syringes, infusion pumps, connections, etc.).

CHECK FINAL STATUS OF MACHINE

- Ensure that power switch if present is in the "on" position, and backup battery is available and being charged.
- Verify vaporizers are mounted and in "off" position.
- Ensure that adjustable pressure-limiting valve is open.

- Ensure that "Man/auto" selector switch is set to "man" position.
- Ensure that all flowmeters fixed to zero.
- Verify the patient's suction level is adequate.
- Ensure breathing system is ready to use.
- Backup ventilation and alternate anesthesia breathing system should be available.
- Check airway equipment.

SUGGESTED READING

1. Association of Anaesthetists of Great Britain and Ireland (AAGBI); Hartle A, Anderson E, Bythell V, Gemmell L, Jones H, et al., Membership of the Working Party: Guidelines, Checking Anaesthetic Equipment 2012, Association of Anaesthetists of Great Britain and Ireland. Anaesthesia. 2012;67:660-8.
2. Merry AF, Cooper JB, Soyannwo O, Wilson IH, Eichhorn JH. International Standards for a Safe Practice of Anesthesia 2010. Can J Anaesth. 2010;57:1027-34.

WEBSITES

1. http://www.asahq.org/resources/clinical-information/2008-asa-recommendations-for-pre-anesthesia-checkout/ Last accessed Oct., 2024.
2. http://onlinelibrary.wiley.com/doi/10.1111/j.1365-2044.2012.07163.x/abstract. Last accessed Oct., 2024.
3. http://onlinelibrary.wiley.com/doi/10.1111/j.1365-2044.2012.07163.x/epdf. Last accessed Oct., 2024.

CHAPTER 9

Electrical Safety, Cautery, and Lasers

Hariharan Seetharaman

ELECTRICAL SAFETY

Electrical Hazards in the Operating Theater Environment

In earlier days, when highly inflammable volatile anesthetic agents such as diethyl ether were being used, most of the anesthetic equipment including the shoes of the anesthetists were required to be "antistatic" to prevent discharge of static electricity. Static electricity is produced by contact of surfaces which builds up an electrical charge. This gets discharged when the surface comes into contact with a conductor. This discharge is sufficient to produce a spark which may cause fire in the presence of highly inflammable anesthetics.

In modern operating theaters, both anesthetic and surgical equipment can contribute to electrical hazards. Electrocautery, patient monitoring equipment such as electrocardiography (ECG), peripheral nerve stimulator, pacemakers, endoscopes, etc., are some examples of equipment which are prone to become faulty and predispose to electrical hazards. Despite stringent safety measures, there have been many reports of electrical malfunctions in the operating theater environment causing fire, explosions, tissue burns, muscle contracture, etc. Hence, it is vital to every practicing anesthetist to understand the concepts of electrical safety to prevent patient's morbidity due to electrical hazards.

What is "Earthing" or "Grounding"?

Figure 1 shows the supply of electricity from a wall outlet which is the source of power for any electrical equipment. Point A is the live terminal of the

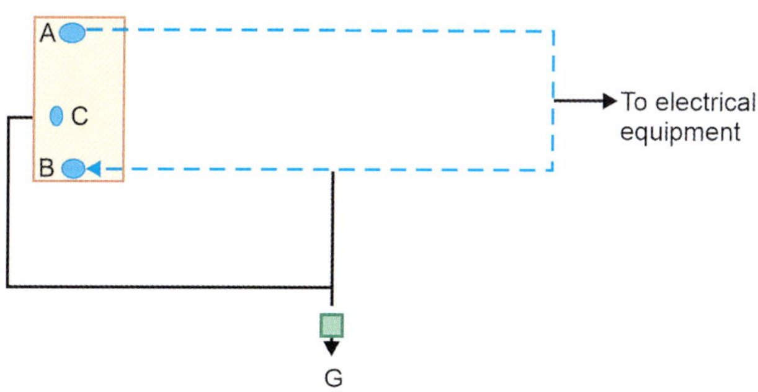

Fig. 1: Grounding.

power source and Point B is the neutral terminal. The circuit needs to be completed from the live terminal until the neutral terminal for the current flow to occur. If the current flows through a human body within this circuit, and if the human body is responsible to complete the circuit to the ground, "electrocution" occurs. In modern equipment, a third point from the wall outlet (Point C) is connected to a reservoir (Point G), which is capable of receiving infinite amount of electrical charge, which is usually the earth. Any charged conductor grounded to the earth loses its charge and assumes a neutral potential as the earth. This is the principle behind "earthing" or "grounding", which is basic in understanding electrical safety. Most modern electrical equipment has the third terminal in order to provide the grounding.

However, it is important to note that if human body comes into contact with the grounding connection, this may still cause harm, since the human body becomes the conductor of electricity to the ground. Therefore, modern electrical circuits in most hospitals isolate the primary electrical source from the power supply of the equipment by a line isolation transformer (LIT) in **Figure 2**. This divides the power supply into a primary source and a secondary supply beyond the transformer. In addition, most electrical equipment in the operating theaters is enclosed by a metal case which is further grounded to the earth.

The line isolation transformers are usually continuously monitored if the secondary power supply from the transformer is isolated from the primary source and if the circuitry is properly grounded. This is done with the help of line isolation monitors (LIM) which is a requirement of the electrical safety standards. The LIM is basically a current meter which detects abnormal flow of current through the circuitry and gives an alarm if there is one.

Electric Shock

An electric shock occurs when human body contacts any source of voltage high enough to cause sufficient current through the tissues.

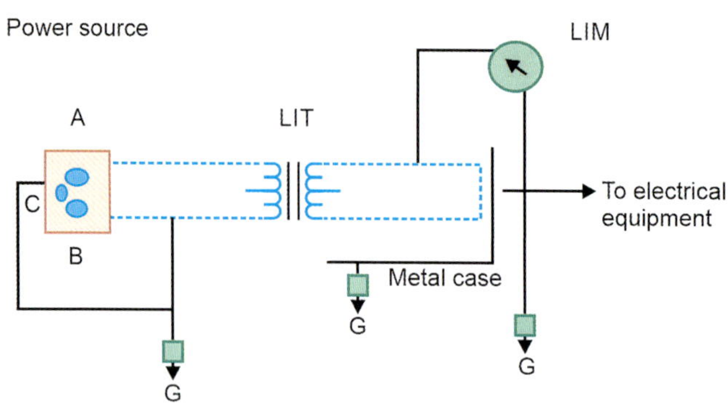

Fig. 2: Electrical line isolation.
(LIM: line isolation monitor; LIT: line isolation transformer)

Macroshock is caused by large voltages or currents applied to the skin or tissues, usually at anatomical locations distant from the heart.

The maximum current a person can tolerate holding a conductor in a hand and still let go of the conductor using the same muscles stimulated by the current is described as the "let-go" current for that individual. The average "let-go" threshold values are between 10 mA and 20 mA (more in males than females). In distinction to the "let-go" current which is a physiological threshold, the "release" current is the maximum current a person can withstand before releasing the conductor electrode which points to the psychological threshold. This has been found as high as 76 mA in volunteer experiments.

The effects of the current passing through human tissue depend upon the strength of the current. Even though one can sense current as low as 300 μA, a current strength of 1–5 mA is considered to be harmless. At the strength of 50–100 mA, there will be pain, exhaustion, blackouts, and mechanical injury. A current strength of 100–2,500 mA will cause ventricular fibrillation. Electrical burns are usually caused by high-density current if the strength is $>100\ mA/cm^2$.

Microshock is caused by small voltages or currents applied directly or in close proximity to the heart. This could be applied intentionally as in pacemaker electrodes; however, when this occurs inadvertently, it leads to life-threatening cardiac dysrhythmias such as ventricular fibrillation.

Saline-filled central venous catheters and arterial lines are potential sources of microshock, if the electrodes are connected to monitors. However, currently, the pressure transducers are connected to the monitors by means of telephone cables with small voltages and hence are relatively safer.

Surface electrodes of the ECG are relatively safer although intravascular and intracardiac ECG may be another potential source of microshock.

With the increasing need of *monitored anesthesia care* for interventional radiology, the potential electrical hazards of these equipment need to be thoroughly understood.

The American National Standards Institute has set 10 μA as the maximum allowable current leakage level in the connections of catheters and electrodes contacting the heart. A LIM will not be able to detect this small leakage because 2 mA is the level at which LIM warns of leakage. Therefore, LIM cannot prevent microshock.

SURGICAL DIATHERMY

Surgical diathermy is utilized in almost all surgical procedures in the modern surgical suite.

Surgical diathermy is a process by which heat generated from an electrical unit is applied to tissues, predominantly for the purpose of achieving hemostasis. The other functions of diathermy include coagulation, dissection (cutting), fulguration, and desiccation of tissues.

Principles

A direct or alternating current is passed through a resistant metal wire electrode in the form of a loop or a pointed tip or needle tip, which generates heat. This heated electrode is applied to the tissue for the aforementioned functions.

The electrosurgical unit (ESU) which generates the process is basically a high-frequency power oscillator. There are two types of oscillators: (1) a solid-state oscillator which generates undamped high-frequency currents useful for cutting; (2) a spark-gap oscillator generating damped high-frequency currents for coagulation.

The usual frequency at which the AC operates ranges from 300 kHz to 3 MHz and the generated temperature ranges between 100 and 1,200°C.

The basic diathermy circuit is schematically shown in **Figures 3 and 4**.

The active electrode is usually a very small size tip in 1–3 mm thickness, which actually generates the heat due to the high-frequency current sourced from the ESU. The passive or neutral electrode completes the circuit from the patient to the ESU, so that the current does not harm the patient. The passive electrode dissipates heat and hence two major factors need to be taken into consideration:

1. The conductivity of the electrode and the patient's body should be high enough.
2. The surface area of this electrode must be large enough to prevent heat concentrating on a small tissue area causing burns.

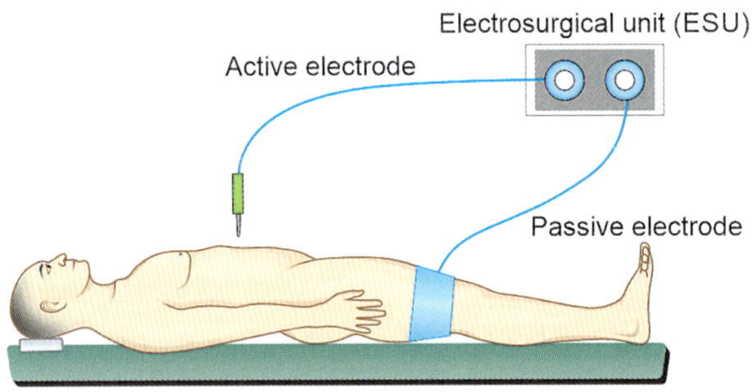

Fig. 3: Basic scheme of unipolar surgical diathermy.

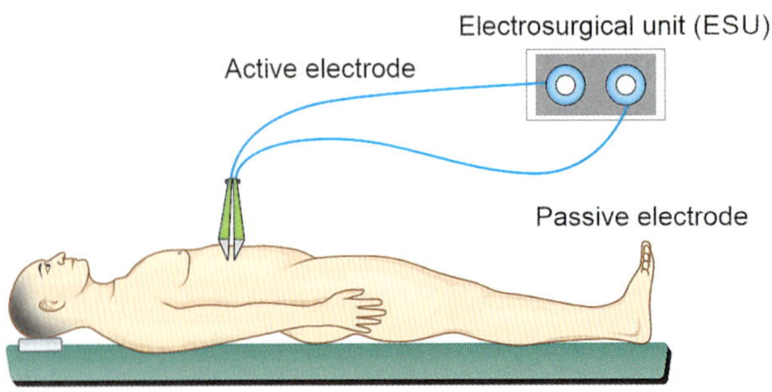

Fig. 4: Basic scheme of bipolar surgical diathermy.

There are two types of active electrodes:

1. *Unipolar: The circuit as shown in **Figure 3***—Current flows from the ESU to the active electrode and then through the patient and passive electrode back to the generator.
2. *Bipolar:* Current flows from the ESU to one arm of the active electrode and then back to the generator through the other arm of the same electrode **(Fig. 4)**.

Electrical Hazards from Surgical Diathermy

Surgical diathermy units discharge high-intensity currents through a pointed tip to a small surface are having a high resistance. The major reported hazards from the diathermy units are explosions and burns, electrocution, cardiac dysrhythmias in patients. When a patient is rendered wet, which commonly happens during surgery, the diathermy current may take different routes other than the grounding pad.

Since the frequency generated by the ESUs is very high, the excitable tissues in human body such as the heart do not get affected by these frequencies and hence do not cause dysrhythmias. However, diathermy produces electromagnetic interference, which can interfere with implanted medical devices in patients such as cardiac pacemakers, implantable cardioverter-defibrillators, and deep-brain stimulators. In such patients, it is advisable to use the bipolar diathermy **(Fig. 4)**. In cases where unipolar diathermy has to be used, it is advisable to place the passive electrode far from the implanted medical device so that the path of the current from the active electrode does not cross the device.

LASERS

LASER is an acronym for *light amplification by stimulated emission of radiation.*

Laser light has some unique properties, which are different to other forms of light. This makes laser significantly more effective than conventional light even if it has the same intensity. The laser light particles are known as photons.

Lasers are usually categorized into three types in accordance with the emission of photons:

1. *Monochromatic:* Laser light consists of a single wavelength or color.
2. *Coherent:* Photons are emitted in phase.
3. *Collimated:* Photons have a parallel alignment, and there is no divergence from the point of origin.

A laser equipment comprises three basic components:

1. *An energy source:* This may be a high-voltage discharge, a chemical reaction, diode, flash lamp or another laser.

2. *A lasing medium:* This may be a solid (crystals and glasses), liquid (dyes or organic solvents), gas (helium and CO_2) or semiconductors. The lasers are usually termed according to the medium.
3. *An optical resonator:* This consists of a cavity containing the lasing medium, with two parallel mirrors on either side. One mirror is highly reflective and the other is partially reflective, which allows a proportion of the light to leave the cavity, which, in turn, becomes the output beam of the laser. This is otherwise known as the output coupler.

How are Lasers Generated?

When energy is applied to an atom, electrons orbiting at low levels of energy may translocate to high-energy orbits causing an excitation of the atom. This process results in "absorption" of energy. Subsequently, when some of the electrons spontaneously return to their low-energy orbits, energy is now released in the form of photons in different wavelengths and directions. This process is known as "emission" of energy. If these random emissions are made to collide by stimulation with the help of the medium and mirrors to form a photon emission of uniform wavelength, direction, phase, and polarity, this process becomes a "stimulated emission" resulting in lasers.

In medicine, lasers are operated in two different modes:

1. Continuous wave where the output is measured as power (watts) and the density is known as "irradiance".
2. Pulsed wave where the output is measured as energy (joules) and the density is known as "fluence".

When the monochromatic laser light comes into contact with the biological tissues, the light can be transmitted, scattered, reflected, or absorbed.

The wavelength of the laser determines its ability to penetrate the tissues—the smaller the wavelength (near the ultraviolet region), the poorer the penetration.

Argon and argon: Fluorine excimer lasers are examples of such smaller wavelength lasers used for ophthalmic procedures.

Some examples of medical lasers are:

- CO_2 laser
- Nd:YAG (neodymium-yttrium-aluminium-garnet) laser
- Ho (holmium):YAG laser
- Diode laser
- Ruby laser
- Argon and argon: Fluorine lasers.

Surgical Lasers

Laser surgery is advantageous in many aspects both to the surgeon and patient. Some of the known advantages include microscopic precision of dissection and a bloodless operative field. However, laser can pose risks to the personnel as well as the patient.

General Safety in Operating Theaters

- Laser surgery should be undertaken only by appropriately and adequately trained surgeons.
- The operating theater should have a prominently visible warning displayed outside during laser surgery and unnecessary traffic should be avoided.
- All theater personnel should wear protective gear including eyewear.
- Training programs should be instituted for theater personnel regarding hazards of laser.
- Laser equipment should clearly display the classification of the hazard; the equipment should be handled only by trained persons and regular maintenance should be in effect.
- Fire extinguisher (nonwater-based) should be available in the theater.

Lasers and Anesthesia

The most commonly reported injury from lasers has been associated with upper airway surgery. Anesthetic agents, oxygen, and the airway equipment as well as the shared airway provide a conducive environment for "airway fires".

There are some recommended measures to avoid airway fires:

Endotracheal Tubes for Airway Surgery

Since laser beams can ignite nonmetallic endotracheal tubes, noncombustible special laser tubes made of stainless steel spiral should be the choice, e.g., Norton tube, Porch tube. If unavailable, regular plastic (PVC) endotracheal tubes should be wrapped with aluminum foil or any similar self-adhesive metal tape.

The cuff of the endotracheal tube should also be filled preferably saline in order to avoid rupture and ignition. Some authors recommend methylene blue to detect rupture. An additional recommendation is to have a twin-cuffed endotracheal tube.

Skin and Eyes for Ophthalmic Surgery

Surgical drapes should not be combustible and the drapes should be flushed to the skin to avoid pockets trapping air or oxidizing agents. Inflammable solutions such as spirit should be avoided for cleaning the skin, or if need to be used, time should be given for complete evaporation.

Moist pads and noninflammable lubricating jellies may be used for eyes as well as facial hair.

Choice of Anesthetic Gases

Although not directly flammable, both nitrous oxide and oxygen support combustion and hence may predispose to laser-induced fire. If oxygen cannot be avoided, FiO_2 of 0.3 with nitrogen and helium may be the best option to use during laser surgery.

Management of Airway Fire

- Inform surgeon to discontinue surgery.
- Discontinue the oxygen supply and use room air for ventilation.
- Remove the "burnt" airway equipment (endotracheal tube, etc.)
- Gently spray or douse water over the burnt tissue in the operating field.
- Endoscopic visualization of the site to remove debris and foreign bodies.
- If there is severe airway edema and inflammation, consider a short course of steroids and/or antimicrobial therapy.
- If severe, consider tracheostomy and critical care support.

SUGGESTED READING

1. Bernstein MS. Isolated power and line isolation monitors. Biomed Instrum Technol. 1990;24:221-3.
2. Buczko GB, McKay WP. Electrical safety in the operating room. Can J Anesth. 1987;34:315-22.
3. Day FJ. Electrical safety revisited: a new wrinkle. Anesthesiology. 1994;80:220-1.
4. Ehrenfeld JM, Hariharan S, Corn SB. Electrical safety. Vacanti's Clinical Anesthesia. Cambridge, United Kingdom: Cambridge University Press; 2010. pp. 149-54.
5. El-Hakim A. TURP in the new century: an analytical reappraisal in light of lasers. Can Urol Assoc J. 2010;4(5):347-9.
6. Fuchshuber P, Jones S, Jones D, Feldman LS, Schwaitzberg S, Rozner MA. Ensuring safety in the operating room: the "fundamental use of surgical energy" (FUSE) program. Int Anesthesiol Clin. 2013;51(4):65-80.
7. Kerr DR, Malhotra IV. Electrical design and safety in the operating room and intensive care unit. Int Anesthesiol Clin. 1981;19:27-48.
8. Litt L. Electrical safety in the operating room. In: Miller RD (Ed). Miller's Anesthesia, 6th edition. Philadelphia: Churchill Livingstone; 2005. pp. 3139-48.
9. Merry AF, Cooper JB, Soyannwo O, Wilson IH, Eichhorn JH. International Standards for a Safe Practice of Anesthesia 2010. Can J Anesth. 2010;57:1027-34.
10. Simpson E. (2012). The basic principles of laser technology, uses and safety measures in anaesthesia. Anaesthesia tutorial of the week 255. [online] Available from http://www.aagbi.org/sites/default/files/255 Basic Principles of Laser Technology.pdf. [Last accessed Oct. 2024].

CHAPTER 10

Equipment for Regional Anesthesia

TVS Gopal

INTRODUCTION

"Regional anesthesia always works, provided you put the right dose of the right drug in the right place" wrote Denny and Harrop-Griffiths in an editorial in the "British Journal of Anesthesia." In pursuit of this simplistic goal, there was reliance on surface anatomical landmarks and paresthesia feedback from the awake patient for successful peripheral nerve blocks. "No paresthesia, no anesthesia," by Danny Moore in 1953, was the prevalent dictum. Multiple attempts to elicit paresthesia, which was perceived as painful, failure rate of nearly 20%, and fears of neurological sequelae prompted search for safer guidance.

The advent of peripheral nerve stimulation (PNS), and later, of ultrasound guidance for regional anesthesia (USGRA) transformed the "art" of nerve blockade into an exact and objective science. While PNS improved reliability by eliciting a muscle twitch to indicate correct perineural placement of the needle, ultrasound guidance offered visualization of needle, nerve, and deposition of local anesthetic solution in real time.

The past few decades witnessed a resurgence in the practice of regional anesthesia and the clinical and economic benefits of nerve blocks have received widespread appreciation. This chapter provides postgraduate students an insight into the equipment utilized for nerve blocks, namely, peripheral nerve stimulators and portable, high-resolution ultrasound.

PERIPHERAL NERVE STIMULATION

History

1912: von Perthes used electrical stimulation for nerve location.

1955: Pearson published a report of a neurostimulator-guided peripheral nerve block with an insulated needle.

1962: Greenblatt and Denson introduced the modern peripheral nerve stimulator.

1969: Koons and Wright modified the Block-Aid monitor for electrical location of peripheral nerves.

Electrophysiology

For optimal use of PNS for nerve blockade, a working knowledge of anatomy and an understanding of related physiology are essential. All human cells have a resting membrane potential of –90 mV. When an electrical charge is applied, nerve and muscle cells are capable of generating an action potential. Nerve stimulation, therefore, implies application of a stimulus in the vicinity of a nerve in order to elicit a twitch of the muscle supplied by that motor nerve, or, paresthesia in case of a sensory nerve.

Strength and Duration of Electrical Stimulus

The minimal current intensity to cause depolarization leading to generation of an action potential in a nerve is defined as *rheobase*. Below this intensity, an action potential is not generated, even if applied for a longer duration. *Chronaxie* is the minimum duration of time current at twice the rheobase must be applied to initiate an impulse. Chronaxie is indicative of excitability of different nerve fibers. Larger and myelinated nerves have shorter chronaxies, hence, easier to stimulate **(Table 1)**.

Electrical stimulation to locate nerves provides for a twitch of effector muscles supplied by motor fibers at lower chronaxie without stimulating unmyelinated, sensory C fibers, thereby avoiding pain.

Frequency

Frequency refers to the number of repeating events per unit time. It is measured as 1, 2, or 3 MHz. The implication is that, at a selected frequency, many stimuli per second will be delivered to the target nerve. For example, at a frequency of 1 MHz, one stimulus per second is delivered from the needle tip. It is imperative to advance the needle toward the target nerve slowly so that the possibility of a stimulus after passing the nerve is minimized.

Pattern of Stimulus

A monophasic stimulus is applied as a square wave with rapid rising time to prevent the phenomenon of accommodation, wherein the application of stimulus which rises slowly reduces excitability of nerve by increasing the threshold for generation of an action potential.

TABLE 1: Chronaxie: indicative of excitability of different nerve fibers.

Nerve	*Function*	*Chronaxie*
Myelinated A α fibers	Motor	50–100 µs
Myelinated A δ fibers	Pain, temperature	150–170 µs
Unmyelinated C fibers	Pain	400 µs

Electrical Polarity

When negative current is applied to the surface of a nerve, there is resultant depolarization leading to generation of an action potential. Conversely, when positive current is delivered, hyperpolarization ensues, with the result that much larger currents are required to bring about an action potential. For electrical location of nerves, the needle and the return electrode, which is attached to the skin, are electrodes. Cathodal (negative) stimulation is preferred, wherein the negative electrode is connected to the stimulating needle. The positive electrode (anode) is attached to the patient, at any distance from the needle insertion site. It is better remembered as: *Negative to needle, + Positive to patient.*

Needle-to-Nerve Distance

Coulomb's law governs the equation between intensity of current to elicit a muscle twitch and distance of needle from the target nerve:

$$I = k\,(i/r2)$$

where (I) is the intensity of current, (k) is a constant, (i) is the minimal current, and (r) is the distance of the needle from the nerve. If this formula is rearranged, it is apparent that (i), the minimum current becomes directly proportional to the square of distance (r). Hence, at a greater distance from the nerve, the minimum current required for excitation is higher. As the needle approaches the nerve, a muscle twitch can be elicited at lower intensity **(Figs. 1A and B)**.

In clinical practice, a current of 1.0–1.5 mA is set initially at a pulse width of 0.1 ms. The needle is gradually advanced toward the nerve till effective muscle twitch is obtained at 0.4–0.5 mA. The current is further reduced to 0.2 mA at which the twitch must disappear. Continued twitch at 0.2 mA is most likely to indicate intraneural placement of needle.

Current Density

This term refers to distribution of current per cross-sectional area. As soon as 0.5–1.0 mL of local anesthetic solution is injected, the muscle twitch ceases, this being appreciated as the positive Raj test. Solutions that conduct electricity such as saline and local anesthetics increase conductive area at the needle tip. This causes lowered density requiring a higher threshold to elicit muscle response. Injection of a nonconductive solution like 5% dextrose in water maintains current density; hence, the muscle response is sustained.

Uninsulated needles being composed of bare metal have a diffuse distribution of current along the entire shaft and tip. The conductive area is large and the density of current at the tip is low necessitating higher intensity of current for effective stimulation. Insulated needles have the entire shaft

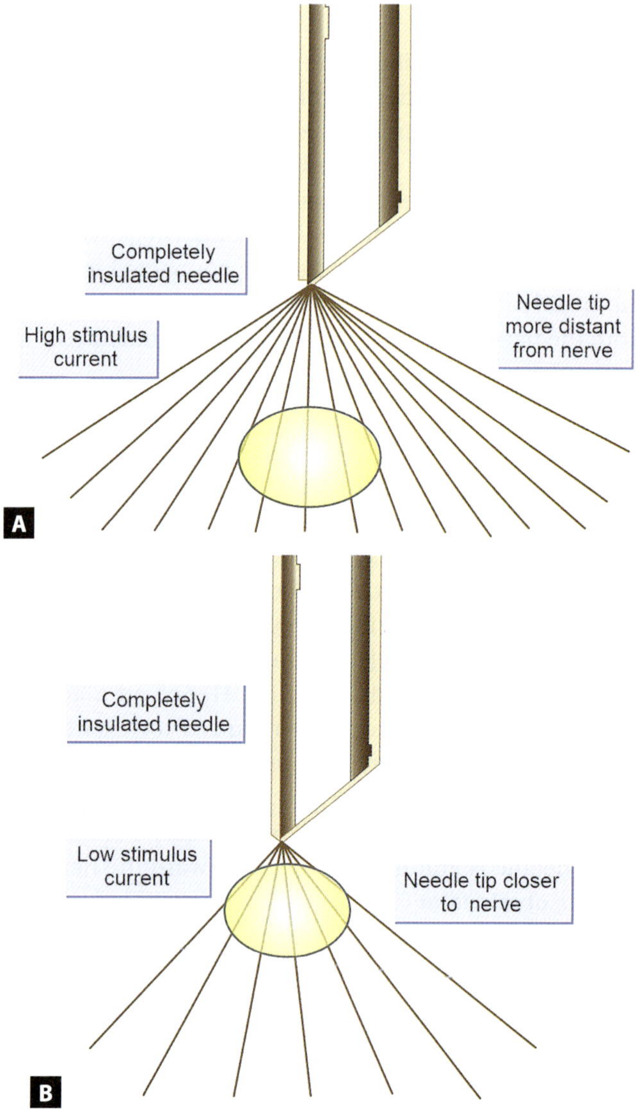

Figs. 1A and B: (A) Peripheral nerve stimulation. Needle away from nerve; (B) Peripheral nerve stimulation. Needle in proximity to nerve.

covered by a layer of nonconductive material such as polytetrafluoroethylene (PTFE) or silicon. The conductive area is concentrated at the uncoated needle tip. As a result, muscle response is achieved at lower currents **(Figs. 2A and B)**.

PERIPHERAL NERVE STIMULATOR

Modern day peripheral nerve stimulators are portable, compact, battery-operated, user-friendly devices that deliver adjustable, low-energy current at

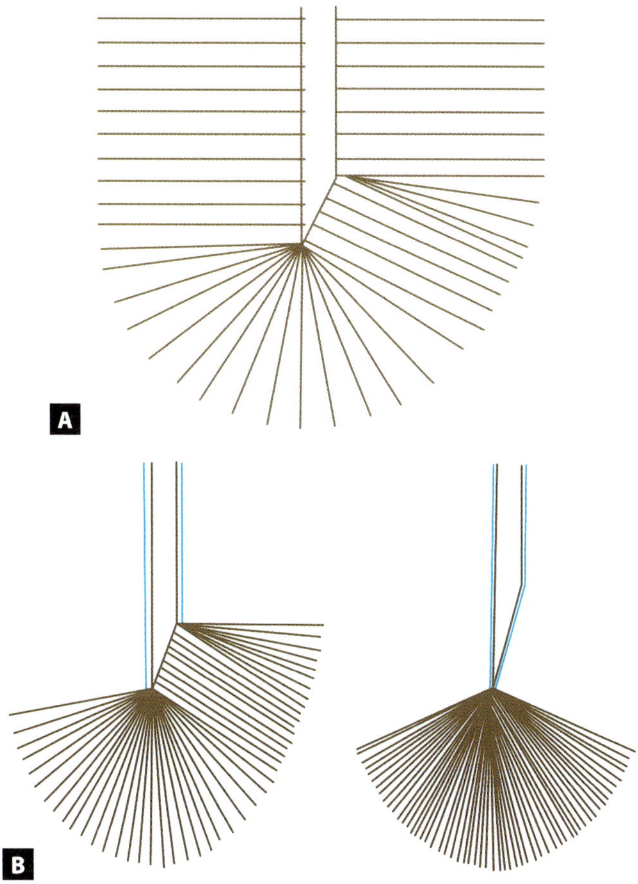

Figs. 2A and B: (A) Uninsulated needle; (B) Insulated needle with bare tip and coated tip.

a set duration, and frequency to facilitate nerve location. The nerve stimulator is broadly composed of the following parts **(Fig. 3)**:

- *Clock reference:* Which synchronizes various functions of the device.
- *Microcontroller:* It is the "brain" of the nerve stimulator. It receives inputs from the controls and adjusts output accordingly.
- *Constant current generator:* Delivers the same current in the face of altering impedance.
- *Display panel:* Bright and liquid crystal display of adjustable variables and safety features.
- *Controls:* Frequency, duration of stimulus or pulse width, and current intensity are placed on the display panel.

Desirable Features of the Peripheral Nerve Stimulator

- *Constant current output:* Ohm's law governs the relationship between current output and resistance offered. Modern nerve stimulators are

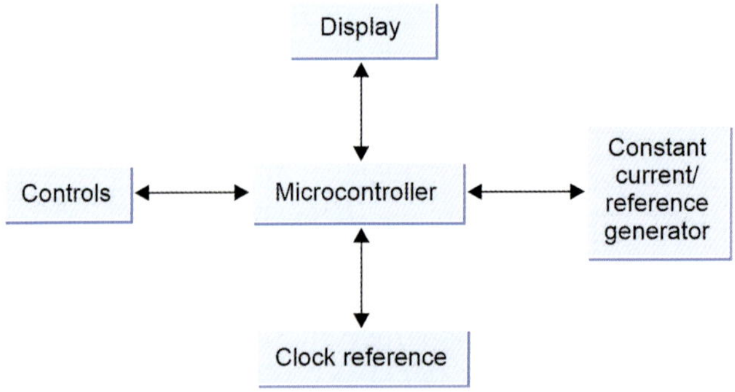

Fig. 3: Basic components of peripheral nerve stimulator.

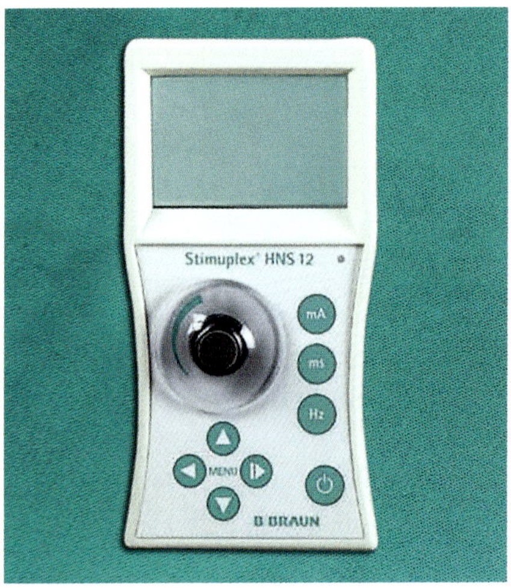

Fig. 4: Peripheral nerve stimulator (HNS 12 B Braun).

engineered to deliver constant current in the face of impedance offered by tissues, needles, connecting wires, and grounding electrodes.

- *Accurate current display:* Of the current delivered to the patient during the procedure.
- *Provision for adjustable stimulus intensity:* Either an analog dial or digital means. The range is from 0.00 mA to 5.00 mA.
- *Duration of stimulus* is adjustable from 0.1 to 1.0 ms.
- *Frequency:* Most new machines offer a choice of 1, 2, and 3 MHz.
- A monophasic, square-wave stimulus is desired.
- *Disconnect indicator:* When the circuit is complete, a green light flashes intermittently. A red flashing light indicates disconnection of the circuit and alerts the operator.
- *Low battery indicator:* A visual/audible alarm is usually incorporated.
- **Figure 4** shows the Braun nerve stimulator and **Figure 5** shows the PNS with complete circuit.

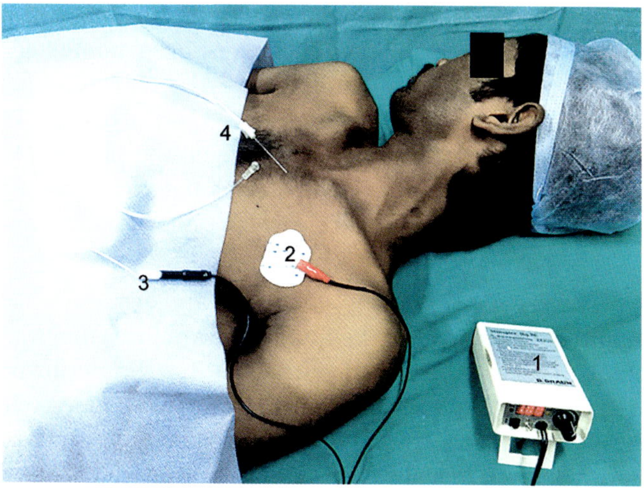

Fig. 5: Complete circuit. (1: Peripheral nerve stimulator; 2: Grounding electrode (Anode); 3: Cathode to needle; 4: Insulated block needle).

Recommended Practice

- Proper patient's positioning
- Aseptic precautions
- Working knowledge of block-related anatomy
- Patient's monitoring and drugs/equipment for resuscitation
- Fifty- or 100-mm insulated block needle depending on depth of nerve from skin
- An initial current of 1.0–1.5 mA as per depth of nerve from skin.
- Frequency of 2 MHz.
- Pulse duration of 0.1 ms.
- Ensure circuit is complete, cathode or negative electrode to stimulating needle, and anode or positive lead to grounding electrode.
- Once muscle twitch is elicited, the current intensity is reduced from 1.0 mA while maintaining twitch at 0.4–0.5 mA.
- When the current is lowered to 0.2 mA, there must not be a twitch. If present, it may indicate intraneural placement of needle. The needle is slightly withdrawn to confirm presence of muscle twitch at 0.4 mA and absence at 0.2 mA.
- The twitch disappears within 0.5–1.0 mL injection of local anesthetic solution (positive Raj test).
- Slow, fractionated injection of local anesthetic with intermittent aspiration while the needle is held steady without inadvertent displacement.

ULTRASOUND-GUIDED REGIONAL ANESTHESIA

Though the objective of eliciting a muscle twitch with electrical stimulation to denote correct perineural location of the needle was often achieved, problems with electrical stimulation did persist. Instances of partial block or failure despite a twitch, or inability to elicit a response, reinforced the credo that blocks with electrical stimulation were essentially blind procedures, and variations in human anatomy contributed to the failure. The advent of ultrasound, as a guidance tool, has redefined the practice of regional anesthesia owing to the ability to visualize nerves and surrounding structures, the advancing needle, and the spread of local anesthetic solution in real time.

History

La Grange and colleagues were the first to use an ultrasonographic blood flow detector to locate the subclavian artery for the performance of a supraclavicular brachial plexus block in 1978. As ultrasound technology at that time was limited, this was, however, an indirect application. The first reported series of direct visualization of the supraclavicular brachial plexus was by Stephen Kapral et al., in 1994. Thereafter, significant improvement in technology increased the popularity of ultrasound among anesthesiologists for peripheral nerve blockade, and, at present, for neuraxial blocks and chronic pain procedures. Today, after more than a decade of widespread use, USGRA is the universal "gold standard."

Basic Physics of Ultrasound

Sound audible by the human ear is in the range of 20–20,000 Hz (20 kHz). Any sound that exceeds 20 kHz is ultrasound. Typically, medical ultrasound machines emit sound waves in a frequency range of 2–20 MHz (1,000 kHz is 1 MHz). Ultrasound is a form of mechanical sound energy that is propagated through a biological medium, i.e., the human tissue, as a longitudinal wave with alternating areas of compression and rarefaction **(Fig. 6)**. The average velocity of ultrasound in human tissue is said to be 1,540 m/s, the slowest speed being 500 m/s through air-filled lung, and the highest is 4,000 m/s through bone.

When an alternating current, i.e., electric signal is applied to the array of piezoelectric crystals that line the patient's end of a transducer, there is distortion and agitation of these crystals, thus, setting off an ultrasound beam. This transduction of electrical to mechanical (sound) energy is the "converse piezoelectric effect." The returning beam, also known as the "echo" is transduced to electrical energy by the piezoelectric crystals, and this

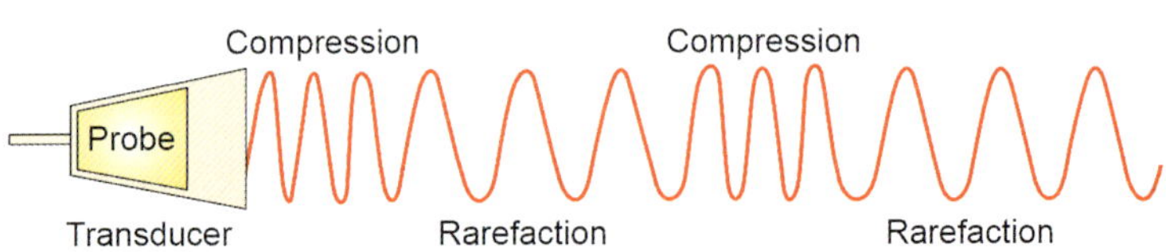

Fig. 6: The ultrasound wave.

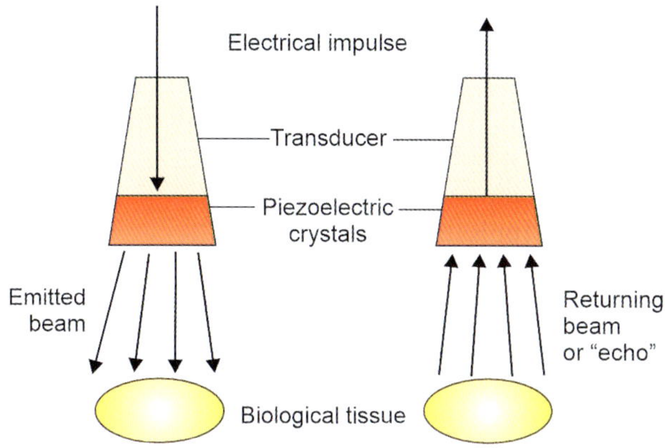

Fig. 7: Transduction of energy.

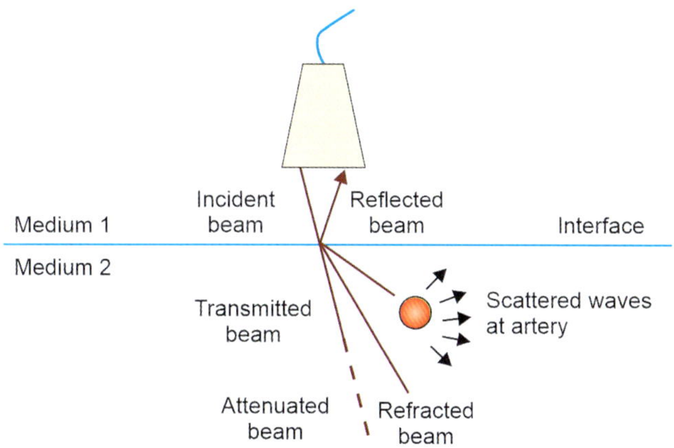

Fig. 8: Interaction of ultrasound beam at tissue interface.

conversion from sound to electrical energy is called the "piezoelectric effect" **(Fig. 7)**. This electric signal is transmitted to the screen to be displayed as a two-dimensional (2D) image in real time. In modern ultrasound machines, this process repeats itself at a rate exceeding 7,000 times per second, so as to give a seamless image.

The ultrasound beam, within the biological tissue, has several interactions **(Fig. 8)**. Any of the following are possible:

- *Transmission:* The beam passes through the tissue. As it progresses, the amplitude of the original signal becomes weaker; this process is known as "attenuation."
- *Refraction:* A change in the direction of the transmitted beam.
- *Scatter:* The beam is weakened and scattered in different directions when it encounters an interface that is small or irregular.
- *Reflection:* Most of the incident beam is reflected back to the transducer by a structure with smooth interface.

Echogenicity is the term used to describe the brightness, or darkness, of tissues relative to other structures in the field of vision. When the structure is brighter than surrounding tissues, it is said to be hyperechoic. If it is darker than surrounding tissues, it is hypoechoic. Blood vessels appear totally dark, i.e., anechoic **(Figs. 9A and B)**.

- *Veins:* Anechoic (compressible with transducer)
- *Arteries:* Anechoic (pulsatile)
- *Muscles:* Hypoechoic tissue with intermittent bright striae
- *Bone:* Hyperechoic curved rim with dark shadow beneath
- *Nerves:* Hyperechoic/hypoechoic.

As a general rule, nerves above clavicle appear as dark, whereas they are bright below the clavicle. Closer to the neuraxis, there is hardly any connective tissue, and as nerves travel farther, more and more connective tissue is added, thereby giving the nerve a speckled and bright appearance. It is obvious that connective tissue imparts brightness to the nerve **(Figs. 10 and 11)**.

The transducer (probe) both emits the ultrasound beam and receives the returning beam (echo) **(Fig. 12)**. The transducer is placed on the patient, and the area of the probe that makes contact with the skin surface is the footprint. Basically, there are high-frequency and low-frequency transducers. High-frequency transducers provide an excellent image quality (spatial resolution) at the cost of limited tissue penetration. Low-frequency probes emit ultrasound waves that penetrate deeper, but the spatial resolution is low, i.e., the quality of image is poorer **(Fig. 13)**. Modern broad bandwidth transducers are capable of generating ultrasound waves at more than one frequency depending on the field of interest, e.g., a curved transducer emits waves between 2 and 5 MHz, and a high-frequency linear transducer between 13 and 6 MHz. With the exception of preprocedural scanning for neuraxial blocks in adults, lumbar plexus and gluteal/subgluteal sciatic nerve blocks, high-frequency transducers will suffice for all other nerve/plexus blocks.

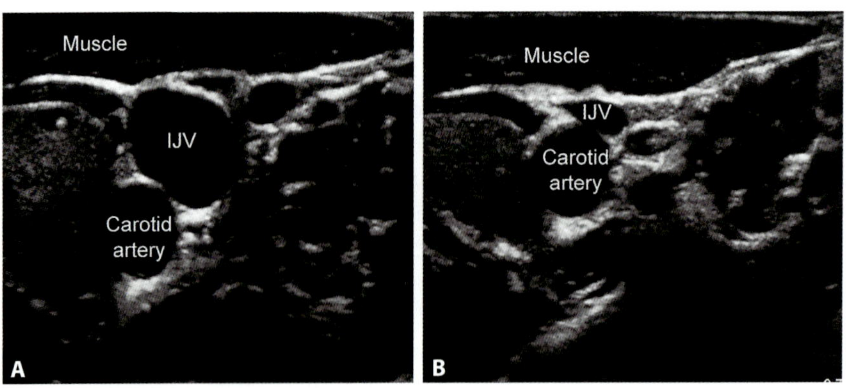

Figs. 9A and B: Artery, vein, and muscle. (IJV: internal jugular vein)

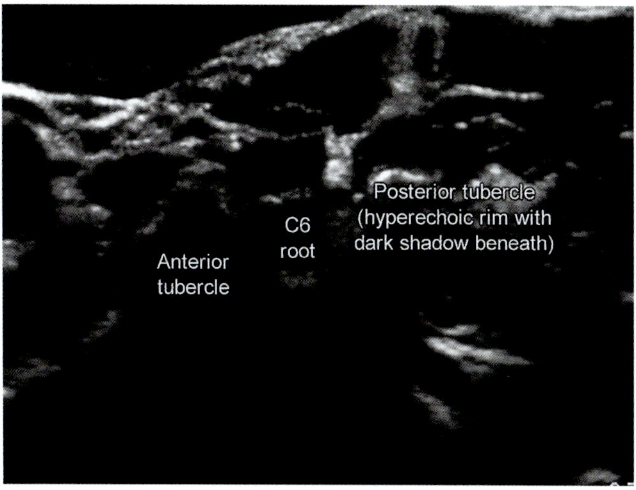

Fig. 10: Nerve above clavicle appearing as dark ring.

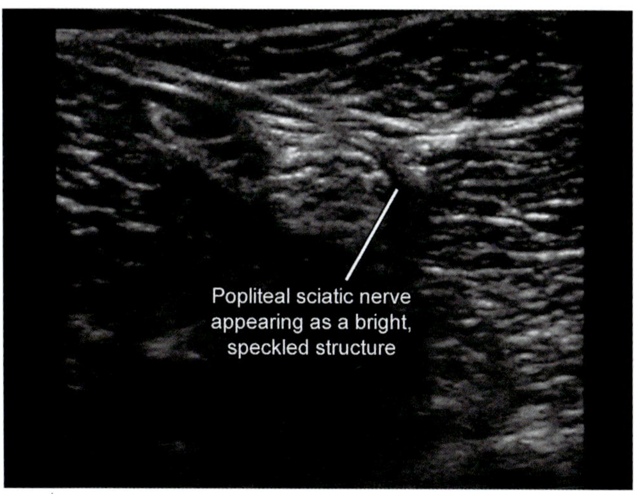

Fig. 11: Popliteal sciatic nerve.

Image resolution refers to the clarity of image, in simple terms. It is defined as the ability of the ultrasound machine to distinguish two closely located structures as distinctly separate. Spatial resolution is governed by axial and lateral resolution. Axial resolution is for structures that lie along the path of the ultrasound beam. Higher the frequency, better the axial resolution. Lateral resolution refers to objects that lie perpendicular to the ultrasound beam. Higher the frequency, shorter the wavelength, and width of the beam and greater the lateral resolution. Lateral resolution is best at the focal zone, where the beam width is most narrow **(Fig. 14)**.

Doppler technology permits identification and quantification of blood flow. When an emitted ultrasound beam strikes red blood cells within a

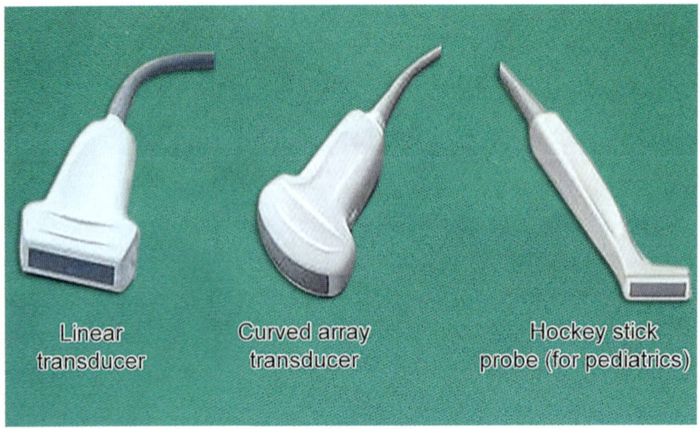

Fig. 12: Types of transducers.

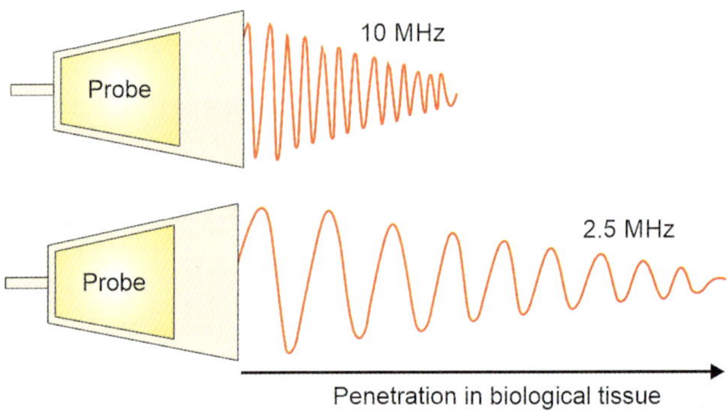

Fig. 13: High-frequency versus low-frequency probes.

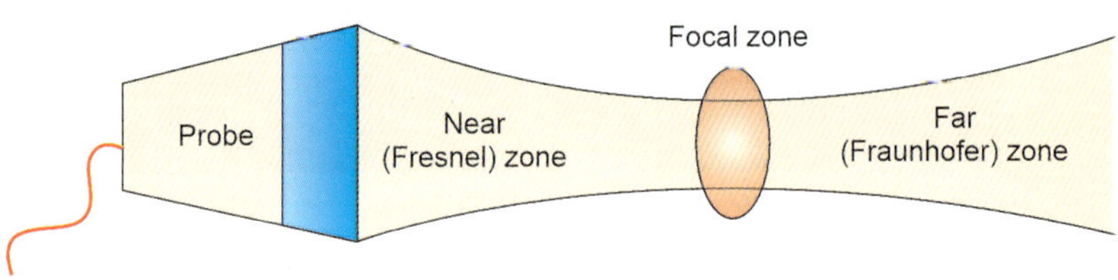

Fig. 14: Typical ultrasound beam.

vessel, the frequency of the returning signal depends on the flow, either toward, or away from the transducer. If the flow is toward the transducer, the frequency of the returning signal is higher, and the vessel appears as red. When the flow is away from the transducer, the frequency of the returning signal is lower, and the vessel appears as blue **(Fig. 15)**. The difference in returning signal frequency, relative to that of the emitted signal, is the Doppler shift. Therefore, all arteries are *not* red, and all veins are *not* blue with color Doppler. It is important for the regional anesthesiologist to identify arteries

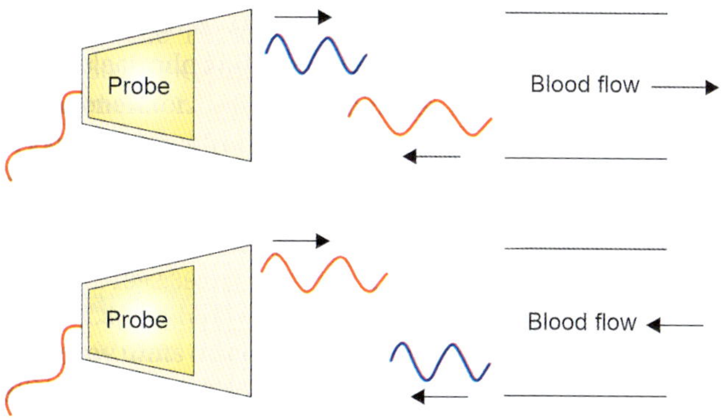

Fig. 15: The Doppler effect.

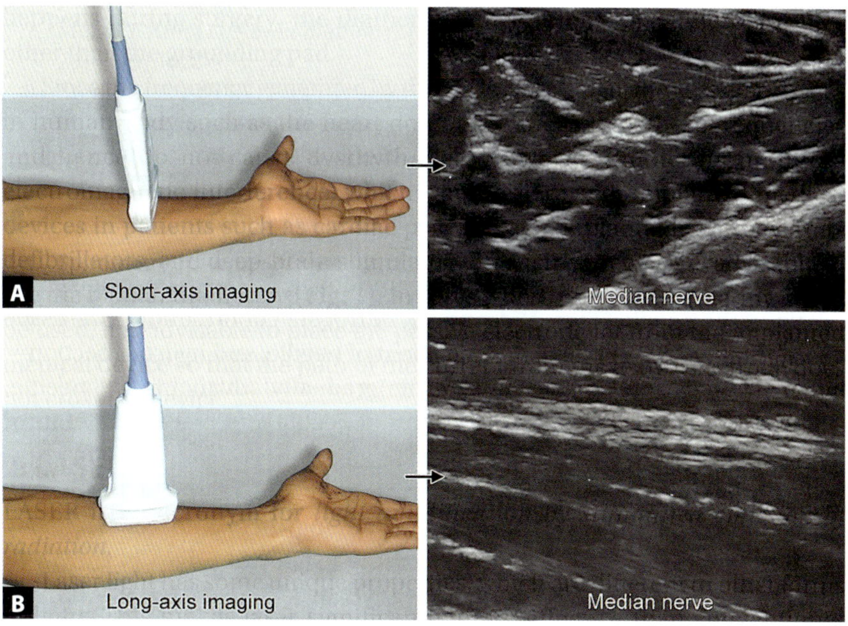

Figs. 16A and B: Planes for nerve imaging.

and veins because nerves often lie in proximity to vessels, "It is useful to remember the pneumonic, BART—Blue Away Red Toward."

Nerves can be imaged either in short (transverse) or long (sagittal) axis **(Figs. 16A and B)**. For all practical purposes, nerves are imaged in short axis. Long axis imaging is useful for confirmation of drug spread along the nerve. Needles may be placed in line with the ultrasound beam—in plane approach, or across the ultrasound beam—out of plane approach. If the needle is aligned along the 1 mm thickness of the ultrasound beam, the entire shaft of the needle should be visible as it is being advanced in plane. With the out of plane approach, only that part of needle that transects the ultrasound

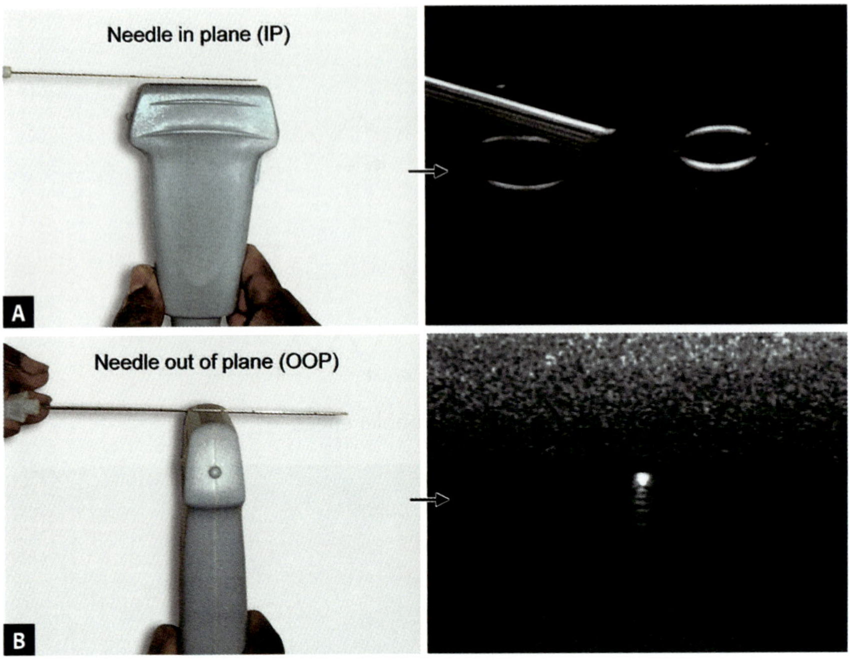

Figs. 17A and B: Image of needle in relation to ultrasound field.

beam is seen on the screen as a hyperechoic dot and is not to be mistaken for the tip of the needle **(Figs. 17A and B)**. Surrogate confirmation, viz., tissue displacement with sharp, short movement of needle, and hydrodissection—injecting small volumes of saline while gradually advancing the needle, is advised to ensure perineural location of needle and placement of local anesthetic solution.

Modern ultrasound machines are lightweight and handheld. In addition to portability that enables "point of care" scanning, there is no fear of ionizing radiation. A portable ultrasound machine (Sonosite Edge) is shown in **Figure 18**. Storage and transmission of data is an advantage that allows these machines to be used as teaching tools, thereby popularizing the practice of regional anesthesia with certainty and precision. Specifically for regional anesthesia, the machines incorporate a "nerve" preset that optimizes settings for better visualization of neural structures.

As mentioned earlier, a linear high-frequency transducer will suffice for most blocks in adults. In certain machines, once a transducer is selected, by toggling with the Resolution, General, or Penetration button, high, mid, or low range of frequency of that particular broad bandwidth transducer may be preferentially selected. All transducers have a prefixed label on one side that corresponds with an orientation marker (a blue dot or the logo of the manufacturer) on the top left corner of the screen. Transducer orientation is essential to maintain uniformity such that sidedness of structures displayed

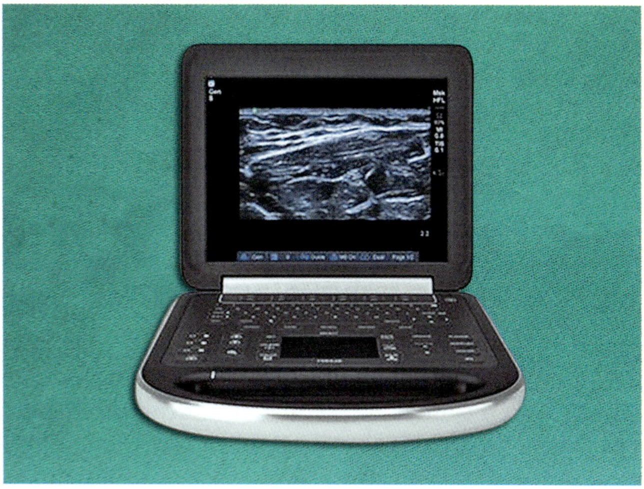

Fig. 18: Portable ultrasound machine (Sonosite Edge).

on screen is constant. Some gel is applied on the transducer and a finger placed on one end to make a movement. If the movement corresponds with the orientation marker, that side of the transducer is placed to the right of the patient in short axis, and head end of the patient in long axis.

The depth is adjusted such that the structure of interest is located at the center of the screen. Time gain compensation (TGC) is akin to contrast function of a television set, and selectively amplifies returning echoes from greater depths, so as to present a homogenous image on the screen. An autogain button facilitates the TGC setting with minimal effort. In machines that have focus setting, focus is set at the structure of interest to maximize lateral resolution. Modern machines have inbuilt software to archive both images and movie clips that can be retrieved and transmitted when necessary.

Peripheral nerve stimulators and ultrasound ensure safety, precision, and reliability of nerve/plexus blocks. Combining the two guidance techniques offers dual endpoints, a muscle twitch to signify exact perineural placement of needle, and visual observation of needle and pattern of drug distribution. There is a learning curve involved for both modalities, more so for ultrasound, because it entails comprehension of terminology alien to anesthetists. However, given the wide range of applications of relevance to anesthesiology, familiarity with ultrasound guidance, especially from the postgraduate level of training, is encouraged.

SUGGESTED READING

1. Brull R, Macfarlane AJ, Tse CC. Practical knobology for ultrasound-guided regional anesthesia. Reg Anesth Pain Med. 2010;35(2 Suppl):S68-73.
2. Frazer RS. Regional blockade: training and the use of nerve stimulators. Reg Anesth. 1993;18(3):199-200.

3. Gray AT. Ultrasound-guided regional anesthesia: current state of the art. Anesthesiology. 2006;104(2):368-73, discussion 5A.
4. Hadzic A, Vloka J, Hadzic N, Thys DM, Santos AC. Nerve stimulators used for peripheral nerve blocks vary in their electrical characteristics. Anesthesiology. 2003;98(4):969-74.
5. Hadzic A. Peripheral nerve stimulators, cracking the code—one at a time. Reg Anesth Pain Med. 2004;29(3):185-8.
6. Klein SM, Melton MS, Grill WM, Nielsen KC. Peripheral nerve stimulation in regional anesthesia—review article. Reg Anesth Pain Med. 2012;37(4):383-92.
7. Marhofer P, Chan VW. Ultrasound-guided regional anesthesia: current concepts and future trends. Anesth Analg. 2007;104(5):1265-9.
8. Marhofer P, Greher M, Kapral S. Ultrasound guidance in regional anaesthesia. Br J Anaesth. 2005;94(1):7-17.
9. Marhofer P, Harrop-Griffiths W, Kettner SC, Kirchmair L. Fifteen years of ultrasound guidance in regional anaesthesia: Part I. Br J Anaesth. 2010;104(5): 538-46.
10. Marhofer P, Harrop-Griffiths W, Willschke H, Kirchmair L. Fifteen years of ultrasound guidance in regional anaesthesia: Part II. Br J Anaesth. 2010;104(6): 673-83.
11. Mehrkens HH, Geiger PM. Peripheral regional anaesthesia—tutorial in the Ulm Rehabilitation Hospital, expanded third edition; 2005.
12. Moore DC. "No paresthesias-no anesthesia," the nerve stimulator or neither? Reg Anesth. 1997;22(4):388-90.
13. Tsui BCH, Hadzic A. Chapter 5: Peripheral nerve stimulators and electrophysiology of nerve stimulation. In: Tsui BCH, Hadzic A (Eds). Textbook of Anesthesia and Acute Pain Management. New York: McGraw Hill; 2007.
14. Pither CE, Raj PP, Ford DJ. The use of peripheral nerve stimulators for regional anesthesia: a review of experimental characteristics, technique and clinical applications. Reg Anesth. 1985;10:49-58.
15. Sites BD, Brull R, Chan VW, Spence BC, Gallagher J, Beach ML, et al. Artifacts and pitfall errors associated with ultrasound-guided regional anesthesia. Part I: understanding the basic principles of ultrasound physics and machine operations. Reg Anesth Pain Med. 2007;32(5):412-8.
16. Sites BD, Brull R, Chan VW, Spence BC, Gallagher J, Beach ML, et al. Artifacts and pitfall errors associated with ultrasound-guided regional anesthesia. Part II: a pictorial approach to understanding and avoidance. Reg Anesth Pain Med. 2010;35(2 Suppl):S81-92.

CHAPTER 11

Central Neuraxial Block (Anesthesia)

Athma Prasanna, Yasodananda K Areti

HISTORY

Although the needle for subarachnoid injection was invented in 1886, the approach to reach cerebrospinal fluid (CSF) in the spinal cord (lumbar puncture) was described in 1896. The first administration of medication (cocaine) into the CSF in humans was performed by Augustus Beir in 1898. Bier used himself as a subject in experimenting with spinals and was first to report headache following spinal. Paraplegia complicating spinal on Albert Woolley and Cecil Roe, healthy middle-aged men, for minor surgery in 1947 and the litigation surrounding the issue had devastating effects in the use of spinal anesthesia in the United Kingdom.

Lumbar epidural anesthesia in humans was first described by Pagés in 1921, the loss-of-resistance technique by Dogliotti in the 1930s, continuous caudal for obstetrics by Hingson in 1941, and lumbar epidural catheterization for surgery by Curbelo in 1947. The use of epidural morphine was first reported by Behar in 1979.

DEFINITION

Regional anesthesia is a broad term used to denote anesthesia affecting a localized part of the body, such as a limb or half of the body and can be divided into central and peripheral techniques. *Central neuraxial anesthesia* comprises spinal anesthesia (subarachnoid block) and epidural anesthesia. The local anesthetics are placed around the nerves, in the subarachnoid space for spinal anesthesia, and in the epidural space for epidural anesthesia/analgesia **(Fig. 1)**. The combined spinal-epidural technique (CSE) has become increasingly popular in recent years. It can be defined as the intentional injection of drug into the subarachnoid space and the placement of a catheter into the epidural space as part of the same procedure. The advantage of the CSE is that neuraxial block can be achieved rapidly using the spinal component while the epidural catheter can be used to prolong or modify the block.

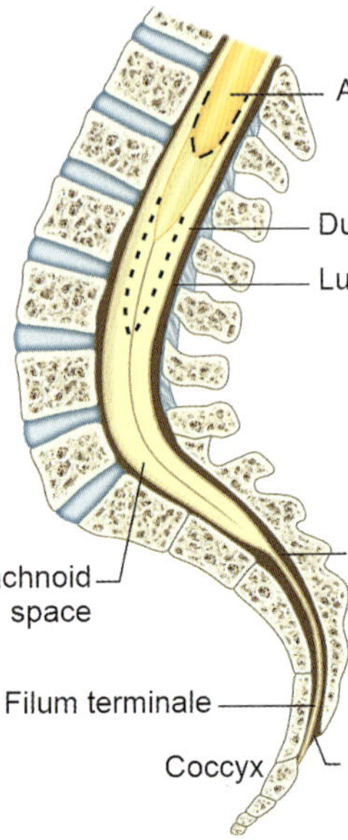

Fig. 1: Diagrammatic representation of epidural and subarachnoid space.

ANATOMY

Subarachnoid Space

The spinal cord is surrounded by pia mater, arachnoid mater, and dura mater. The subarachnoid space is the anatomic space between the arachnoid mater and pia mater. It surrounds the brain in the cranial cavity and extends up to S1–S2 level in the vertebral canal. The spinal cord originates at the foramen magnum of the skull and the brainstem and extends caudally to the conus medullaris. The distal termination varies from the level of the 3rd lumbar vertebrae (L3) in infants to the lower border of L1 in adults. The subarachnoid space is occupied by spongy tissue consisting of trabeculae (delicate connective tissue filaments that extend from the arachnoid mater and blend into the pia mater) and intercommunicating channels in which the CSF, the spinal nerves and blood vessels supplying the spinal cord are confined.

The total volume of CSF is 150 mL and it buoys the central nervous system (CNS) protecting it from injury. The CSF is formed by the choroid plexus (50%) and directly from the walls of the ventricles (50%) at a rate of approximately 500 mL/day.

Epidural Space

This is the space between dural sheath and spinal canal. It is bounded cranially by the foramen magnum, caudally by the sacrococcygeal ligament covering the sacral hiatus, anteriorly by the posterior longitudinal ligament, laterally by the vertebral pedicles, and posteriorly by both the ligamentum flavum and vertebral laminae. The epidural space is a potential space (with ability to expand) with rigid confines and contains fat, extradural veins, lymphatics, and segmental arteries. The epidural anesthesia can be divided into cervical, thoracic, lumbar and sacral or caudal epidural depending on the vertebral space selected. The division applies to all age groups.

Blood Supply

Arterial

The blood supply to the spinal cord is divided into anterior and posterior spinal arteries in addition to radiculospinal arterial branches. All these branches arise from vertebral artery. Sometimes, the radiculospinal artery branches may arise directly from the aorta. Of these, the largest is the artery of Adamkiewicz, which supplies much of blood flow to anterior spinal artery. The anterior spinal artery supplies to the anterior two-thirds of the spinal cord. The two posterior spinal arteries supply to the posterior one-third of the spinal cord. The radicular arteries enter every intervertebral foramen and supply the spinal nerve roots.

Venous Drainage

There are two veins, anterior spinal and posterior spinal veins to the spinal cord which drain into the vertebral veins.

INDICATIONS FOR NEURAXIAL BLOCKS

Both subarachnoid and epidural techniques can be used within the operating room as a sole anesthetic or in combination with general anesthesia (GA), providing optimal anesthesia for procedures involving lower limbs, pelvis, perineum, and lower abdomen. In addition, epidural technique is also often used for surgeries on thorax and sometimes on cervical regions. The spinal segments to be blocked for various surgical procedures are indicated in **Table 1**.

Epidural analgesia can be used outside the operating rooms to reduce the postoperative pain following surgery of the lower limbs, perineum, pelvis, abdomen, and thorax or in chronic pain management of certain intractable pains including pain due to cancer.

The epidural anesthesia is commonly used as a continuous anesthesia by the placement of an epidural catheter, making it suitable for surgical procedures of long duration. Subarachnoid block is commonly performed as a single injection technique, and continuous spinal anesthesia (CSA) is used relatively infrequently. CSE is a combination of single shot spinal with continuous epidural catheter technique.

TABLE 1: Spinal segments to be blocked for various surgical procedures.

Cervical	C-3 to T-1
Thoracic	T-2 to T-12
Upper abdominal	T-4 to L-1
Lower abdomen	T-10 to L-1
Perineum	T-10 to S-4
Lower limbs	T-12 to S-4
Renal	T-6 to L-1
Hip	T-12 to L-3
Lower abdominal and gynecology	T-10 to L-5

CONTRAINDICATIONS

The contraindications for neuraxial blocks are classified as *absolute* (cannot be performed, also called rule of thumb) and *relative* (requiring the discretion of the performer).

Absolute

- *Patient's refusal:* The success of this technique is dependent on the cooperation of the patient in conjunction with communication and technical skill of the performer.
- *Sepsis and local infection:* Patients with either generalized or local area sepsis or infection may be prone to develop meningitis.
- *Coagulopathy:* Patients with deranged coagulation are at risk of developing hematoma with or without neural compression.
- *Raised intracranial pressure:* Patients are at risk of herniation of brain.
- *Hypovolemia, shock, and myocardial dysfunction:* Patients with these conditions may be at risk of exaggerated cardiovascular response.

Relative

- *Undocumented preexisting neurological disease:* Patients with these conditions may pose a medicolegal problem to the performer.
- *Vertebral skeletal anomaly or deformities (congenital/acquired/documented):* Patients with these conditions pose a technical problem and depend on the skill of the performer.
- *Postvertebral skeletal surgery (post laminectomy):* Patients with these conditions pose a technical problem and depend on the skill of the performer.

TECHNIQUE OF PERFORMING NEURAXIAL BLOCKS

The success of administration of subarachnoid anesthesia is dependent on meticulous following of the *four principles (Ps)*: *Preparation* (patient and performer), *position* (patient and performer), *projection* (equipment and asepsis), and *puncture.*

Preparation

Patient

Proper selection of patient is of utmost importance. It is mandatory to discuss the details of subarachnoid procedure with the patient, including the risks and benefits prior to obtaining consent. The consent is to be obtained from the patient preoperatively either at the preanesthesia evaluation clinic or during the preanesthetic evaluation on the previous evening of surgery. *At the time of obtaining consent, the patient should have a chance to understand the procedure and hence, it is not a good practice to obtain consent in the preoperative preparation room just prior to the administration of the procedure.*

In case of minors or mentally challenged and very elderly patients, the discussion and consent should be made by the parent or the guardian. It is advisable to explain the sequence of events that may happen while performing the technique to patients of all age groups including the mentally challenged with the help of the parent or the guardian. This will not only allay the fear complex but facilitates the cooperation of the patient.

Performer

It is advisable to plan in advance, the technique of providing surgical anesthesia, spinal or epidural, single shot or continuous catheter technique. It is also important to plan ahead as to whether the drug is to be deposited as intermittent boluses or through continuous infusion.

The patient is to be wheeled into preanesthesia preparation room or operating room, depending on the institutional practice after premedication with an anxiolytic. It is mandatory to document the baseline hemodynamic monitoring prior to obtaining an intravenous access in the nondominant hand for infusion of an appropriate electrolyte solution.

Position

Patient

It is well documented that the success of the block is dependent on the proper positioning of the patient. Some of the factors which would influence the difficulty of positioning may be lack of understanding the rationale of proper position by the assistant, inability of the patient to follow the instructions properly, or sedation administered to allay anxiety.

The technique of subarachnoid anesthesia can be performed either in the lateral decubitus or sitting positions. Epidural anesthesia technique can be performed in the lateral decubitus, sitting or prone positions. The choice of the position is dependent on the comfort level of the performer and the patient. The position adopted could be maintained with the help of an operating room assistant. In the absence of an assistant, commercially available mechanical aids may be useful.

Lateral Decubitus Position (Fig. 2)

The left or right decubitus position is adopted depending on the comfort of the patient, performer, and the surgical requirement. This position allows the anesthetist to administer sedation with less dependence on an assistant for positioning. It also is comfortable to the majority of patients except in obstetrics undergoing lower segment cesarean section. The patient is positioned with their back parallel to the side edge of the operating table. Both the thighs of the patient are flexed up to the abdomen, with neck flexed over the anterior chest wall to assume fetal position. It is essential to support the neck and head with a pillow in this position. The decubitus position is preferred in children, since the technique is often performed under GA.

Sitting Position (Fig. 3)

Sitting position is advocated in obese, morbidly obese, full-term obstetric patients, and in patients with abnormal anatomical curvatures of the spine. The pendulous pad of fat in obese and morbidly obese patients poses a challenge to identify the landmarks in decubitus position. It is recommended to support both the feet on a firm surface (e.g., a stool), and does not allow

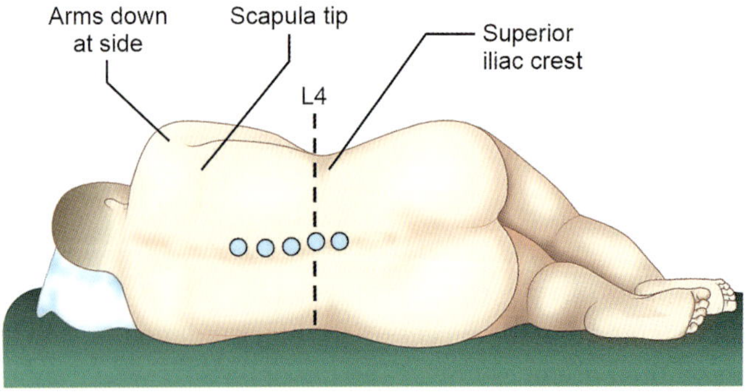

Fig. 2: Lateral position and landmarks for neuraxial blocks.

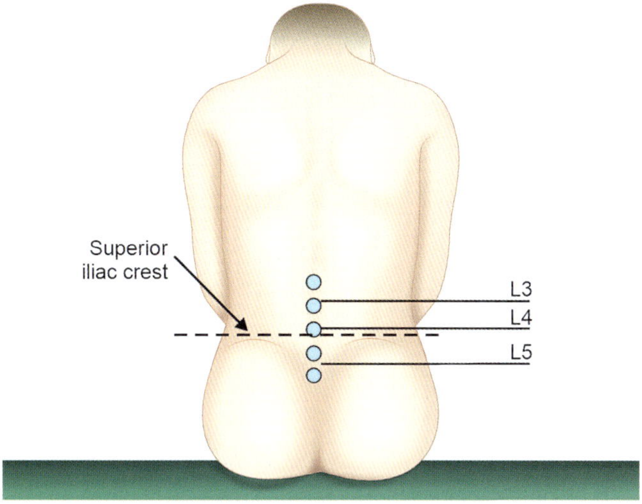

Fig. 3: Sitting position and landmarks for neuraxial blocks.

the patients' feet to dangle without support. The patient hugs a pillow or a mechanical support in front and the head is flexed over the support. A description to arch the back to resemble the English alphabet C may help the patient to understand the position to assume. This maneuver will maximize the "opening" of the vertebral interspaces. The proper position is important as it influences the spread, onset, and density of subarachnoid anesthesia, unlike epidural anesthesia. The onset of anesthesia is faster and denser in the dependent areas.

Prone Position (Fig. 4)

The prone position is commonly used for caudal epidural anesthesia in adults while this position for lumbar epidural is used in the radiology room under imaging techniques for interventional pain relief procedures.

Performer

The comfort of the performer during the technique influences the success of the block. The performer should be seated appropriately.

Projection

It is essential to assemble and check equipment for monitoring (ECG, pulse oximeter, and blood pressure monitor) and resuscitation (oxygen, bag and mask, and suction). The medications required for resuscitation should be available and ready to administer without any delays when required.

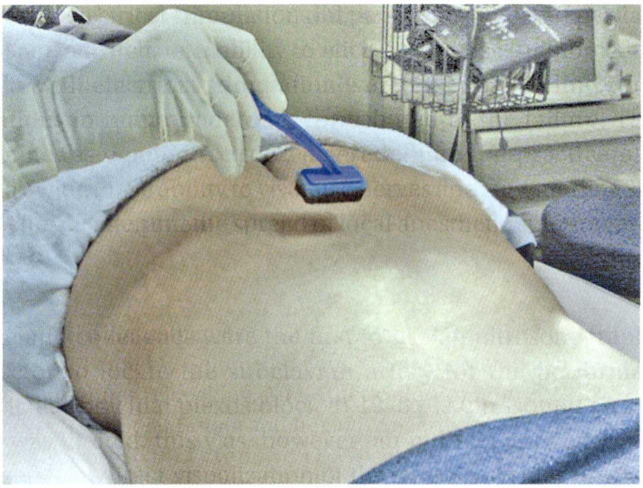

Fig. 4: Prone position for epidural blocks. Position the patient prone on the procedure table with a pillow under the waist to decrease the lumbar lordosis.

The required equipment and medications (appropriate syringes and drugs) for performing the procedure can be assembled by the performer in the institution or obtained commercially depending on the institutional practice.

The equipment for sterile preparation should include appropriate aseptic solution, sterile gauze swabs, and sponge-holding forceps. A small 2 mL dry syringe (glass or plastic with rubber bush) with Leur slip for local anesthetic for skin infiltration with small (25 or 30 gauge) hypodermic needle, and suitable local anesthetic should be available.

Puncture

Identification of the Puncture Site and Preparation

It is advisable to confirm the level of insertion of the needle and mark the spines and iliac crest prior to aseptic preparation of the patient. The imaginary line joining the highest point of iliac crests is at L3/4 and is called Tuffier's line. A sterile field is established with an antiseptic solution depending on the institutional practice applied with three basic sponges. The solution is applied starting from the injection site moving outward in a circular fashion. Some of the performers use 95% alcohol (commonly called spirit) to clean the iodine solution (if used) prior to the application of a fenestrated drape. The spirit or the povidone-iodine solution is cleared from the injection site through the fenestrated drape with a sterile gauze to prevent the possibility of chemical neuritis. The puncture site should be reconfirmed after the preparation.

SUBARACHNOID BLOCK

Subarachnoid (spinal) anesthesia is very commonly performed regional technique because of ease of performance, fast onset, return of gastrointestinal function faster than with GA, ability of patient to maintain airway, and fewer pulmonary complications compared to GA.

Equipment Specific for Subarachnoid Block

There are a variety of spinal needles available commercially for the performance of subarachnoid anesthesia **(Fig. 5)**. The available needles are grouped based on their tips, under dura cutting (Quincke) and dura noncutting needles (Whitacre and Sprotte needles). The Quincke needles are the first commercially available spinal needle and are most commonly used needle. The spinal needles are available in various lengths of 7.5, 10 (standard), 12.5, and 15 cm, and are of different sizes varying from thicker 18 G to thinner 29 G. The choice of the needle is dependent on the performer and the body mass index of the patient. The common length required in an adult male or female is 10 cm. The thinner 25–29 G are generally preferred

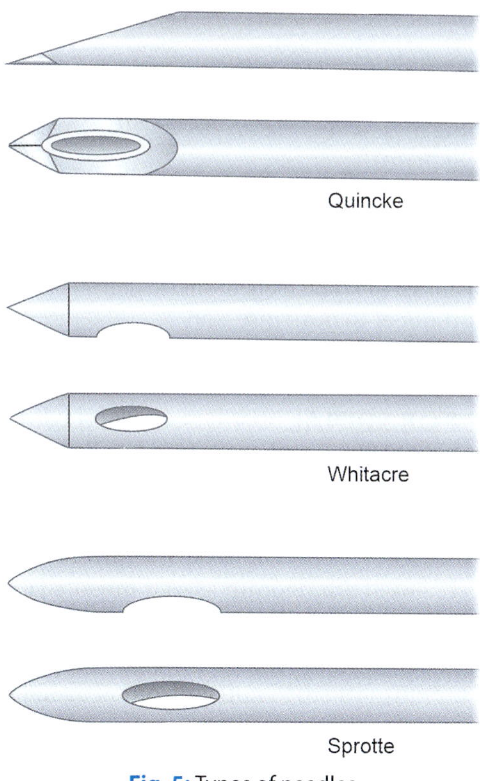

Fig. 5: Types of needles.

in younger patients to reduce the incidence of postdural puncture headache (PDPH).

Advantage of Different Needles

Quincke (cutting needle):

- Ease of flow of CSF through the needle
- Introducer may not be necessary depending on length and gauge of needle.

Whitacre and Sprotte (pencil point needles):

- Designed to spread the dural fibers
- Reduced incidence of PDPH
- Yields a distinct "pop" as the pencil point penetrates the dura.
- Offers increased "tip strength" to minimize bending or breakage.
- Precision-formed side hole enables directional flow of anesthetic.
- Reduces the possibility of straddling the dura.
- Tracks straight when advancing through ligaments toward the dura.
- Minimal damage to the nerve fibers during injection.

Disadvantages of Different Needles

Quincke (cutting needle):

- Dural "pop" is less likely to be appreciated due to the sharper tip.
- Increased trauma to the dura mater
- Increased risk of PDPH
- Damage to the nerve fibers during injection.

Whitacre and Sprotte (pencil point needles):

- Difficult to introduce through skin
- Requires an introducer to puncture skin
- Flow of CSF is slow.

TECHNIQUE FOR SPINAL

There are several approaches to introduce the spinal needle to reach the subarachnoid space. The performer should raise a skin wheal with 1% lidocaine at the predetermined site of insertion of spinal needle under aseptic precaution, following, the sterile preparation of the skin. The local anesthetic infiltration should be furthered into subcutaneous tissue after informing the patient. It is advisable to have a lapse period of 2/3 minutes between infiltration of the local anesthetic and insertion of the needle.

Midline Approach (Fig. 6)

In this approach, the performer should insert a 17 G introducer (when thinner spinal needles are used) with a slight cephalad angle of 10–15° through the subcutaneous tissue, supraspinous ligament, interspinous ligament, and into ligamentum flavum. Next the spinal needle is passed through the introducer which goes through ligamentum flavum, epidural space, dura mater, and subarachnoid mater in order to reach the subarachnoid space. Resistance changes as the spinal needle passes through each level on the way to the subarachnoid space. When the spinal needle goes though the dura mater, a "pop" is often appreciated. Once this pop is felt, the stylet should be removed from the introducer to check for flow of CSF. For spinal needles of small gauge (26–29 gauge), this usually takes 5–10 seconds; but in some patients, it can take a minute or longer. The needle should not be introduced beyond in the subarachnoid space for the possibility of spinal cord injury. If there is no flow rotating the needle by 90° may be helpful or the needle should be repositioned.

Once the space is reached, a 3–5 mL syringe with the local anesthetic to be administered in the subarachnoid space is attached and mixing lines are identified as local anesthetic and CSF mix in the syringe due to a change in baricity and temperature. The predetermined calculated dose is slowly injected. Some of the performers, although debatable, aspirate the CSF during administration of the local anesthetic (barbotage).

The needle and the drug injecting syringe should be removed together exerting sustained pressure on the piston with the palm of the dominant hand by the performer prior to removal of the introducer needle and positioning.

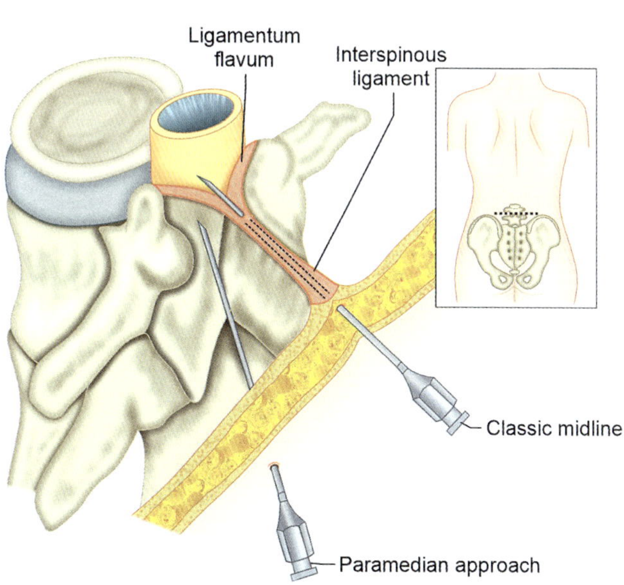

Fig. 6: Different approaches to subarachnoid block. Tuffier line illustrated in the insert.

Paramedian Approach

Paramedian approach is indicated in patients who are unable to adequately flex the vertebral column due to pain, structural abnormalities, or ossification of ligaments. The spinal needle is placed 1.5 cm laterally and slightly caudal to the center of the selected interspace. The needle is aimed medially and slightly cephalic and passed lateral to the supraspinous ligament. If the lamina is contacted, the needle is redirected and "walked off" in a medial and cephalic direction.

Taylor or Lumbosacral Approach (Fig. 7)

This approach is useful in patients with calcified or fusion of higher intervertebral spaces. The injection site is 1 cm medial and 1 cm caudal to the posterior iliac spine. The needle is directed 45° medial and 45° cranial to contact the lamina of S1. Following this, needle is walked upward and medially to enter the L5–S1 interspace.

MEDICATIONS USED FOR SUBARACHNOID BLOCK

Local Anesthetics

The choice of a local anesthetic for subarachnoid anesthesia depends on the potency, fast onset, duration, and requirement for postoperative analgesia. The local anesthetics used for subarachnoid block can be classified on the basis of duration of action as short-acting (procaine), intermediate-acting

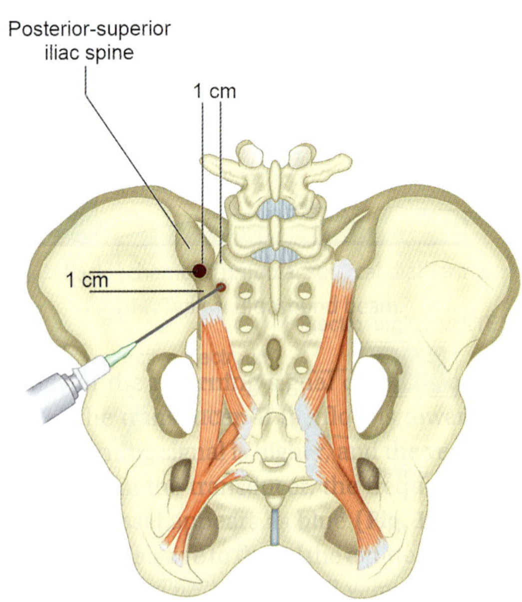

Fig. 7: Taylor approach.

TABLE 2: Different local anesthetics used for subarachnoid block. Procaine is short-acting, lidocaine is intermediate-acting, and the rest are long-acting.

Local anesthetic	*Concentration*	*T10 level lower abdomen*	*T4 level upper abdomen*	*Duration of action plain*	*With epinephrine*
Procaine	10%	125 mg	200 mg	45 min	60 min
Lidocaine	5% in 7.5% glucose	50–75 mg	75–100 mg	60–75 min	60–90 min
Bupivacaine	0.5% or 0.75% in 8.25% dextrose	12–14 mg	12–18 mg	90–120 min	100–150 min
Tetracaine	1% in 10% glucose	10–12 mg	10–16 mg	90–120 min	120–240 min
Ropivacaine	0.2–1%	12–16 mg	16–18 mg	90–120 min	90–120 min

(lidocaine), and long-acting (bupivacaine, ropivacaine, and levobupivacaine). Different local anesthetics used, their doses and characteristics are given in **Table 2**. It is recommended that only preservative-free solutions are used in subarachnoid space.

Lidocaine used to be the most frequently used agent for subarachnoid block. However, it is replaced by bupivacaine because of its dubious distinction of producing cauda equina syndrome and transient neurological symptoms (TNS). Lidocaine is compatible with adjuvants to be administered in subarachnoid space for surgical anesthesia.

Bupivacaine, a long-acting amide local anesthetic, used for epidural anesthesia is 0.5–0.75% concentrations. Bupivacaine in concentrations of 0.75% is strictly not recommended for obstetric anesthesia, since inadvertent intravenous. Injections have resulted in several cardiac arrests. *Levobupivacaine* is the S-enantiomer of bupivacaine used in the same concentrations as bupivacaine. It is less cardiotoxic than bupivacaine and often recommended for obstetric anesthesia.

Ropivacaine is a long-acting amide local anesthetic, used in concentrations of 0.5–1% for anesthesia. It is similar to bupivacaine in onset, duration, and quality of blockade, provides excellent sensory blockade with minor motor blockade, less cardiotoxic than bupivacaine, and is often recommended in obstetric and pediatric anesthesia.

Additives (Adjuvants)

The commonly used adjuvants are vasopressors and opiates. Other types of adjuvants such as α-2 agonists (clonidine and dexmedetomidine), anticholinesterases (neostigmine), and phencyclidines (ketamine) have also been tried. This chapter will discuss the use of vasopressors and opiates.

Epinephrine will increase the duration of action for all local anesthetics administered in the subarachnoid space. Differences exist in the extent of increase among individual local anesthetics. The greatest increases are found with lidocaine, mepivacaine, and 2-chloroprocaine. It is less effective for bupivacaine, levobupivacaine, and etidocaine. Epinephrine is not added to ropivacaine due to its inherent vasoconstrictive effects.

Compared to phenylephrine, epinephrine has been found to be more effective in reducing peak blood levels of local anesthetics. The small doses of epinephrine added to local anesthetics in the subarachnoid space are also responsible for analgesia unlike in epidural space. Epinephrine reduces the absorption of local anesthetics and opioids allowing for a prolonged exposure at the site of action resulting in a prolonged and intense effect.

Opioid drugs: Currently, preservative-free morphine and fentanyl are used commonly. A small dose of 0.5 mg of morphine to bupivacaine would enhance the duration of the sensory block by 27%. Addition of morphine to the local anesthetic does not enhance the onset time unlike fentanyl and its analogs. Short-acting opiates such as fentanyl and its analogs provide faster onset and segmental analgesia of shorter duration. The maximum dose of fentanyl required in the subarachnoid space is 25 μg for hastening the onset time. The use of 2.3 mL of 0.5% levobupivacaine with fentanyl 15 μg has been recommended in spinal anesthesia for urological surgery, and has been found to be as effective as 2.6 mL of 0.5% levobupivacaine alone.

Mode of Action of Local Anesthetics and Opioids in Subarachnoid Block

Local anesthetic binding to nerve tissue disrupts nerve transmission, resulting in neural blockade. The target binding sites are located within the spinal cord (superficial and deep portions), and on the spinal nerve roots in the subarachnoid space. *The spinal nerve roots and dorsal root ganglia* are considered the most important sites of action. Nerves in the subarachnoid space are highly accessible and easily anesthetized, even with a small dose of local anesthetic.

The addition of opioids as adjuvants increases the duration of action by acting at the opioid receptors in the spinal cord. In combination with local anesthetics, they provide prolonged blockade.

The sensitivity of different nerve fibers varies depending on their size. Autonomic fibers are blocked first, followed by sensory fibers. Motor and proprioception are most resistant. The intensity of sensory and motor block depends on the concentration of local anesthetic drug used, and the amount available at site. Because of this differential block, there may be a difference of 2–4 segments in each block, the level of autonomic block being highest, followed by sensory level and then motor level. This may result in vasodilation and a drop in blood pressure with the patient being aware of touch.

Onset Time and Duration of Subarachnoid Block

The onset time of sensory block is the period of time from deposition of the anesthetic solution in subarachnoid space to loss of pain sensation to pinprick over the surgical area. The onset time of motor block is the time to loss of voluntary movement of involved part. The onset of the subarachnoid block is dependent on the chemical characteristics of the local anesthetic drug. Lignocaine acts from 1 to 5 minutes. Hyperbaric bupivacaine can take up to 15 minutes. The pKa of the local anesthetics and tissue pH influences the action at site, however, with minimal practical implication in subarachnoid block. The most commonly used adjuvants like opioids hasten the onset time. Epinephrine (1:200,000 or 5 µg/mL) usually reduces the rate of absorption, prolonging the duration of action, whereas its physical properties may delay the onset slightly. The duration of action also depends on the clearance of the drug from the site of deposition and the vascularity of the site.

Factors Affecting the Spread of the Local Anesthetic Solution

Baricity: The baricity [specific gravity (sp.gr.)] of the local anesthetic solution is always compared with that of CSF. Accordingly, they are grouped according to the baricity as hyperbaric (sp.gr. > CSF), hypobaric (sp.gr. < CSF) and isobaric (sp.gr. = CSF). The baricity determines the direction of flow of the local anesthetic within the CSF and the position of the patient to be adopted before injecting into CSF to achieve a desired level of block. The hyperbaric solution flows down to the caudal region, hypobaric raises cephalic while the isobaric solution is dependent on the equal balance. Addition of 7.5% dextrose not only results in hyperbaric local anesthetic but also reduces the rate of diffusion by facilitating a uniform mixture with the CSF. Isobaric and hyperbaric solutions produce reliable blocks. The level of the subarachnoid block can be manipulated by the combination of hyperbaric solution and patient's position.

Position: Position of the patient influences the intensity of the block. The dependent area is affected with a denser block compared to the nondependent area.

Concentration: The intensity of sensory and motor block depends on the amount (concentration) of local anesthetic drug available at site and size of the nerve fiber. The concentration required is dependent on the thickness and type of the nerve fiber. Thus, motor fibers require higher concentrations compared to sensory and autonomic fibers.

Volume: The volume of local anesthetic plays a crucial role in the level of block achieved. The volume should be decreased by 30–50% in patients with suspected increased intra-abdominal pressure since there is a decrease in compliance in subarachnoid space.

Puncture site: Higher puncture site may lead to high-level blocks. However, the puncture site is chosen usually.

Speed: The speed of injection is important as it influences the height of the block achieved. It is advisable to inject the drug slowly over a 10–15-second period.

Purging (barbotage): Purging is a unique technique of administration of the local anesthetic where the performer repeatedly alternates between aspiration of small aliquots of CSF into local anesthetic syringe and injects back the mixture. This technique causes ripple effect resulting in higher level of blockade. However, this technique may also result in patchy block.

Age of patient: The local anesthetic required to achieve certain level of blockade decreases as age advances. This is largely due to changes in the size and compliance of the subarachnoid space.

Height of patient: The amount of local anesthetic required is smaller in a patient who is shorter in height. This is largely due to changes in the distribution of the volume of the solution in the subarachnoid space.

Gravity: There is influence on the spread and level of block achieved due to positioning of the patient after injection of local anesthetic. The block is most intense in the dependent position. Sitting, reverse Trendelenburg, or Trendelenburg positions can be used to manipulate the block.

Disadvantages of Subarachnoid Anesthesia

- Not suitable for surgeries above umbilicus.
- The occurrence of long-term complications like PDPH, meningitis, neurological sequelae following even minor surgical procedures will be devastating.
- Potential to place wrong intrathecal medications which can lead to death.
- Rapid hemodynamic variations.

EPIDURAL BLOCK

Equipment Specific for Epidural

The equipment required may be assembled, but more commonly commercially available kits **(Fig. 8)** are used. In addition to the cleaning tray, several other items of equipment that are essential should be available.

- *Epidural needle:* Tuohy type needle is provided with clear depth marking for accurate insertion depth reading.
- *Epidural catheter:* It is especially designed for short-term and long-term anesthesia and detectable by radiology.
- *Epidural catheter adapter:* This adapter is for safe and secure attachment to the catheter for convenience of the procedure.
- Loss of resistance (LOR) devices that is especially designed for clear identification of epidural space **(Fig. 9)**. The LOR syringes can be glass or plastic.

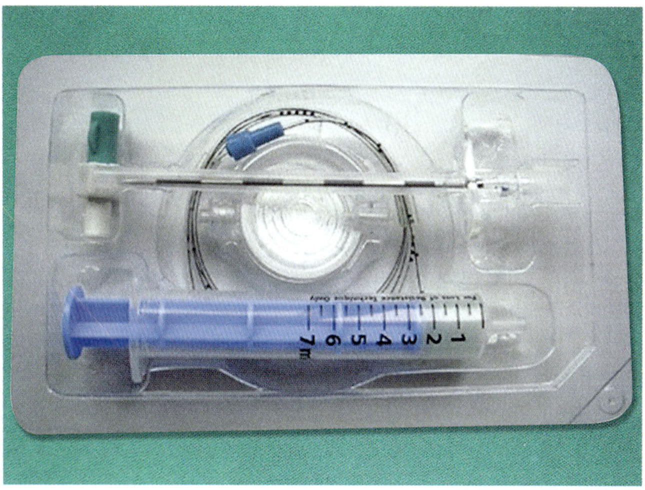

Fig. 8: Epidural set.

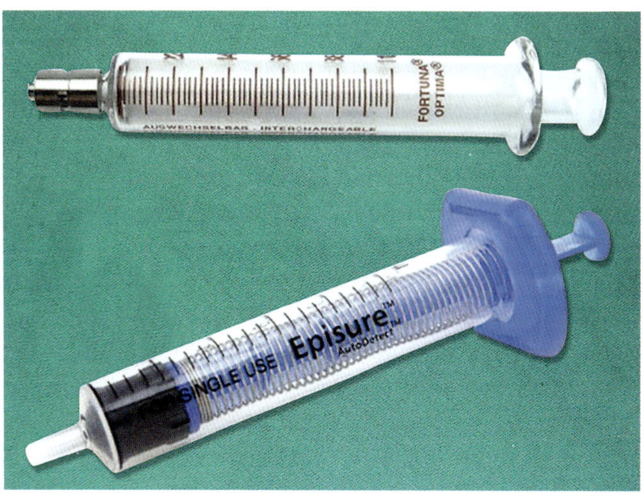

Fig. 9: Loss of resistance syringes (glass and plastic).

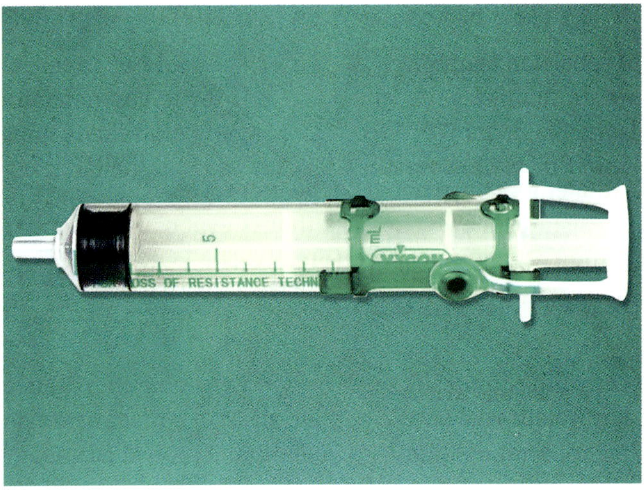

Fig. 10: Epimatic syringe. There is continuous positive pressure applied on the barrel of the syringe by elastic strip.

- Special devices such as Epimatic syringe allows automatic location of the epidural space due to the continuous positive pressure applied on the plunger by an elastic strip. Syringe can be used either with liquid or air **(Fig. 10)**.
- *Hydrophobic filter:* A 0.2-μ filter is available for additional safety and control against microbial infection.

Technique for Epidural Block

Under aseptic precautions, a skin wheal is raised with 1% lidocaine at the predetermined site of insertion of Tuohy needle. The local anesthetic infiltration should be furthered into subcutaneous tissue after informing the patient. A period of 2/3 minutes should elapse between infiltration of the local anesthetic and insertion of the Tuohy needle. The approaches for surgical anesthesia can be either midline or paramedian. The direction of the insertion of the Tuohy needle differs in thoracic and lumbar regions due to the direction of the spines. The epidural needle that is correctly placed into the ligamentum flavum remains straight and stays without swaying. In an average-built adult male/female patient, the depth of ligamentum flavum from skin measures approximately 4 cm in the lumbar area. The average thickness of the ligamentum flavum is 5–6 mm. Hence, the ligamentum flavum offers resistance to the insertion of the needle as it cuts through the ligament and gives a distinct tactile feel when the needle is placed in it. The stylet is then removed epidural space is identified by LOR device or demonstration of negative pressure. Currently, ultrasound-guided techniques are becoming more popular.

Identification of Epidural Space

Loss of resistance technique is the most commonly used technique. There are several LOR devices. Once the epidural needle is inserted into ligamentum flavum, the stylet is withdrawn, and a LOR device of choice is attached to the needle. The needle should be held steady by the nondominant while the dominant hand supports the LOR device **(Fig. 11)**. A steady pressure is applied to the plunger to compress the air/saline by the *dominant hand*. The needle is inserted slowly and steadily by the *nondominant hand* with a steady push until LOR is noted by a sudden give away sensation (like a knife going through a block of butter) as the needle tip (bevel) reaches epidural space.

The performer should stop at this juncture since the needle will be in the epidural space. The give way sensation after initial resistance of the needle piercing the ligament is called "*loss of resistance*." The control of the needle is important to avoid dural puncture and risk of spinal cord injury. This is of special importance in the thoracic area. If the needle is not placed in the ligamentum flavum, the anesthesia provider may experience false positives with the LOR technique. It is important for the performer to know that the dominant hand should not be removed from the plunger to assist the insertion of the needle through the ligamentum flavum.

As far as use of "air" or "saline" for LOR technique, the current evidence favors *saline*. Use of *air* may lead to pneumocephalus, spinal cord and nerve root compression, and venous air embolism. Additionally, inadequate analgesia and paresthesia have been reported with the use of air. The simultaneous administration of nitrous oxide, and positive pressure ventilation have also been reported to expand localized collections of air, resulting in heightened symptoms. A meta-analysis in obstetric population

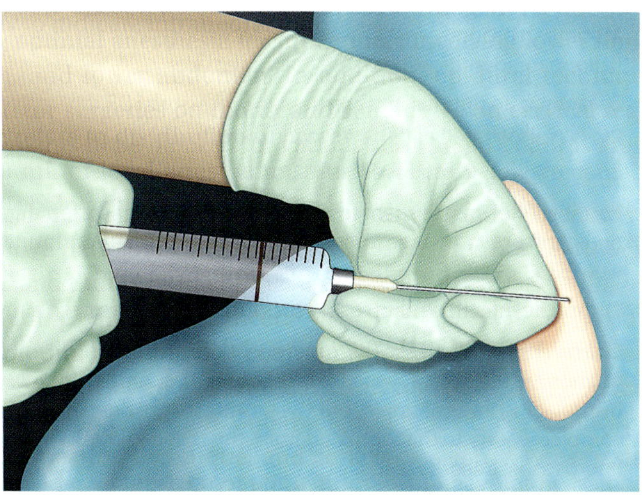

Fig. 11: Technique of identification of epidural space.

revealed reduced incidence of PDPH, when "saline" was used. These reports suggest that use of "saline" may be superior.

Hanging Drop Technique

A drop of preservative-free normal saline is applied to the hub of the needle which has been inserted into ligamentum flavum. A slow and steady pressure is applied to the Tuohy needle, similar to the technique described above (LOR technique) until the hanging drop gets "sucked" in. The intrathoracic negative pressure transmitted to the epidural space helps in this mechanism. This technique is preferred in identifying epidural space at thoracic and cervical levels. This technique is of little value in identifying epidural space at lumbar level.

Confirmation with Mechanical Aids

There are various mechanical aids to facilitate the identification of the epidural space. Although they aid in identification, the manual skill and dexterity required should not be compromised to prevent complications. **Table 3** gives a list of some such devices; however, the use of some is relatively uncommon. Some of them are trying to define the directions for the future.

Ultrasound-guided Technique

There is a growing interest in ultrasound imaging to guide neuraxial blockade in difficult subjects. Simultaneous ultrasound imaging and needle placement for neuraxial procedures are difficult in adult patients. The two

TABLE 3: Devices for identification of epidural space.

Sl. No.	*Name of the aid*
1.	Macintosh balloon Balloon for identification of the epidural space
2.	Epidrum is an optimal and constant low-pressure LOR device. It gives positive visual signal that the needle has entered epidural space
3.	Episure spring-loaded syringe
4.	Portable intelligent system for optical-technology-based epidural space detection optical needle fiber (http://www.amepc.org/qims/article/view/5333/6249)
5.	CompuFlo injection pump using pressure measurement
6.	*Optical epidural catheter:* This optical epidural needle has the potential to improve the accuracy of needle placement during epidural injections by providing information about the location of the needle tip that is complementary to that obtained from the LOR technique and from fluoroscopic images

(LOR: loss of resistance)

ultrasound-guided techniques are offline technique (skin markings prior to needle insertion), or online technique (simultaneous use of epidural needle and ultrasound probe). When using ultrasound to guide neuraxial blocks, a visual confirmation of access of Tuohy needle to the epidural space is received, because ultrasound can accurately identify the intervertebral levels, the midline spinous process, the midline interspinous window, and the paramedian interlaminar window. Bone does not permit ultrasound beam transmission, thus casting a hypoechoic (dark) shadow on the image. Conversely, passage of the ultrasound beam through the interspinous and interlaminar windows allows visualization of the hyperechoic dura (a bright line), the subarachnoid space, and the posterior aspect of the vertebral body **(Fig. 12)**. Visualization of the ligamentum flavum and epidural space is often more difficult. Successful transverse or longitudinal scan facilitates identification of the optimal location for proper needle insertion during neuraxial block and an estimation of the skin-to-dura distance. This is particularly useful in patients with difficult surface anatomic landmarks (e.g., obesity), spine pathology (e.g., scoliosis), and previous spine surgery (e.g., laminectomy). Several outcome studies have confirmed the utility of ultrasonography when neuraxial block is performed by the novice and in patients with difficult anatomic landmarks.

Radiological Technique Using C-arm

Radiological guidance is used for interventional epidural steroid injection for chronic pain due to nerve root compression. A midline approach is used to introduce epidural catheter in cervical, thoracic, and caudal epidural spaces.

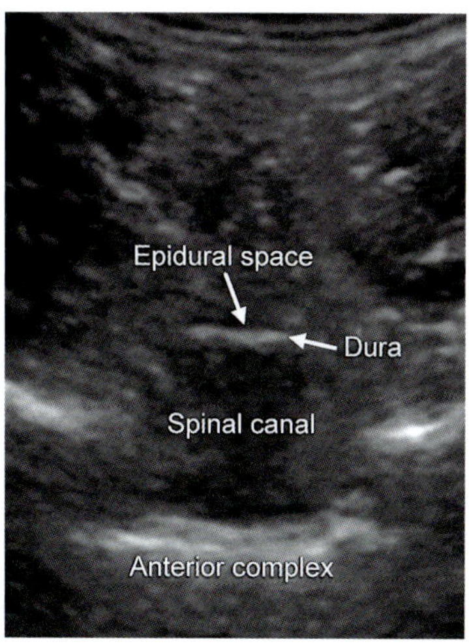

Fig. 12: Identification of epidural space using ultrasound. The echoes from the ligamentum flavum and posterior dura (the posterior complex) are visualized in longitudinal paramedian view.

The correct placement of the catheter is confirmed radiologically after injecting radio-opaque dye. In patients with multiple nerve root compressions, leading to sciatica, multiple transforaminal epidural steroid injection can be administered using radiological guidance. Patient is positioned prone and an oblique view reveals confluence of shadows resembling "scotty dog" **(Fig. 13 and Box 1)**. Epidural is accessed through this transforaminal approach below the eye and medial to the chin of the "scotty dog". The space is confirmed by radio-opaque dye and steroid solution is used, which can relieve the pain for several months.

Epidural Catheter Insertion

Once the space is identified, further advancement of the Tuohy needle by 1–2 mm is advocated by some to ensure that the insertion of the catheter is not obstructed by tissue at the tip of the Tuohy needle. This has the potential to increase the risk of inadvertent dural puncture. An alternative technique

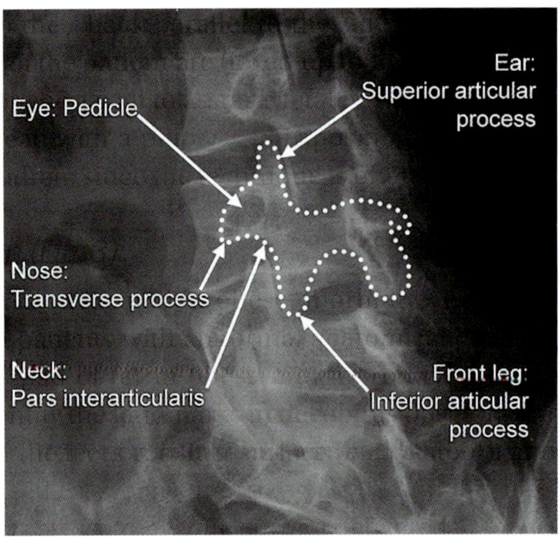

Fig. 13: Oblique radiological view demonstrating "scotty dog" appearance.

BOX 1: The scotty dog sign refers to the normal appearance of the lumbar spine when seen on oblique radiographic projection.

On oblique views, the posterior elements of vertebra form the figure of a scotty dog with:
- The transverse process being the nose
- The pedicle forming the eye
- The inferior articular facet being the front leg
- The superior articular facet representing the ear
- The pars interarticularis (the portion of the lamina that lies between the facets) equivalent to the neck of the dog

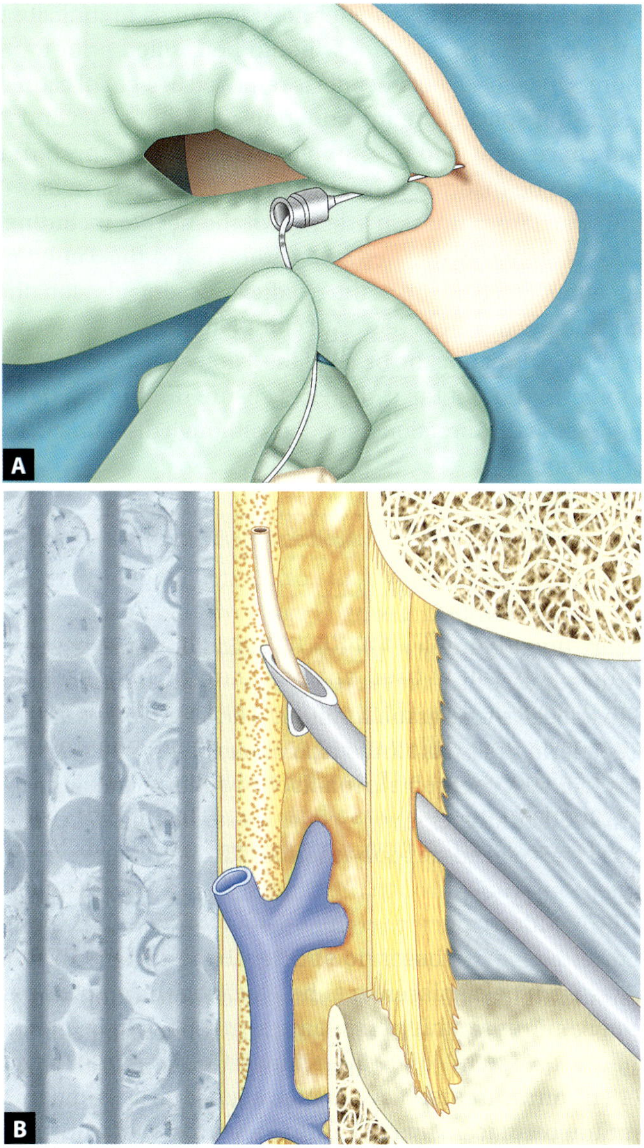

Figs. 14A and B: Technique of epidural catheter insertion. Schematic representation of direction of the bevel and the direction of catheter.

is to administer an additional 2–3 mL of preservative-free normal saline, expanding the epidural space and assume that the obstructing structure is pushed away. Despite these maneuvers, the performer may encounter difficulty during insertion of the catheter if the needle is partially in the epidural space. The techniques of insertion of catheter and directing the catheter are illustrated in **Figures 14A and B**.

Both epidural needle and catheter have markings to indicate the depth in the tissues. The relative markings should be verified prior to the start of the procedure. Once the Tuohy needle is removed 3–4 cm of catheter should be in the epidural space. The introduction of catheter beyond 3–4 cm in the epidural space may lead to a unilateral block. The appropriate length of the catheter to be inserted is calculated (3–4 cm in the space + depth of the epidural space from the skin + length of the needle including the hub) and once this distance is reached, the catheter and the Tuohy needle are removed together. Once the tip of the needle is just outside skin, the catheter is stabilized, and the needle is removed completely.

The concept of directing the bevel of the Tuohy needle either cephalad or cauded before insertion of the catheter to ensure the smooth passage of the epidural catheter in the direction intended, although disclaimed, is practiced in clinical situation.

Fixation of Catheter

The catheter is fixed on the skin at the calculated length (marking) with the help of sterile transparent dressing (Tegaderm) by looping to prevent the direct pressure on the catheter while positioning or transporting which may displace or alter the depth of the catheter placement. The rest of the catheter is fixed with an adhesive tape at the shoulder. The length of the catheter exiting from the Tegaderm dressing till the fixation at the shoulder is supported by the vertebral column of the patient and is covered by the adhesive plaster. The outer end of the catheter is covered with a sterile gauze or cover **(Fig. 15)**.

If the catheter is placed correctly, there should be no resistance to saline or local anesthetic injection through the catheter. If any flow of fluid or blood is noticed in the epidural catheter, it is mandatory to confirm the position of the catheter. Lowering the catheter below the level of the operating table for CSF flow indicates intrathecal placement and elevating the epidural catheter for flow of blood confirms intravascular placement. The correct placement must be confirmed by using 3 mL of 2% lignocaine with 1 in 200,000 adrenalines as a test dose. The intravascular placement produces tachycardia in 3 minutes, whereas intrathecal placement can result in a sensory block up to T10 level. In the event of intravascular placement of the catheter, it is advisable to perform the technique all over again ensuring that the needle is in the midline.

After confirmation of the correct placement and fixation of the catheter, the patient is repositioned in the supine posture prior to the administration of the anesthetic solution. The performer should not forget to perform a negative aspiration with syringe before each injection to ensure inadvertent migration of the catheter, although it may not always detect intravascular or subarachnoid placement of a catheter. This is to ensure that there is no inadvertent migration of the catheter at any time. A high index (level)

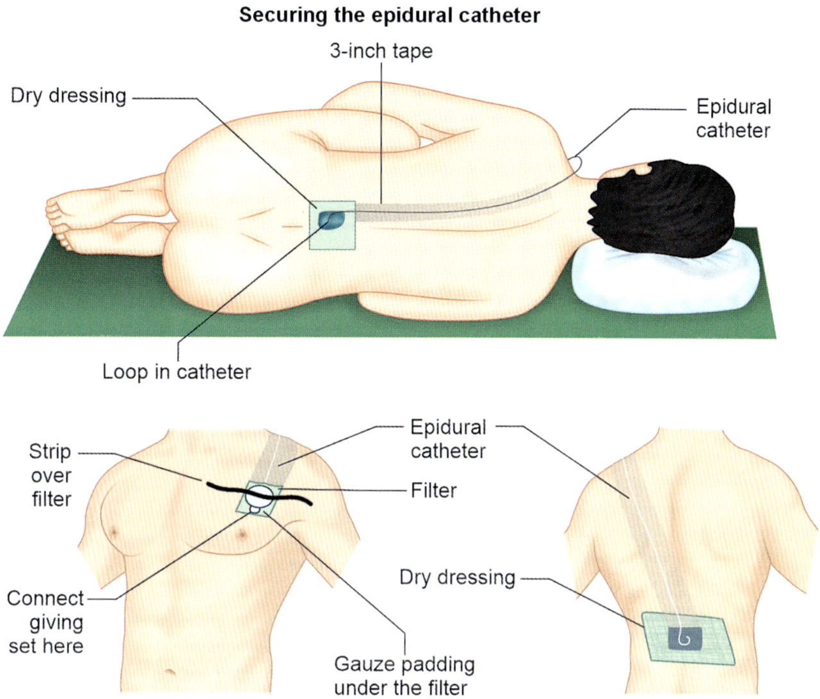

Fig. 15: Fixing epidural catheter.

of suspicion may be necessary while administering the total dose of the anesthetic drug. The total calculated dose of the local anesthetic should be administered in incremental doses of 5 mL at an interval of 5 minutes, with continuous monitoring. This volume is adequate to cause symptoms of intravascular injection without seizures and/or cardiovascular collapse. Once adequate level is achieved, smaller boluses may be repeated every 1–2 hours, or a constant infusion is administered using syringe pumps if surgical procedure is expected to last long. Patients' comfort should be achieved by administering sedation. Once surgical procedure is completed, the catheter can be used to provide postoperative analgesia. The local anesthetic should be sufficiently low concentration to provide analgesia without motor block. Opioids like fentanyl may also be added for this purpose. During epidural anesthesia, the target binding sites, as with subarachnoid block, are located within the spinal cord (superficial and deep portions) and on the spinal nerve roots in the epidural spaces. The spinal nerve roots and dorsal root ganglia are considered the most important sites of action. Nerves in the epidural space are not easily anesthetized because they are often ensheathed by dura mater (the "dural sleeve"). Generally, used local anesthetics and opioids for epidural and their doses are as shown in **Tables 4 and 5**.

TABLE 4: Local anesthetics for epidural block.

Drug	*Conc. %*	*First dose (mg)*	*Duration (min)*
Prilocaine	1–3	150–300	6–180
Lidocaine	1–2	150–300	60–180
Bupivacaine	0.25–0.75	37.5–100	180–300
Levobupivacaine	0.25–0.75	37.5–100	180–300
Ropivacaine	0.5–1	75–300	180–300

TABLE 5: Opioids as adjuvants during epidural block.

Drug	*Initial bolus*	*Basal infusion (per hour)*	*Breakthrough dose (every 10–15 mins)*
Morphine	2–3 mg	0.5–0.8 mg	0.2–0.3 mg
Hydromorphone	0.8–1.5 mg	0.15–0.3 mg	0.15–0.3 mg
Fentanyl	0.5–1.5 mcg/kg	0.5–1.5 ag/kg	10–15 ng
Sufentanil	0.3–0.7 mcg/kg	0.1–0.2 ag/kg	5–7 lag

TECHNICAL PROBLEMS DURING NEURAXIAL BLOCKS

The techniques of performing neuraxial blocks are quite subjective and depend on high levels of manual skill and dexterity and require specialist training. Epidural blocks are more challenging than subarachnoid blocks. Faulty techniques can lead to failed blocks and serious complication. Patient's factors may also contribute to technical challenges.

Skills of the performer: The performer must learn to differentiate the various structures by the feel at the pulp of the fingers of dominant hand as the needle pierces various structures before reaching the epidural or subarachnoid space.

Patient's factors: Problems may arise due to obesity, skeletal abnormalities, and improper position of the patient. In the event of technical challenges, a thorough reassessment of the site of puncture, direction of the needle, and the position of the patient must be checked. Occasionally, despite the needle being in correct location, there can be patchy analgesia, or one may experience difficulty in inserting the epidural catheter. These can be due to anatomical abnormalities or presence of sepia. These problems are encountered more often in elderly patients.

Needle strikes bone: Sometimes, the needle hits bone when attempting a spinal anesthetic. When this occurs, note the depth of the needle at bone contact, and place the needle more cephalad. If bone is contacted on reinsertion of the needle, the depth should be compared. If the needle contacts bone deeper on reinsertion, then likely the inferior spinous process is being contacted and the needle should be inserted even more cephalad. If the bone contact is shallower, then likely the superior spinous process is being felt and the needle needs to be redirected in a caudal fashion. If the depth of bone contact is the same, then likely the vertebral lamina is being contacted.

Technical Problems Specific to Subarachnoid Block

No Cerebrospinal Fluid Flow through the Spinal Needle

It is not uncommon to encounter the lack of flow of CSF through the spinal needle, despite the placement of the needle being in the subarachnoid space. The flow of the CSF might be delayed with higher gauged thin needle. Some of the measures to be adopted are:

- To exercise patience for a period of at least 30 seconds
- Rotation of the needle by 90°
- Ensure that the needle is not blocked by purging the needle with 0.5–1 mL of air
- Gradual and slow withdrawal of the spinal needle. The withdrawal is stopped as soon as CSF flow is visualized at the hub of the needle.

Blood Flow from the Spinal Needle

The performer may sometimes notice the flow of blood in the spinal needle. This may be due to the presence of the needle in a vein in either the subarachnoid or in the epidural space. It is advocated to confirm the flow of blood through the needle for a few seconds. The partial presence of the needle in the vein, in subarachnoid space is confirmed by the dilution of the blood flowing through the needle as it gets mixed with CSF. The performer should be patient to confirm a clear flow of cerebrospinal fluid before administering the local anesthetic. If blood continues to drip, it is probable for the needle tip to be in an epidural vein. It can be advanced further or angled more medially to pierce the dura mater.

Complaint of Sharp and Stabbing Leg Pain

If the patient complains of a paresthesia, during insertion, it may be because the needle touches the nerve, or spinal cord. If the pain persists despite minor manipulation, the needle should be withdrawn and procedure repeated at the same level or at different space.

Technical Problems Specific to Epidural Block

Flow of Fluid through the Needle or Catheter

It is not uncommon to notice a small amount of fluid flowing back through the needle. This is possible when preservative-free normal saline is used for

LOR technique for identification of the epidural space, or the test dose of the local anesthetic administered through the needle. In order to differentiate with CSF, a few drops of dripping fluid are collected on the dorsum of the nondominant gloved hand, and add a drop of thiopentone sodium. The resultant mixture shows precipitation with local anesthetic.

If there is a continuous flow, and intrathecal placement is confirmed, two approaches may be used:

1. Proceed as a CSA, or
2. The epidural is placed at another level and monitored for the development of a PDPH.

If the flow of fluid stops, the catheter is inserted and a test dose is administered to ensure that the needle/catheter has not crossed the dura mater.

Pain during Performance

Some patients may complain of pain (paresthesia) upon insertion of the needle if it is not in the midline. It is mandatory to remove the needle and reassess the site of insertion and position of patient. It is not unusual to get transient pain upon insertion of the epidural catheter as a brief shock-like symptom or sensation. The persistence of the symptom warrants removal of the catheter as it may be in contact with a nerve root.

If the patient complains of pain or paresthesia, the catheter should be withdrawn by a few millimeter. If the paresthesia persists, the catheter should be withdrawn and the procedure is repeated.

CAUSES OF FAILURE ENCOUNTERED WITH NEURAXIAL BLOCKS

Technical problems can occur in both with spinal and epidural anesthesia leading to failure or inadequate blocks. The endpoint is more clear-cut in subarachnoid, when compared to epidural block and hence lesser incidence of failure.

Failed or Patchy Block

This could be due to false tactile feeling or loss of resistance. Due to this, the local anesthetic may be misplaced. Relatively uncommon occurrence is depositing the drug in *subdural space.* The presence of the spinal needle in the subdural space with free flow of CSF may give a false impression of the needle being in subarachnoid space. Deposition of drug in subdural can lead to patchy analgesia, lack of motor block, and inadequate height of block.

Subarachnoid may be repeated if there is a total failure. However, having administered the initial total dose epidural should not be repeated.

Unilateral Block

A planned hemiblock is attempted for providing surgical anesthesia for one limb. However, autonomic block is mostly bilateral. Unilateral block as a technical failure seldom occurs. However, unilateral block may be produced during epidural, if the catheter is too far inside the epidural space, migration out of the epidural space or pointed laterally. Pulling the catheter back in increments and with a steady movement by 1–2 cm may move the catheter back into a midline position.

Segmental Sparing

This may occur due to anatomical conditions (septa) within the epidural space or subarachnoid space. The larger size of L5–S2 nerves may result in these nerves not being affected by the local anesthetic resulting in sacral sparing. Administering an extra volume of local anesthetic may help to alleviate this condition during epidural technique. The rate of segmental sparing and failure is very low during subarachnoid block compared to an epidural block. If block failure occurs, one should be prepared to induce GA.

Visceral Pain

The inability to block the visceral pain should not be considered as a failure of neuraxial block. Visceral afferent fibers travel with the vagus nerve and are difficult to block. An intravenous supplementation with opioid analgesics and sedatives may be required to get the patient through "uncomfortable" portions of the surgical procedure. If unable to adequately treat the discomfort, it is advisable to induce GA.

ASSESSMENT OF THE NEURAXIAL BLOCK

The assessment is to be performed to ensure adequate motor and sensory blocks. Sensory *autonomic* block is assessed by loss of temperature discrimination using a damp alcohol swab. Level of *pain* block is tested using a 25-G hypodermic needle. The assessment is performed after ascertaining the ability of the patient to appreciate cold sensation to the damp alcohol swab or the pain sensation to the pinprick over a nonanesthetized area of the body (where sensation is normal). This should be followed by assessment from anesthetized area to nonanesthetized area until the patient is able to appreciate the cold sensation to the alcohol swab or the pain sensation to the pinprick.

It is not uncommon to encounter difficulty in eliciting the level of sensory block and more so for motor block. The assessment of motor block may be extrapolated with objective signs (modified Bromage scale; **Table 6**). This scale grades the motor power by testing the patients' ability to raise legs at the hip from the operating table.

TABLE 6: Modified Bromage scale.

Grade	*Criteria*	*Degree of block*
1	No motor block	Nil (0%)
2	Can flex knee, move foot, but cannot raise leg	Partial (33%)
3	Can move foot only	Almost complete (66%)
4	Cannot move foot or knee	Complete (100%)

The assessment is to be repeated at 5-minute intervals for a 15-minute period and again at the end of 30-minute period of injecting the local anesthetic. The increase in the level of the block is confined to sensory and autonomic fibers sparing the motor fibers. This is due to the fact that the level of the block ascends until the concentration of the drug in the subarachnoid space is diluted to the minimum to have effect on the nerve fibers.

EFFECTS OF NEURAXIAL BLOCKS ON DIFFERENT SYSTEMS

Most of the hemodynamic and respiratory effects are similar for both subarachnoid and epidural blocks and are based on the segmental level of block. However, the onset depends on the type of block. Local anesthetics injected into the subarachnoid or epidural space result in sympathetic and motor blockade.

Cardiovascular System

A block at the level of T5–L1 provides ideal conditions for abdominal surgery due to blockage of splanchnic sympathetic supply, maintenance of intact parasympathetic tone, contracted bowel, relaxed sphincters, and good muscle relaxation. High sympathetic block along with paralysis of calf muscles may lead to decrease in preload. The decrease in arterial tone leads to decrease in afterload. With or without parasympathetic effects, patients develop bradycardia. These effects lead to an unusual situation where hypotension is accompanied by bradycardia. If this hypotension produces evidence of tissue hypoperfusion, immediate management should consist of oxygen, atropine, vasopressors, and IV fluids. Measurement of end-tidal CO_2 levels using appropriately adopted nasal cannula is a usual adjunct to evaluate total perfusion of tissues.

Respiratory System

Generally, regionals are considered superior to GA in patients with respiratory diseases. A block below T10 has minimal effects on respiratory system. Higher blocks can cause intercostal paralysis which may not affect gaseous exchange. However, the vital capacity will be reduced, leading to secretion retention and increased chances of aspiration. Accidental injection of large dose, intended for epidural, can lead to total spinal. Pulse oximetry and apnea monitors are very useful to monitor such situations.

Central Nervous System

Generally, there is no altered level of consciousness during neuraxial blocks except when inappropriate sedation was produced. If a total spinal occurs, patient may develop nausea and altered sensorium due to cerebral hypoxia. One must watch out for such ominous signs.

Stress Response

Neuraxia blocks obtund hormonal and metabolic response and modify stress response during intraoperative and postoperative periods. Though this effect appears exciting, the evidence that there is overall benefit in outcomes is not very strong.

Genitourinary

Normally, these patients develop urinary retention, which is similar in duration of the block. Hence, there may be prolonged block when opioid adjuvants are used. A prolonged lower block (S2–S4) can also lead to bladder atony.

COMPLICATIONS OF NEURAXIAL BLOCKS

The complications may be grouped as immediate, delayed, and long-term.

Immediate Complications

These complications occur during administration, or intraoperatively.

Cardiovascular system (CVS): Severe hypotension can occur if the block is high. Cardiac arrest is one of the rare complications encountered. This is secondary to unrecognized total spinal or the preoperative comorbid condition of the patient or intraoperative surgical causes.

Respiratory system: Respiratory arrest, although very rare, is mainly due to hypoperfusion of respiratory center. This may also occur as a part of the complication in *total spinal.*

Total spinal: Although this is not so common, it is advisable to be knowledgeable about the possibility. High spinal or total spinal can occur both during subarachnoid block and epidural block. Accidental rapid injection or rise of the injected drug volume in subarachnoid space causes the drug to depress the brain. This complication is termed as *total spinal.* Accidental total spinal causes profound hypotension, bradycardia, respiratory arrest requiring fluids, vasopressor, atropine, and ventilatory support.

Local anesthetic toxicity: This is a rare complication in subarachnoid block, and is relatively more common with epidural blocks. Toxic manifestations are generally due to migration of epidural catheter resulting in accidental intravascular injection rather than absorption from epidural space. The chief complications affect cardiovascular, respiratory, and central nervous system. Toxic blood concentrations depress cardiac conduction and excitability, which may lead to atrioventricular block, ventricular arrhythmias and cardiac arrest, sometimes resulting in fatalities. In addition, myocardial contractility is depressed and peripheral vasodilation occurs, leading to decreased cardiac output and arterial blood pressure. Adrenaline-containing local anesthetic solutions have modest increase in heart rate, cardiac output, decreased peripheral vascular resistance, and mean arterial pressure. Toxic levels can produce CNS stimulation, depression or both and may be manifested as restlessness, tremors and shivering, which may progress to convulsions, followed by coma and ultimately to respiratory arrest. Local anesthetics like lidocaine are more toxic to CNS, whereas bupivacaine produces more CVS toxicity.

Pruritus is relatively common and is associated with administration of intrathecal opioids. Pruritus is effectively treated by using naloxone.

Delayed Complications

Following subarachnoid back after a day or two, patients may develop headache. This could be due to chemical meningism, infective meningitis, or low-pressure headache which is termed as PDPH. PDPH is caused by CSF leak resulting in continuous headache, aggravated by standing, sitting, and coughing. It is relieved by lying down. The condition is one of the common complications with a reported incidence of as high as 25%. The incidence decreases if smaller needles with noncutting tip are used. PDPH is reported to be as low as 1.5% when 24-G noncutting is used. Hence, it is recommended that noncutting needles of 25 G be used for subarachnoid blocks in young patients. In elderly patients, larger needles from 22 G to 25 G may be used. PDPH is conservatively treated with bed rest, caffein, analgesics, and adequate hydration. In refractory conditions, epidural blood patch may be used. There seems to be no role for prophylactic blood patch.

Late Postoperative Complications

Transient radicular syndrome/transient neurological syndrome is a self-resolving pain thought to be related to the use of lidocaine, lithotomy position, and early ambulation in the postoperative period.

Low backache: It is the commonly attributed symptom by the medical profession. The back pain is secondary to the increased lordosis or improper positioning following the subarachnoid or epidural anesthesia. This is due to the relaxation of the muscles and ligaments maintaining the protective posture under anesthesia. The vigilant performer should be able to take precautionary measures to prevent this complication.

Cauda equina syndrome: Cauda equina syndrome is a major complication in the postoperative period. It is attributed to the type of local anesthetic administered, trauma to the spinal cord during subarachnoid puncture, and posture. Unlike transient radicular syndrome, transient neurological syndrome is not a self-resolving pain.

Serious neurological deficits are rare; the most common injuries are persistent paresthesia, and limited motor weakness. Direct trauma by the subarachnoid needle causes nerve root lesions, rarely cord injury. Severe hypotension may cause ischemia of the cord. Subarachnoid hematomas and abscess do occur as a complication. Though rare, paraplegia or death due to injection of cleaning chemical or wrong drug is devastating to the patient and performer.

Urinary retention is not uncommon in the postoperative period with opioids as an adjuvant or as a reflex mechanism in lower abdominal surgery.

POSTOPERATIVE CARE

The postoperative recovery begins at the end of surgery, i.e., on the operating table. During recovery from an anesthetic, the patient should receive the same vigilant care as the patient recovering from GA. The patient should be assessed for block regression at the end of surgery before transportation to the postanesthesia care unit. The patient should be assessed for urinary retention in the absence of a urinary drainage catheter. The discharge from the recovery room should not occur until vital signs are stable with regression of the subarachnoid block. It is important to follow the postanesthesia care protocols before transfer. The patient should remain in bed until full sensory and motor functions have returned. It is mandatory for the concerned performer to visit the patient in the postanesthesia care unit before transfer and again the following postoperative day.

Monitoring

It is essential to monitor the respiration, pulse, and blood pressure repeatedly at each stage of the technique. The blood pressure can fall precipitously following induction of spinal anesthesia, in patients with delicate hemodynamic balance, particularly the elderly. The signs that are of concern of dropping blood pressure include pallor, sweating, nausea, or feeling generally unwell.

It is mandatory to ensure that the block is adequate for the surgical procedure and does not progress further high by continuous monitoring for numbness of the arms or hands and difficulty with breathing which may indicate a higher spread of the block. An aggressive management of the blood pressure is required with a fall of >20% of the baseline blood pressure, and is associated with bradycardia which may progress to cardiac arrest.

It is not uncommon to notice the occurrence of bradycardia immediate to the administration and positioning requiring urgent remedial measures, indicating a high spread of block. It is also not uncommon to have bradycardia in the intraoperative period during manipulation of the structures of the foregut and the genitalia in both sexes. The need for immediate corrective measures is dependent on the well-being of the patient, and hemodynamic stability. A drop in the heart rate (below 50 beats/min) or associated hypotension may require corrective measures with intravenous anticholinergic (atropine 300–600 μg) drug in addition to intravenous fluid therapy.

It is generally considered a good practice, although debatable, for all patients undergoing surgery under subarachnoid (spinal) anesthesia to be administered supplemental oxygen by Hudson mask at a rate of 2–4 L/min or 1–2 L/min with nasal spectacle, especially if sedation has also been administered.

It is mandatory to monitor the patient continuously for block progression and complications after a successful placement of an epidural catheter and administration of the anesthetic. A continuous noninvasive hemodynamic monitoring of heart rate, pulse oximetry, at 5-minute interval initially for 30–45 minutes after administration of the anesthetic drug, followed by a 15-minute interval is essential throughout the surgical procedure. The patient should be monitored throughout the surgical period for signs and symptoms of toxicity of the local anesthetic on the CNS by continuous monitoring of the level of consciousness, breathing, and voice production.

It is mandatory to ensure that the block is adequate for the surgical procedure and does not progress too high by continuous monitoring for numbness of the arms or hands and problems with breathing which may indicate that the block is too high. An aggressive management is required if the blood pressure fall is >20% of the baseline blood pressure, and also bradycardia since it may progress to cardiac arrest.

NEURAXIAL BLOCKS IN PATIENTS ON ANTICOAGULANTS

Although the incidence of neurological dysfunction, resulting from hemorrhagic complications associated with neuraxial blockade, cited in the literature is estimated to be <1 in 150,000 epidurals and <1 in 220,000 spinal anesthetics, recent epidemiological surveys suggest that the frequency is increasing and may be as high as 1 in 3,000 in some patient populations.

SUMMARY OF CURRENT RECOMMENDATIONS

Antiplatelets

- Neuraxial blocks can be performed on patients taking aspirin or nonsteroidal anti-inflammatory drugs.
- It is safe to perform neuraxial blocks on patients taking cyclooxygenase (COX)-2 inhibitors.
- For the thienopyridine drugs, the American Society of Regional Anesthesia (ASRA) recommendation is that clopidogrel be discontinued for 7 days and ticlopidine for 10–14 days before a neuraxial injection.
- Epidural catheters can be removed safely and neuraxial injections can be performed 5 days (not 7 days, as once advised) after clopidogrel is discontinued.

Oral Anticoagulants

The current ASRA guidelines recommend an INR value of ≤1.4 as acceptable for the performance of neuraxial blocks.

Intravenous Heparin

The following considerations are in order for IV heparin:

- There should be at least a 1-hour delay between needle placement and heparin administration.
- The catheter should be removed 1 hour before subsequent heparin administration and 2–4 hours after the last heparin dose.
- The partial thromboplastin time or activated clotting time should be monitored to avoid excessive heparin effect.

Patients Receiving Low-molecular-weight Heparin

- The administration of other anticoagulant medications with low-molecular-weight heparins (LMWHs) may increase the risk of spinal hematoma.
- The presence of blood during needle placement and catheter placement does not necessitate postponement of surgery. However, the initiation of LMWH therapy should be delayed for 24 hours postoperatively.
- The first dose of LMWH prophylaxis should be given no earlier than 24 hours postoperatively and only in the presence of adequate hemostasis.
- In patients who are on LMWH, needle/catheter placement (or catheter removal) should be performed at least 12 hours after the last prophylactic dose of enoxaparin or 24 hours after higher doses of enoxaparin (1 mg/kg every 12 hours), and 24 hours after dalteparin (120 U/kg every 12 hours or 200 U/kg every 12 hours) or tinzaparin (175 U/kg daily).

- The LMWH can be administered 2 hours after the epidural catheter is removed.
- Monitoring of anti-Xa level is not recommended.

Thrombolytic Therapy

Except in highly unusual circumstance, patients who received fibrinolytic or thrombolytic drugs should be cautioned against receiving spinal or epidural blocks. There is no definite recommendation on the timing of removal of neuraxial catheters in patients who unexpectedly receive fibrinolytics or thrombolytics. Measurement of fibrinogen levels may be helpful in guiding the decision to remove epidural catheter.

Herbal Therapy

At this time, there appears to be no specific concerns as to timing of neuraxial block in relation to the dosing of herbal therapy.

Fondaparinux

- Rapidly absorbed, it reaches maximum concentration within 1.7 hours of administration. Its half-life is 17–21 hours, allowing once-daily dosing.
- The ASRA recommends against the use of fondaparinux in the presence of an indwelling epidural catheter.
- Avoid indwelling catheters.

Thrombin Inhibitors

The most recent ASRA guidelines recommend against the performance of neuraxial techniques in patients who received thrombin inhibitors.

Newer Anticoagulants

Dabigatran Etexilate

Dabigatran is an oral direct thrombin inhibitor. Its bioavailability is only 5%, peak plasma levels occur at 2 hours, and its halflife is 8 hours after a single dose but up to 17 hours after multiple doses. 48-hour interval is recommended before a neuraxial injection.

Rivaroxaban

- Rivaroxaban is an oral factor Xa inhibitor. Its peak effect occurs after 1 hour; the duration of effect is 12 hours, and it has a halflife of 9–13 hours.
- No reported incidence of spinal hematoma
- In the studies reviewed apparently, a 24-hour interval (2 x halflife) was observed between the rivaroxaban dose and epidural catheter placement

or removal; subsequent dosing of the drug was 6 hours after removal of the catheter.

Prasugrel

- Prasugrel is an oral anticoagulant and its mechanism of action is similar to clopidogrel.
- Prasugrel and clopidogrel are prodrugs.
- Prasugrel has a quicker onset of action, a longer duration and is 10 times more potent.
- A 7–10-day interval is recommended before a neuraxial injection.

SUGGESTED READING

1. Brull R, Macfarlane AJR, Chan VWS. Spinal, epidural, and caudal anesthesia. In: Miller RD (Ed). Miller's Anesthesia, 8th edition. Philadelphia: Elsevier Churchill Livingstone; 2015. pp. 1684-720.
2. Burkard J, Lee Olson R, Vacchiano CA. Regional anesthesia. In: Nagelhout JJ, Zaglaniczny KL (Eds). Nurse Anesthesia. St. Louis: Elsevier Saunders. 5th Edition, 2014.
3. Carron M, Freo U, Veronese S, Innocente F, Ori C. Spinal block with 1.5 mg hyperbaric bupivacaine: not successful for everyone. Anesth Analg. 2007;105: 1515-6.
4. Desjardins AE, Hendriks BH, van der Voort M, Nachabé R, Bierhoff W, Braun G, et al. Epidural needle with embedded optical fibers for spectroscopic differentiation of tissue: *ex vivo* feasibility study. Biomed Opt Express. 2011;2(6):1452-61.
5. Drasner K. Local anesthetic neurotoxicity. Clinical injury and strategies that may minimize risk. Reg Anesth Pain Med. 2002;27:576-80.
6. Evron S, Gurstieva V, Ezri T, Gladkov V, Shopin S, Herman A, et al. Transient neurological symptoms after isobaric subarachnoid anesthesia with 2% lidocaine: the impact of needle type. Anesth Analg. 2007;105:1494-9.
7. Ghelber O, Gebhard RE, Vora S, Hagberg CA, Szmuk P. Identification of the epidural space using pressure measurement with the compuflo injection pump—a pilot study. Reg Anesth Pain Med. 2008;33(4):346-52.
8. Glaser C, Marhofer P, Zimpfer G, Heinz MT, Sitzwohl C, Kapral S, et al. Levobupivacaine versus racemic bupivacaine for spinal anesthesia. Anesth Analg. 2002;94(1):194-8.
9. Gray AT. Neuraxial blocks. In: Gray AT (Ed). Atlas of ultrasound guided regional anesthesia, 2nd edition. Philadelphia: Saunders, Elsevier Inc; 2013. pp. 249-56.
10. Kleinman W, Mikhail M. Spinal, epidural, and caudal blocks. In: Butterworth JF, Mackey DC, Wasnick JD (Eds). Morgan and Mikhail's Clinical Anesthesiology, 5th edition. New York: Lange Medical Books; 2013. pp. 937-74.
11. Lee YY, Muchhal K, Chan CK, Cheung AS. Levobupivacaine and fentanyl for spinal anesthesia: a randomized trial. Eur J Anesthesiol. 2005;22(12):899-903.
12. Luck JF, Fettes PD, Wildsmith JA. Spinal anesthesia for elective surgery: a comparison of hyperbaric solutions of racemic bupivacaine, levobupivacaine, and ropivacaine. Br J Anaesth. 2008;101(5):705-10.

13. Neustein SM. The use of lidocaine for spinal anesthesia. Anesth Analg. 2008;106:1586-7.
14. Niemi G, Breivik H. Epinephrine markedly improves thoracic epidural analgesia produced by small-dose infusion of ropivacaine, fentanyl, and epinephrine after major thoracic or abdominal surgery: a randomized, double-blind cross-over study with and without epinephrine. Anesth Analg. 2002;94:1598-605.
15. Saberski LR, Kondamuri S, Osinubi OY. Identification of the epidural space: Is loss of resistance to air a safe technique? A review of the complications related to the use of air. Reg Anesth. 1997;22(1):3-15.
16. Samhan YM, El-Sabae HH, Khafagy HF, Maher MA. A pilot study to compare epidural identification and catheterization using a saline-filled syringe versus a continuous hydrostatic pressure system. J Anesth. 2013;27(4):607-10.
17. Schier R, Guerra D, Aguilar J, Pratt GF, Hernandez M, Boddu K, et al. Epidural space identification: a meta-analysis of complications after air versus liquid as the medium for loss of resistance. Anesth Analg. 2009;109(6):2012-21.
18. Warren DT, Neil JM, Bernards CM. Neuraxial anesthesia. In: Longnecker DE, Brown DL (Eds). Anesthesiology. New York: McGraw-Hill Medical; 2012. pp. 786-807.
19. Waxler B, Mondragon SA, Patel SN, Nedumgottil K.. Intrathecal lidocaine and sufentanil shorten postoperative recovery after outpatient rectal surgery. Can J Anaesth. 2004;51:680-4.

WEBSITES

1. http://www.proceduresconsult.com/medical-procedures/. Last accessed Oct., 2024.
2. http://www.rxlist.com/. Drugs used for subarachnoid block. Last accessed Oct., 2024.
3. http://www.drugs.com/. Professionals' prescribing information. Last accessed Oct., 2024.
4. http://www.nysora.com/index.php?news=3425. Spinal anesthesia. Last accessed Oct., 2024.
5. http://www.frca.co.uk/article.aspx?articleid=100126. Last accessed Oct., 2024.
6. http://www.exmoorinnovations.co.uk/index.php?option =com_content&view= article&id=1&Itemid=42. Epidrum. Last accessed Oct., 2024.
7. http://www.hospira.com/en/products_and_services/drugs/index. Last accessed Oct., 2024.
8. http://www.hindawi.com/journals/bmri/2014/437679/. Fiber optic-based epidural anesthesia. Last accessed Oct., 2024.
9. http://www.amepc.org/qims/article/view/5333/6249. Portable intelligent system for optical-technology-based epidural space detection optical needle fibre. Last accessed Oct., 2024.
10. http://radiopaedia.org/articles/scotty-dog-sign. Scotty dog sign. Last accessed Oct., 2024.
11. https://www.asra.com/advisory-guidelines/article/1/anticoagulation-3rd-edition. Horlocker TT, Wedel DJ, Rowlingson JC, et al. ASRA practice advisory. Last accessed Oct., 2024.

CHAPTER 12

Disinfection and Sterilization

Karisha Hinkson-LaCorbinière

INTRODUCTION

As healthcare providers, we well know the mantra of "first, do no harm" (*Primum non nocere—in Latin*). Healthcare-associated infections are the leading cause of preventable disease. Disinfection and sterilization therefore become an essential tool in infection control.

Oliver Wendell Holmes and Ignaz Semmelweis independently, in 1843, proposed the germ theory that infection could be spread from one patient to another by medical personnel and/or the instruments used for patient care and successfully implemented prophylactic measures of handwashing and washing of instruments before patient handling which led to a marked decrease in morbidity and mortality of patients under his care and many millions of others to follow. He used then a solution of chlorine in limewater with good success. Almost 2 centuries later, this simple mantra holds true that handwashing **(Fig. 1)** and adequate antiseptic measures still are our most effective weapons in the ongoing war against transmission of infection. All reusable items are subjected to some form of decontamination. Sterilization, disinfection, and antisepsis are all forms of decontamination **(Table 1)**.

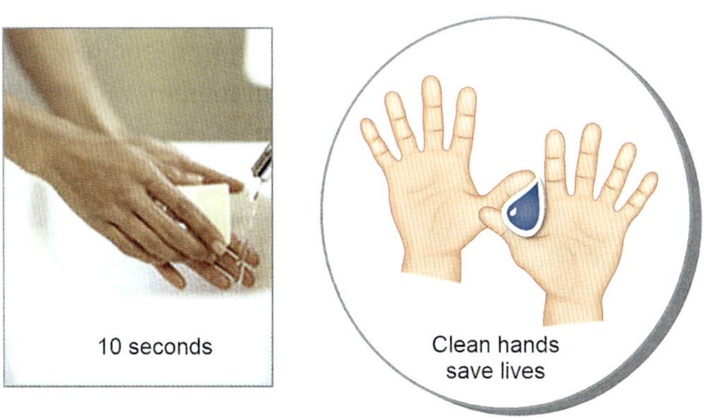

Fig. 1: Washing hands properly prevents transinfection from patient to healthcare worker and vice versa.

TABLE 1: Cleaning, disinfection, and sterilization.

Cleaning	*Disinfection*	*Sterilization*
Cleaning is the removal of visible soil (e.g., organic and inorganic material) from objects and surfaces	Disinfection describes a process that eliminates many or all pathogenic microorganisms on inanimate objects with the exception of bacterial spores	Sterilization is the complete elimination or destruction of all forms of microbial life
It is normally accomplished by manual or mechanical means using water with detergents or enzymatic products	It is usually accomplished by the use of liquid chemical and heat (washer disinfector)	This is accomplished in healthcare facilities by either physical or chemical processes
Cleaning does much to reduce risk of vCJD		

(vCJD: variant Creutzfeldt-Jakob disease)

BOX 1: Sterilization and levels of disinfection.

Sterilization:
- Kills all microbial life including highly resistant spores and prions

High-level disinfection:
- Kills all bacteria including tubercle bacilli, fungi and viruses, but a small number of bacteria spores may survive

Intermediate-level disinfection:
- Kills most bacteria, most fungi and most viruses, but tubercle bacilli and bacterial spores survive

Low-level disinfection:
- Kills most bacteria, some fungi and some viruses, but mycobacteria and bacterial spores survive

LEVELS OF DISINFECTION

Disinfection can be further subclassified into high, intermediate, and low levels according to which organisms may survive the process. The levels of disinfection and techniques used to achieve them are as shown in **Box 1**.

SPAULDING CLASSIFICATION

Whether a specific piece of equipment should be disinfected, sterilized, or used after cleaning alone depends on its intended use. In 1968, Earl Spaulding and colleagues categorized these devices into critical, semicritical, and noncritical **(Table 2)**.

TABLE 2: Spaulding's classification of various medical devices.

Critical devices	
Syringes, needles, stopcocks, IV tubing, percutaneous cardiac interventional catheters, surgical instruments, and urethral catheters	Use disposable equipment or cleaning followed by sterilization techniques that destroy all endospores, viruses, and vegetative bacteria
Semicritical devices	
Gastrointestinal endoscopes, esophageal echocardiography and temperature probes, laryngoscope blades, endotracheal tubes, laryngeal mask airways, and nasopharyngeal and oropharyngeal airways	Use disposable equipment or cleaning followed by HLD. Sterilization is not necessary
Noncritical devices	
Patient's care items: Laryngoscope handles, stethoscopes, blood pressure cuffs, facemasks, etc. *Environmental surfaces:* Stretcher side rails, mattresses, walls and surfaces within the immediate patient's care area	• ILD or LLD • Regular cleaning

(HLD: high-level disinfection; ILD: intermediate-level disinfection; LLD: low-level disinfection).

Critical devices are instruments that are introduced into the blood or any sterile area in the body. *Semicritical devices* are items that come into contact with but do not penetrate mucous membranes and/or nonintact skin. *Noncritical devices* are items that only come into contact with intact skin. The Spaulding's system has limitations, and oversimplification is both its strength and its weakness. The recommended guidelines for the level of decontamination are as shown in **Table 2**.

CLEANING

The first step in decontamination is cleaning. It serves to rid the device of large quantities of microbes that are attached to organic material. This foreign material may serve to protect microbes from the chemical or physical antimicrobial agents, or may protect them by diluting or inactivating these agents. Hence, *all* items requiring disinfection or sterilization must undergo proper cleaning beforehand. Equipment should be fully dismantled to ensure proper cleaning of all its surfaces, especially those that have a lumen. This process can be achieved by:

- Chemical action (use of detergents or enzymatic agents)
- Thermal action (mildly warm water)
- Mechanical action (mechanical or ultrasound washers)

Delicate instruments (optical equipment) should be cleaned with caution. After cleaning, the devices should be rinsed and dried. The operator should protect themselves against exposure to chemical agents.

METHODS OF DISINFECTION

Physical Methods

Boiling: Devices are exposed to boiling water (≥100°C) in a container for 15–25 minutes. The devices should be completely covered by the boiling water and the container itself is also covered, with no breaks during the boiling cycle, e.g., addition of other devices during a cycle.

Flushing and washer disinfectors or water-jet disinfectors: These are automated machines that flush, clean, rinse, and disinfect. It uses water at temperature 80–90°C and cycles from 1 minute to 25 minutes.

Pasteurization: These devices are exposed to hot water at 77°C for 30 minutes. This process will offer high-level disinfection (HLD) but does not destroy bacterial spores. It is suitable for most airway devices even in the presence of drug-resistant bacteria.

Irradiation

Ultraviolet radiation: These devices use ultraviolet radiation (210–328 nm), which has maximum antimicrobial action in the 240–280 nm range. The radiation causes the denaturation of nucleic acids and seems more effective on bacteria and viruses than spores. Multiple factors affect its germicidal activity: the potency of the UV tubes; the degree of organic burden; the wavelength and the intensity of the UV. UV radiation has been used to disinfect surfaces of the operating theater environment. One must ensure that patients and exposed persons are protected against keratoconjunctivitis.

Liquid Chemical Agents

These agents are the most commonly used form of disinfection in the hospital setting. Multiple agents and multiple commercial formulations that are available to make it necessary that the manufacturer's guidelines for each agent be adhered to for the sake of efficacy. Many of the liquid chemicals are quite toxic, and the process of disinfection is carried out manually. Hence, proper precautions such as protective gear (gloves, masks, etc.) and adequate ventilation should be in place.

Alcohol (Ethyl or Isopropyl)

Sixty to ninety percent alcohol in water is bactericidal to most bacteria, tuberculocidal, fungicidal, and virucidal to most viruses [including hepatitis B virus (HBV) and human immunodeficiency virus (HIV)]. Spores are spared. They are used to disinfect stethoscopes, thermometers, and external surfaces. The Centers for Disease Control and Prevention (CDC) recommends exposure to 70% ethanol for 15 minutes to inactivate HBV, but 1 minute should be adequate for HIV.

Glutaraldehyde

It comes in concentrations of 2, 2.4, and 3.4% and is popularly known as Cidex Plus®. Alkaline solutions are more efficient than acidic solutions. Once activated, it has shelf-life up to 4 weeks. It is most commonly used for HLD of endoscopes, anesthesia and respiratory equipment, dialyzers, and transducers when sterilization is not possible.

Orthophthalaldehyde

It is commonly known as Cidex orthophthalaldehyde (OPA) and is effective for HLD. It is bactericidal, fungicidal, virucidal, and sporicidal when contaminated devices are soaked for 10–20 minutes. Disinfection with OPA is indicated for semicritical instruments that come into contact with mucous membranes or broken skin, such as specula, laryngeal mirrors, and internal ultrasound probes.

Formaldehyde is generally not used nowadays due to its pungent odor and carcinogenicity.

Liquid Bleach

Sodium hypochlorite solution has antimicrobial effect and is an inexpensive, fast-acting, easy-to-store high-level disinfecting agent. 1 mL household bleach when diluted with 1,000 mL water yields 50 ppm solution and is effective against vegetative bacteria and HIV. Many viruses are inactivated with 200 ppm solution. 500 ppm solution is effective against HBV. Chlorinated agents are used for the decontamination of environmental surfaces following spills (bodily fluids on floor). They can be used for disinfecting mannequins, laundry, mattresses, and nurses' station.

Hydrogen Peroxide

Six to ten percent hydrogen peroxide exhibits bactericidal, mycobactericidal, fungicidal, virucidal, and sporicidal activity. It is nontoxic, does not damage glass or plastic articles, and is a good choice of HLD for ventilators, tubing, fabrics, soft contact lenses, endoscopes, and laparoscopic equipment.

Phenols

Phenols are present in commonly used hospital disinfectants and are considered intermediate to low-level disinfectants. Most phenolic detergents are tuberculocidal, fungicidal, and bactericidal when used as directed.

Certain viruses, including those associated with widespread common respiratory illnesses, are resistant to these compounds. Commercial 3% phenols are bactericidal, kill some viruses, and kill most fungi but they do not kill *M. tuberculosis* or small viruses, e.g., poliovirus and echovirus.

Iodophors

These are iodine with a solubilizing agent in solution. The latter allows free iodine to be available; it is the free iodine that is the active antimicrobial agent with this type of disinfecting agent. The most common example in the healthcare setting is povidone-iodine. Iodophors are used for low-level disinfection and as a skin antiseptic.

Regardless of the type of disinfecting agent used for HLD, adequate monitoring of the critical parameters for each agent should be adhered to, that is, the concentration of the agent, temperature, and exposure time. Also, the validity and recommendations as provided by the manufacturer should be adhered to.

STERILIZATION

Sterilization is any method that will destroy all microbial life including spores. Strictly speaking, sterilization is a relative term and represents the probability of a single living microorganism occurring on a product after undergoing a sterilization process. This is commonly referred to as the *sterility assurance level or SAL* and expressed as 10-n; for example, if the probability of finding a live micro-organism is one in a million then the corresponding SAL would be 10-6. SAL then would also describe how lethal a particular sterilization method is, where one that gives a SAL of 10-6 would be more lethal than one that gives a SAL of 10-3. In the USA, there are two SAL standards, 10–3 for drainage bags, blood collecting tubes and the like, and 10-6 for more critical devices, e.g., scalpels, implants, etc. Both these SAL numbers were chosen arbitrarily according to patient's risk and have a wide margin of error.

The various methods may be subclassified below **(Flowcharts 1A to C)**.

Dry Heat

This form of sterilization employs exposure of material to hot dry air. Exposure times at given temperatures are shown in **Table 3**.

Mechanism of Action

Death occurs due to energy transfer and by oxidative mechanisms too. Dry heat sterilization may be employed for items that are heat-resistant but cannot undergo the process of moist heat (oils, silicone, paraffin, creams, and talcum powder). This technique is less corrosive with metals (exception are copper-based ones); it is relatively inexpensive, and no hazardous

Flowcharts 1A to C: (A) Different methods of sterilization; (B) Physical methods of sterilization; and (C) Chemical methods of sterilization.

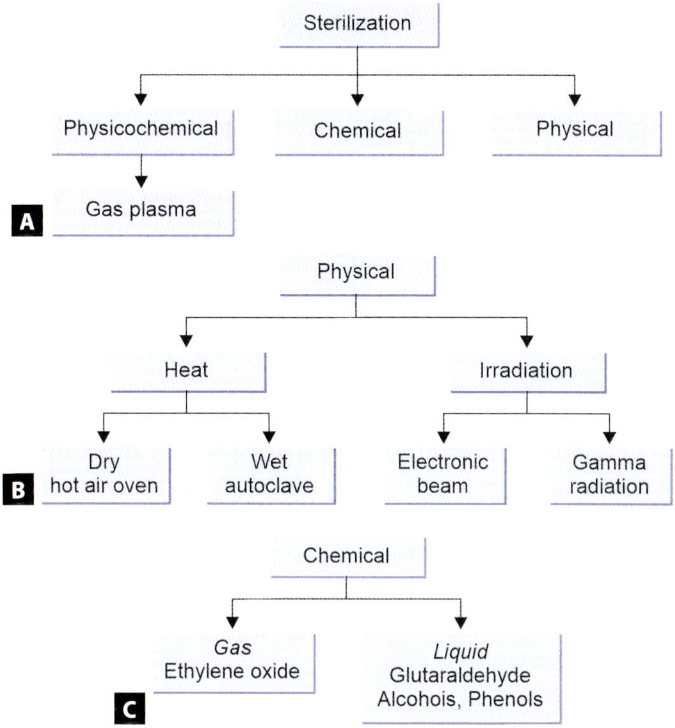

TABLE 3: Dry heat and steam sterilization with temperature and time.

Dry heat sterilization				
Temperature	150°C	160°C	170°C	
Exposure time	150 min	120 min	60 min	
Autoclave: Steam under pressure (>15 psi)				
Temperature	121°C	126°C	(Flash) 134°C	150°C
Exposure time	15 min	10 min	3–4 min	A few seconds

material or waste is produced. Other items that may be considered for dry heat sterilization include sharp stainless steel instruments (scissors, needles, and blades), crystal syringes, glass tubes, etc.

Steam Sterilization (Autoclaving)

Steam sterilization is the most commonly used form of sterilization and is recommended for all items that are heat- and moisture-resistant. It is the use of heated steam under pressure in a specialized chamber called an autoclave. Autoclaving should be considered the gold standard in sterilization. It involves the exposure of the device or item to be sterilized to saturated steam at high temperatures (120–135°C), under pressure (≥15 psi), for a specified period of time **(Table 3)**. Pressure per se does not destroy the organism; rather it is necessary to produce steam at higher temperatures. The mechanism of action is the destruction of proteins by the moist heat. Sterilization by steam affords the advantage of having short sterilization times, relatively affordable and safe, no associated toxic agents or toxic waste and least affected by organic or inorganic material. Disadvantages include: It is neither suitable for heat or moisture-sensitive devices nor flammable or volatile chemicals; residual moisture may encourage rusting and corrosion; delicate or microinstruments may be damaged over time; it may affect the light port and/or viewing port for some pieces of equipment, e.g., laryngoscopes, and burns (of staff or patients) are possible.

Autoclave

The basic components of an autoclave include a high-pressure chamber where water is heated to steam and pressurized, a pressure control valve and a fail-safe system that prevents buildup of very high pressures. Lastly, there is also a mechanism for air-expulsion to prevent dilution of the saturation of steam.

Flash Sterilization

This is a modified version of steam sterilization, designed to process instruments for urgent use. There are flash autoclaves especially designed for this purpose and operate at temperatures of 134oC for 3–4 minutes. Flash sterilization may be used for cleaned patient care devices that cannot be sterilized, packaged, and stored before use and for items for urgent use. It is particularly useful if stationed in or near the operating theater so that transfer of the uncovered sterilized device is as short as possible and in a clean environment. The longer the device is in contact with air, the greater the risk of recontamination. Routine use of this form of steam sterilization should not be encouraged since the devices that are sterilized are unwrapped, and the cycle eliminates drying so that the risk of recontamination is greatly increased. Generally speaking, flash sterilization should not be used for implants.

Monitoring Steam Sterilization

Mechanical, chemical, and biological controls are used to monitor the steam sterilization process.

Mechanical: An example of this is a printout or graph of temperatures reached during the cycle and a record of the time at the appropriate temperature and pressure.

Chemical: May be used both externally and internally into the pack to monitor the temperature and/or time.

Bowie-Dick test: It is used to detect air leaks and/or inadequate air removal in the system. A Bowie-Dick test sheet is placed in the center of a test pack of 100% cotton-folded surgical swabs that are clean and preconditioned. The pack is then very specifically placed in the sterilizing chamber by itself as the first load of the day. If the test sheet shows a uniform color change, then the autoclave performance is adequate. The appearance of any spots means that entrapped air was present and the test has failed. Autoclaves that have failed the Bowie-Dick test should be checked by a technician and not be used until a subsequent Bowie-Dick test has been passed **(Figs. 2 and 3)**.

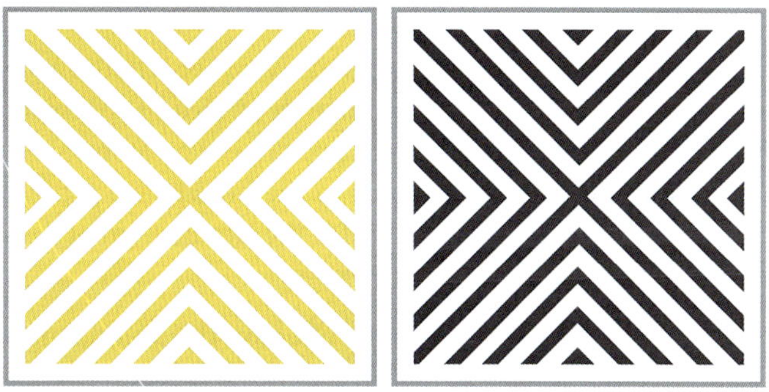

Fig. 2: Adequacy of autoclave. Unprocessed disposable test pack on left and a successful test on right (all turned black without any yellow patches).

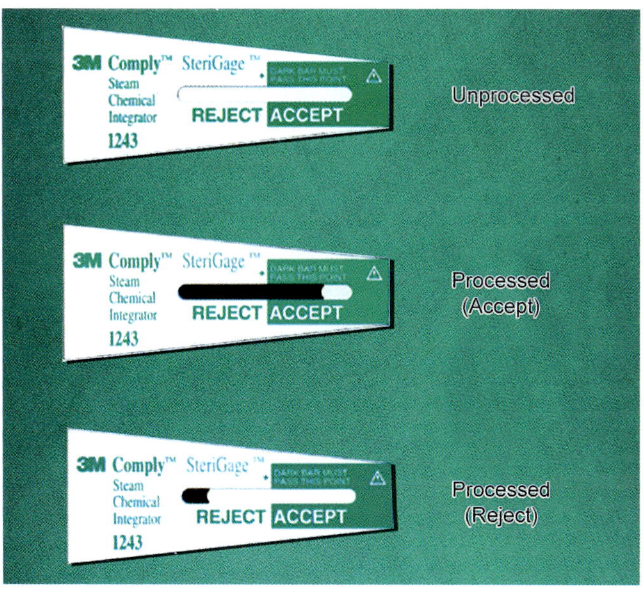

Fig. 3: 3M Comply™ SteriGage™ which assesses adequacy of the autoclave process.

Biological (spore test): This may be monitored by the introducing a commercially prepared biological indicator containing *Geobacillus stearothermophilus* spores into the autoclave, which is otherwise empty, placed in an area of the sterilization chamber which may be least accessible by steam and a full cycle is performed. The tester is then sent to the laboratory and analyzed for presence of surviving spores. A positive spore test is a rare but important event, and use of the respective autoclave is discontinued until a technician evaluates it and a negative spore test is obtained. Usual causes include inaccurate operation, inadequate steam delivery, or equipment malfunction.

CHEMICAL STERILIZATION

Ethylene Oxide

Ethylene oxide (EtO) is a colorless and faintly sweet-smelling gas at room temperature. It is a toxic substance, which is irritant, flammable, and explosive with known mutagenic and carcinogenic potential in humans. It has been used as a chemical sterilant in the healthcare profession since 1950 and is a commonly used alternative for the sterilization of delicate heat-sensitive and moisture-sensitive devices.

There are four parameters that determine effective operational use:

1. Concentration (450–1,200 mg/L of gas)
2. Temperature (37–63°C)
3. Exposure time (1–6 hours) **(Table 4)**
4. Humidity (40–80%; EtO needs H_2O to carry it)

Ethylene oxide sterilizer may come as pure EtO cartridges or as a mixed gas. The chamber pressure is usually subatmospheric when pure EtO is used but the EtO mixtures require higher than normal atmospheric pressures.

The stages of the EtO sterilization cycle include:

- Preconditioning and humidification
- Introduction, exposure, and then evacuation of the gas
- Aeration

The last part of the process is vital and is the longest part of the process. The aeration process may be done automated or by air drying, but the latter

TABLE 4: Times for ethylene oxide sterilization.

Method of EtO aeration	*Temperature in °C*	*Duration in hours*
Air drying	20	168
Automated (mechanical)	50	12
Automated (mechanical) drying	60	8

(EtO: ethylene oxide)

takes a much greater time as lower temperatures decrease the desorption process.

With the exception of metals, EtO adsorbs to materials (including the paper and the metal instruments are wrapped in) and if not properly aerated to allow for desorption of the chemical, residual EtO may be introduced to both patient and staff causing serious health concerns. This is particularly so for indwelling devices. Some manufacturers have issued warnings explicitly advising users not to sterilize their laryngeal mask airways using EtO as the material used seems to adsorb the gas for longer periods (despite usual aeration times) and would have a higher risk of life-threatening reaction than other devices used elsewhere in the body. Acute exposure to EtO may result in irritation to skin, eyes, gastrointestinal and respiratory tracts, and central nervous system depression. Symptoms include chemical burns, headaches, nausea and vomiting, dyspnea, cyanosis, pulmonary edema, weakness, and ECG abnormalities. Chronic exposure has been associated with cataracts, cognitive impairment, neurologic dysfunction, polyneuropathies, hematologic changes, an increased risk of spontaneous abortions and various cancers. EtO should be considered a known human carcinogen. Hence, multiple brands of product exist to aid with monitoring of EtO exposure in the workplace, for example, passive monitors **(Fig. 4)** such as the 3M 3551 and Amsco EtO Self-Scan which must be worn by personnel and act as indicators of exposure, or environmental exposure devices such as gas chromatographs (Envirogard III) and detector tubes (Draeger).

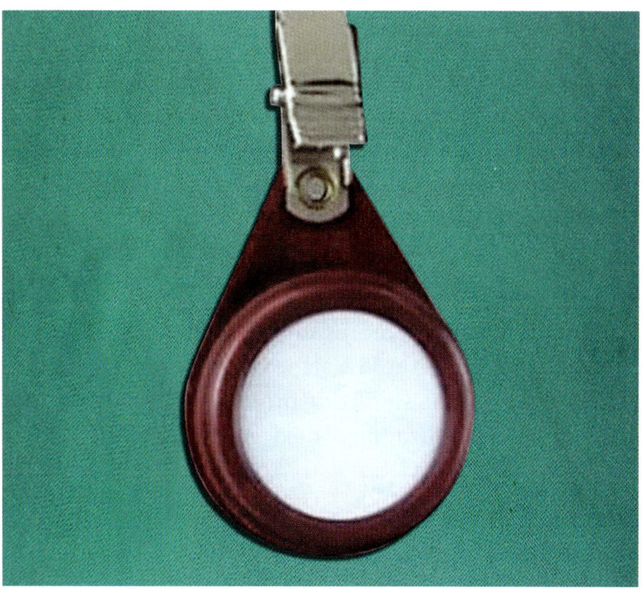

Fig. 4: Example of a passive ethylene oxide (EtO) (personal) monitor (3M).

The EtO chemical is highly reactive and causes the death of microbes by alkylation of functional groups on structural proteins and enzymes as well as on DNA and RNA, so interfering with both cellular metabolism and reproduction.

Until the mid-1990s, the carrier gas was a chlorofluorocarbons (CFCs); however due to environmental concerns, these types of EtO preparations are no longer available for use. Their immediate replacement EtO with hydrochlorofluorocarbon (HCFC) mixture is less damaging than the CFCs but still a hazard and their use is scheduled for regulation and review 2015 with a planned discontinuation altogether by year 2030.

Liquid

Sterilization by immersion in liquid sterilants is not ideal and should only be reserved for those devices that are not compatible with other forms of sterilization. The process is difficult to control and has a much greater risk of recontamination afterward during the rinsing or drying process and, of course, the devices cannot be prepackaged. There are also environmental and health concerns with the use of many of the chemical agents currently in use for sterilization of medical materials.

Most of the liquid chemical agents aforementioned are also used for sterilization but with either longer immersion times and/or more concentrated agent.

Steris System

Steris 20 is a patented product for sterilizing fibrotic scopes. The active ingredient is a concentrate of 35% peracetic acid solution. The equipment needs to be cleaned, but there is no need for drying. It is then placed securely in a special container. The tray is sealed and loaded into the processor. Diluted sterilant is circulated on the equipment at 50°C for about 12 minutes. Then, the equipment is raised and rinsed with sterile water and taken for use. The whole cycle may take 20–45 minutes.

Physicochemical Methods

Hydrogen peroxide plasma is an example of this. Hydrogen peroxide is vaporized in aqueous solution at 58% of the plasma state. The unique property of this method is that it offers sterilizing properties at lower temperatures, so making it useful for the sterilization of devices that have only a low resistance to heat.

The parameters that determine effective operational use:

- Temperature (<50°C)
- Exposure time (45–75 minutes)
- Pressure (subatmospheric)

Mechanism of action: Along with the oxidation action expected of the hydrogen peroxide, there is also alkylation activity of free radicals.

There are other methods of sterilization available; however, these are usually reserved for mass sterilization and some are still not yet officially approved for sterilization of medical equipment. Examples include ozone sterilization, infrared or ionizing radiation, microwave radiation, peracetic acid vapor and filtration. **Table 5** compares the most common types of in-hospital sterilization techniques.

TABLE 5: Comparison of various methods of commonly used sterilization.

Method of sterilization	*Advantages*	*Disadvantages*
Steam (autoclave)	• Nontoxic • Easy to control and monitor • Fast cycle time • Penetrates package material and lumens • Compatible with most devices	• Not appropriate for heat-sensitive instruments • Microsurgical instruments damaged by repeated exposure • May cause rusting • Potential for burns
Hydrogen peroxide gas plasma	• Nontoxic • Used for heat and moisture-sensitive devices (temp. less than 50°C) • Relatively short cycle time (28–75 min) • No aeration necessary • Compatible with most devices • Easy installation	• Low penetration power • Cellulose items are not compatible (e.g., paper and cotton) and special packaging materials are required • Items with very narrow and/or long lumen may be incompatible
EtO (pure and mixtures)	• Good penetration • Simple to operate and monitor • Compatible with most medical materials	• Requires aeration time to allow desorption of EtO • It is toxic, flammable, and carcinogenic • Hazardous to staff and patients • Long cycle time (including aeration)
Liquid chemical agents (e.g., Cidex OPA or Cidex Plus)	• Good for heat sensitive and delicate equipment • Flows through lumen, so providing more reliable sterilization of long narrow devices, e.g., endoscopes and bronchoscopes	• May be toxic/hazardous • Irritant to skin/eyes/respiratory tract • May require extensive flushing after (so compromising sterility) • No packaging and no storage • Some materials may be incompatible

CLEANING, DISINFECTION, AND STERILIZATION OF ANESTHESIA EQUIPMENT

Disposable equipment should be used when possible. High-efficiency particulate air (HEPA) filters may be used to prevent contamination of equipment. Develop strategies to reduce the risk of cross-contamination caused by anesthesia and respiratory equipment **(Table 6)**. Manufacturers'

TABLE 6: Disinfecting anesthesia equipment.

Environmental surfaces that may contribute to secondary cross-contamination (work environment, workstation, operating tables, etc.)	Cleaning; liquid antiseptics; dilute bleach for HIV and HBV
Noncritical items (monitoring cables, electrodes, skin probes, etc.)	Cleaning and LLD; use of germicidal sprays or swipes
Face masks (one of the heavily contaminated equipment)	Cleaned and HLD; liquid agents; EtO sterilization or autoclaving may be used depending on level of contamination
Breathing circuits	• Filters • Disassembling; cleaning and LLD. Metal pieces can be autoclaved. Rubber and plastic parts may undergo gas or plasma sterilization
Anesthesia cylinders	Unwrapped, washed with water, and detergent sprayed with germicides
Ventilators, tubes, bags and bellows, UDV, and APL valves	Clean surfaces. Tubes and bellows can be sterilized by EtO UDV can be disassembled and cleaned. Some APL valves can be autoclaved or pasteurized
Absorbers are rarely contaminated.	Newer machines have cassettes that can be easily removed and autoclaved
LMA	Autoclaved
Rigid laryngoscopes (precaution to be taken to prevent contamination of clean area after use)	Clean outside of handle and blade. Blades may be sterilized by liquids, EtO or autoclave
Flexible systems	Liquid disinfection; Steris system
Stylets	Immerse in liquid disinfectant
Endotracheal tubes	Clean immediately after use; rinse thoroughly and prevent drying of secretion. EtO is used most often. Spiral latex tubes should not be EtO sterilized with vacuum. Liquid chemical disinfection should be used in such equipment

(APL: adjustable pressure-limiting; HLD: high-level disinfection; LLD: low-level disinfection; UDV: unidirectional valve)

BOX 2: Risk to healthcare professional.

Strategies to reduce the risk of infectious disease transmission from patients to anesthesia professionals

- When following standard precautions:
  - Use barriers: Gloves, masks, face shields, safety glasses, and waterproof gowns to limit exposure
  - Practice timely and appropriate hand hygiene
- When caring for patients on airborne precautions:
  - Wear a well-fitting N95 mask
  - Ensure appropriate air-handling measures (negative-pressure rooms and HEPA filtration) are in effect in the patient's care location
  - Use a HEPA filter within the breathing circuit to prevent discharge of airborne infectious particles into the ambient environment
- When caring for patients on droplet precautions:
  - Wear a mask when working in close proximity (within 3–6 feet) of the patient
  - Use airborne precautions when performing aerosolizing procedures such as endotracheal intubation or suctioning or bronchoscopy
- When following principles of injection safety:
  - Do not recap or disassemble syringe and needle units prior to disposal
  - Locate puncture-resistant, leak-proof sharps containers where they can easily be accessed during patient care
  - Whenever possible and practical, use safety-engineered sharps devices (e.g., self-sheathing needles, safety catheters, scalpels with blade covers), and use needleless systems (e.g., stopcocks and valved access ports) for delivering parenteral medications and fluids and for performing anesthesia procedures.
  - Use a one-handed and scoop technique to recap needles, if recapping cannot be avoided
  - Avoid shearing or breaking needles
  - Use curved needles and needle holders for suturing (vis-à-vis straight needle) and forceps to hold tissue during suturing
  - Consider "double gloving" when performing procedures associated with a risk of needle-stick injury
- If a sharp injury occurs, wash the wound thoroughly with soap and water as soon as possible after the incident and report promptly to employee health or an infection prevention specialist for evaluation for possible prophylactic oral antiretroviral therapy
- Actively participate in periodic health assessments and infectious disease screening programs (e.g., periodic surveillance for tuberculosis infection)
- Get vaccinations recommended for healthcare professionals
- If you are suffering from a flulike or febrile illness, a severe respiratory infection, a weepy rash, or symptoms or signs of a highly transmissible disease (e.g., herpes zoster), refrain from patient's care activities until you are no longer contagious

(HEPA: high-efficiency particulate air)

instruction should be followed. Each institute must also develop strategies to prevent infectious disease transmission from patients to anesthesia professionals **(Box 2)**.

SUGGESTED READING

1. Acosta-Gnass SI, Stempliuk VA. Sterilization manual for health centers. Washington, D.C., United States: Pan American Health Organization; 2009.
2. Bucx MJ, Veldman DJ, Beenhakker MM, Koster R. The effect of steam sterilization at 134 degrees C on light intensity provided by fibrelight Macintoch laryngoscopes. Anaesthesia. 2000;55:185-6.
3. Canadian Standards Association (CSA). Decontamination of reusable medical devices. Mississauga, Ont.: Canadian Standards Association; 2008. pp. 1-87.
4. Owings MF, Kozak LJ. Ambulatory and inpatient procedures in the United States, 1996. Vital Health Stat 13. 1998;(139):1-119.
5. Juwarkar CS. Cleaning and sterilization of anaesthesia equipment. Indian J Anaesth. 2013;57(5):541-50.
6. Miner NA, Ross C. Clinical evaluation of ColdSpor, a glutaraldehyde-phenolic disinfectant. Respir Care. 1991;36:104-9.
7. Rutala DR, Rutala WA, Weber DJ, Thomann CA. Infection risks associated with spirometry. Infect Control Hosp Epidemiol. 1991;12:89-92.
8. Rutala WA, Weber DJ. Disinfection and sterilization in health care facilities: what clinicians need to know. Clin Infect Dis. 2004;39:702-9.

WEBSITES

1. http://www.cdc.gov/handhygiene/CDC. Guideline for hand Hygeine in Health-Care Setting. Last accessed Oct., 2024.
2. https://www.usciences.edu/safety/bimanual/decon.htm. Decontamination, Sterilization, and Disinfection. Last accessed Oct., 2024.
3. https://explorable.com/Semmelweis-germ-theory. Semmelwis germ theory. Last accessed Oct., 2024.
4. http://www.cdc.gov/hicpac/pdf/guidelines/Disinfection_Nov_2008.pdf. Guideline for Disinfection and Sterilization in Healthcare Facilities, 2008. Last accessed Oct., 2024.
5. https://www.osha.gov/pls/oshaweb/owadisp.show_document?p_table=STANDARDS&p_id=10051. Last accessed Oct., 2024.
6. http://www.cdc.gov/hicpac/pdf/InfectControl98.pdf. Guideline for infection control in health care personnel, 1998. Published in American Journal of Infection Control (1998; 26:289-354). Last accessed Oct., 2024.

CHAPTER 13

Simulation in Anesthesia

Ramkumar Venkateswaran

INTRODUCTION

Teaching in medicine has traditionally followed the path of classroom lectures and tutorials followed by laboratory exercises or demonstrations that complement the knowledge that is imparted in the classroom. While this method works well for some areas of medical learning, it falls miserably short in many other spheres of medical education. Unlike mathematics, two plus two does not always equal four in medicine as human beings are inherently different even in health. The presence of disease complicates the picture further because of the myriad ways in which disease can manifest depending on the way in which the individual responds to the illness. The diagnosis of a medical condition is often akin to solving a mystery thriller where a detective pieces bits of carefully unearthed information together to eventually determine who committed the murder. Medical diagnosis involves several steps such as obtaining a detailed history, performing a close physical examination and obtaining relevant laboratory data. Some of these steps involve “prying” into the personal life of the patient. In addition, the examination often involves close physical contact which at times can become very personal. Taken in this perspective, bedside teaching of medical skills to a large group of medical students could pose a number of hurdles. Therein lies the strength of simulated learning.

Medical emergencies occur with varying frequency and in a totally unpredictable manner. The number of times patients with such emergencies present to a hospital could range from several times every day to may be once in the lifetime of a physician’s or surgeon’s career. Though the frequency of presentation of these possibly life-threatening emergencies varies, when such an emergency does present (often at a time and place that is least expected!), the physician’s actions need to be not only appropriate for the occasion but also perfect to the letter in execution. Now that is like telling an airline pilot that the chances of the landing gear getting stuck during landing may be only 1 in 100,000 but when it happens, he/she must land the aircraft safely with no harm to anyone on board. When such a safe outcome is not possible even in the highly efficient 6-sigma aviation industry, the scenario is understandably worse in medicine.

WHAT MAKES ANESTHESIA UNIQUELY SUITED FOR SIMULATED LEARNING?

Anesthesia stands apart from many other medical/surgical specialties in that a major part of the knowledge that one accumulates at the end of the training period and beyond is applied in everyday practice. It is also unique in the sense that it involves a series of basic psychomotor skills that can be learnt outside the environment of a hospital within the safe precincts of a simulation center. Finally (and most importantly), a large part of anesthetic practice is based on the logical application of treatment algorithms. This is especially true of anesthetic emergencies that can be easily replicated and repeated in the safe environs of a simulation center.

WHAT IS REQUIRED TO MAKE A SIMULATION EXERCISE SUCCESSFUL?

The first step in planning for a simulation exercise is to clearly enunciate the learning objectives that need to be achieved at the end of the exercise. Simulators that are needed to achieve this learning objective should then be identified. Simulators come in a wide range of capabilities. They also come in a matching wide range of cost. Simple task trainers that are used to impart training in basic psychomotor skills are essentially low-fidelity mannequins. Examples of such simple task trainers include intravenous cannulation arm, airway management trainer, urinary catheterization trainer, cardiopulmonary skills trainer, and many more.

The more realistic or high-fidelity mannequins are capable of simulating more complex medical scenarios. They are able to create normal and pathological heart and breath sounds; vary heart rate/rhythm, blood pressure and pulse oximetric saturations; alter pupillary size and reaction; and produce appropriate sounds and verbal responses when interrogated by the treating team as would happen in a real-life situation. High-fidelity simulators also include those that allow endoscopic procedures such as laryngoscopy, bronchoscopy, upper gastrointestinal scopy, colonoscopy, and surgical/gynecological laparoscopies. These high-fidelity endoscopic simulators provide realistic images and true-to-life tactile appreciation of the passage of the endoscope. They also allow one to vary the complexity of the procedure and are inclusive of steps such as creating adequate topical anesthesia before performing the procedure. Simulators with capabilities that lie between these two extremes are also available as, for instance, those meant for training in arterial access and central venous access, pediatric procedures, and labor and delivery.

While good simulators positively impact the quality of a simulation exercise, it is the imagination of the simulation instructor that delivers the final punch. Physicians and surgeons who are excellent bedside clinicians and teachers need not necessarily be good simulation instructors. An imaginative instructor who plans the unfolding of a clinical scenario in a realistic manner is likely to be very successful in the simulation environment. Good simulation instructors should have the ability to create minor modifications to the scenario as it unfolds without losing sight of the overall learning objectives. They should have a clear idea as to what they are aiming to teach and be capable of changing the simulation methodology while the group being trained is actually performing the exercise so that the teaching objective is eventually realized.

Once the simulation exercise is complete and a scenario has been called off, the debriefing that follows is often the most educative part of the entire exercise. Debriefing is an art that will be described at the end of this chapter. But before that, let us take a look at the range and capabilities of the simulators that are used in anesthesia.

AIRWAY MANAGEMENT TRAINERS

By design, this simple task trainer allows the trainer to impart to the trainee the skills of opening the airway by *head tilt-chin lift* method or the *jaw thrust* method. It also permits the trainee to insert airway adjuncts such as the oropharyngeal airway and nasopharyngeal airway for overcoming airway obstruction caused by a relatively large tongue falling onto the posterior pharyngeal wall. The adult airway management trainer has two independent lungs with a basic tracheobronchial tree **(Fig. 1)**. The mannequin also comes with an esophagus and stomach that will get distended if the trainee does not open the airway well enough. It could even simulate regurgitation and vomiting. Airway management trainers often come with an accompanying model of the larynx that helps the trainee in understanding the structures

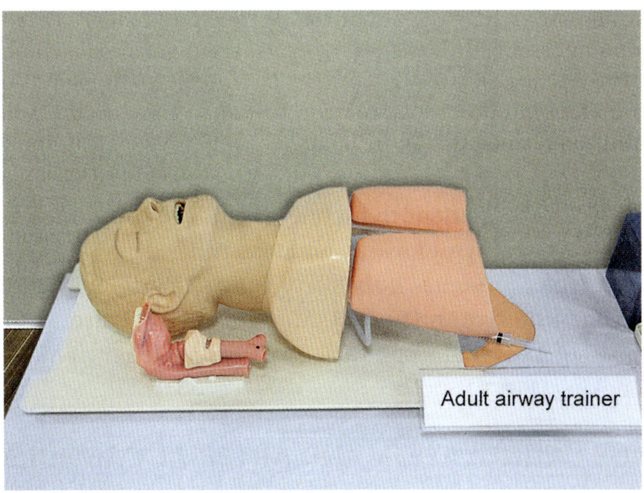

Fig. 1: Adult airway management trainer with open model of larynx.

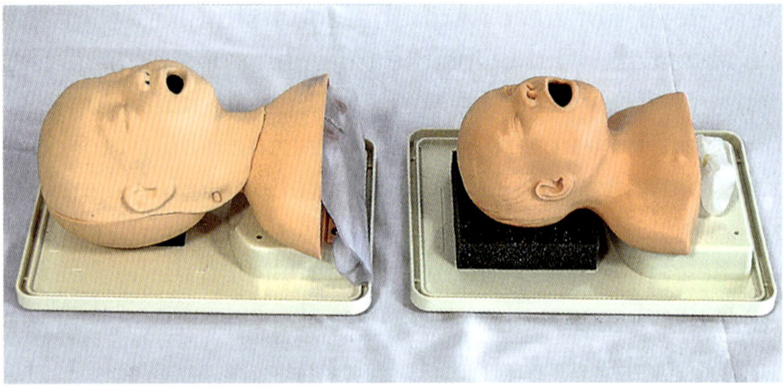

Fig. 2: Infant and neonatal intubation trainer.

that will be seen while performing a laryngoscopy and intubation. The classic airway management trainer is designed to mimic the normal airway. Mannequins especially designed to simulate a difficult airway can create limited neck movements, a large tongue, and an edentulous patient. Intubation trainers are also available that address the skills of endotracheal intubation in infants and neonates **(Fig. 2)**.

With increasing use of supraglottic airway devices in routine as well as emergency management of the airway, the need has been felt for mannequins that are especially designed to facilitate the placement of a supraglottic airway device. The classic airway management trainers that were designed prior to the widespread use of supraglottic airway devices did not have an "anatomy that was favorable" for the placement of such devices. Companies that sell supraglottic airway devices now provide special airway mannequins that have a specially designed roomy upper airway that not only facilitates the placement of the device but also gives the operator an idea of how newer-generation supraglottic airway devices provide better airway seal and near-complete protection from passive regurgitation and aspiration of gastric contents.

Advanced airway simulators have an anatomically correct tracheobronchial tree that allows the trainee to pass the fiberoptic intubation scope while the trainer describes the views obtained via a video camera that constitutes an inherent part of the setup. The cricoid stick trainer is especially designed to train the student to identify the cricothyroid membrane and perform surgical cricothyrotomy (an emergency lifesaving procedure) when faced with a *cannot intubate-cannot oxygenate* scenario during the process of endotracheal intubation **(Fig. 3)**. Mannequins are also available that can demonstrate lifesaving techniques such as the Heimlich maneuver in a victim of choking **(Fig. 4)**.

VENOUS CANNULATION AND ARTERIAL CANNULATION

Peripheral venous access is an important skill that all doctors should master, particularly the anesthesiologist. Training arms meant for peripheral

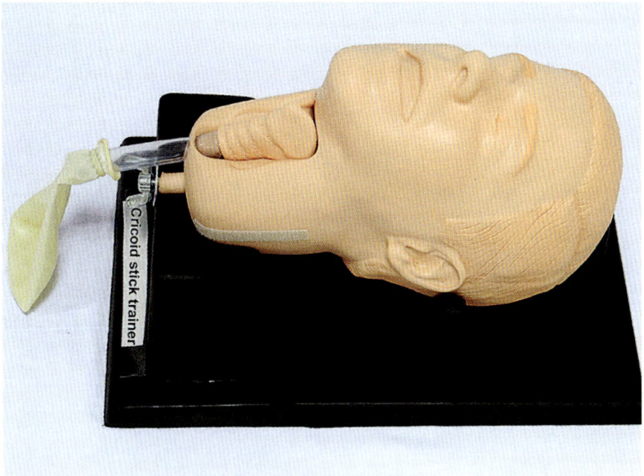

Fig. 3: Cricoid stick trainer for teaching surgical cricothyrotomy.

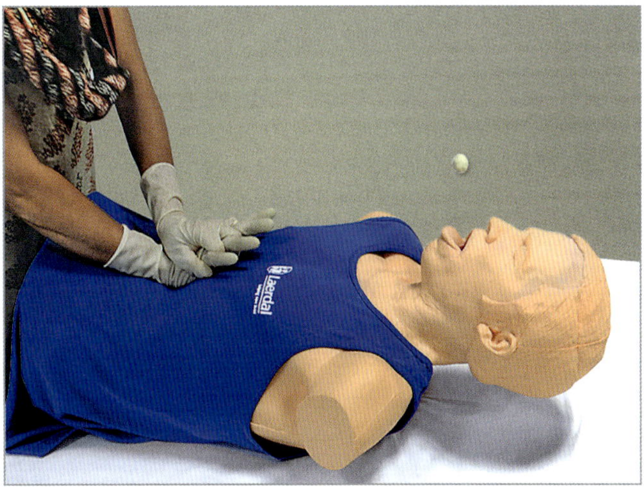

Fig. 4: Heimlich maneuver demonstrating successful dislodgment of foreign body.

venous cannulation have a realistic venous pattern that can be distended by connecting the "subcutaneous" artificial venous channels to a bag of red-colored liquid that simulates blood **(Fig. 5)**. The bag with simulated blood is hung from an intravenous stand, the height of which is adjusted so as to create the right amount of pressure within the venous network. A mildly-pressurized venous system such as this will ensure that there is a flashback of simulated blood the moment the venous puncture is made. Intravenous cannulation can be repeated several times at different sites on the same arm and the puncture points sealed off with a sealant liquid provided by the manufacturer. The skin and venous channels will eventually need to be replaced once a certain recommended number of uses have been completed.

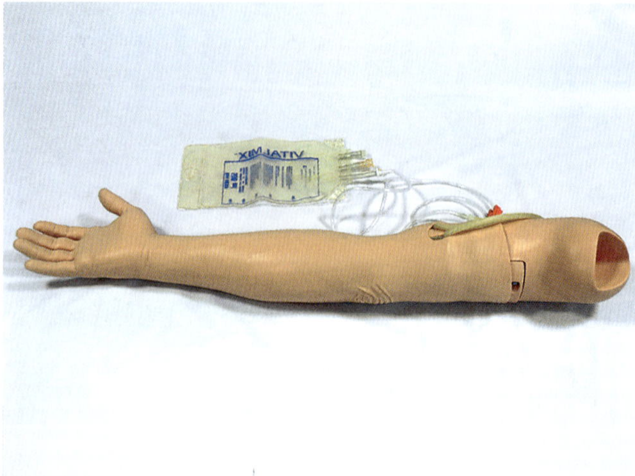

Fig. 5: Adult venous cannulation arm.

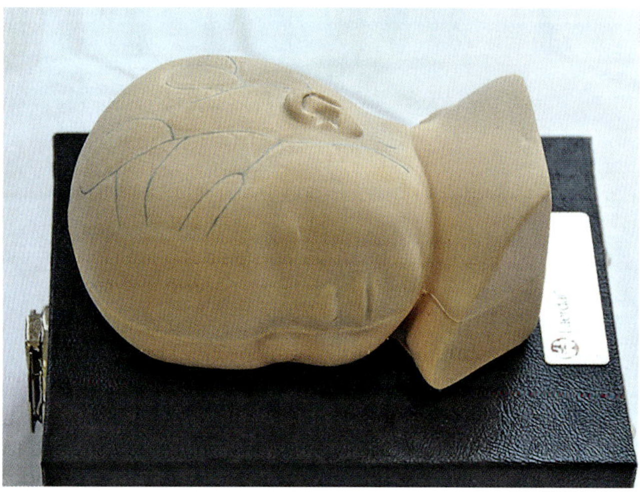

Fig. 6: Pediatric scalp vein trainer.

Venepuncture is technically more difficult in the child. Special task trainers are available for pediatric intravenous cannulation including a customized head for training in the art of scalp vein cannulation **(Fig. 6)**.

An adult arm with the radial artery pressurized to an appropriately higher level is available for training in arterial cannulation **(Fig. 7)**. These pressurized vessels can also be made to pulsate by means of a bulb that is periodically squeezed by the trainer to simulate arterial pulsations. Puncture of the artery is thus accompanied by a pulsatile flow out of the cannula.

Central Venous Cannulation

Central venous cannulation is a skill that is needed not only for the anesthesiologist but also for the emergency medicine and intensive care

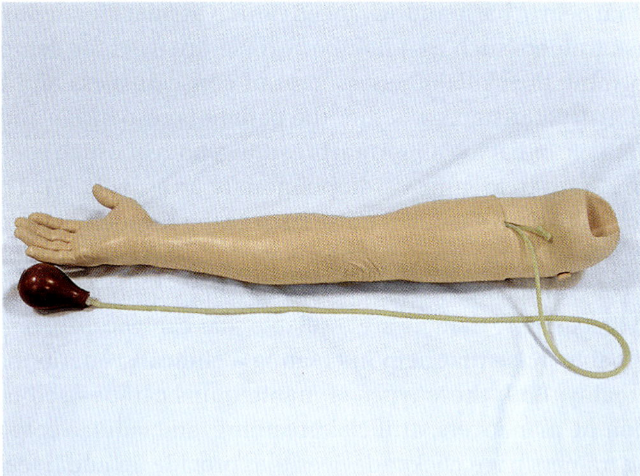

Fig. 7: Adult arterial cannulation arm.

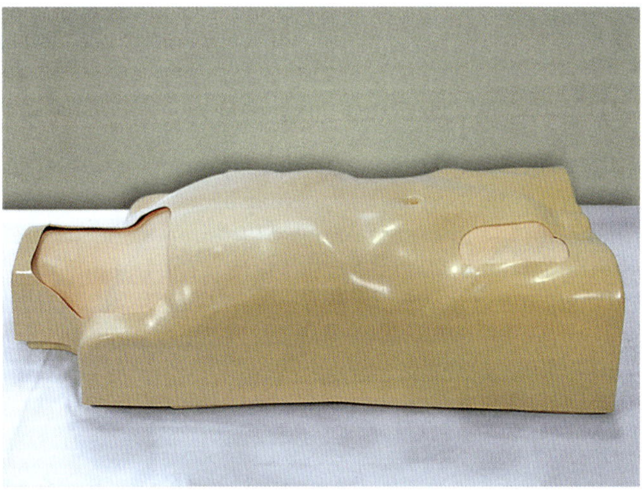

Fig. 8: Central venous cannulation mannequin.

specialist. The training unit for central venous cannulation usually allows training in the commonly used access routes such as the internal jugular, subclavian and femoral routes **(Fig. 8)**. The units have mildly-pressurized reservoirs filled with simulated blood to identify successful cannulation of the respective major central veins. Mannequins with subcutaneously implanted reservoirs for drug administration and preplaced peripherally inserted central lines are also available for training healthcare workers in the proper care of such long-term venous access routes.

LIFE SUPPORT TRAINING UNITS

If there is one area that has found maximum application in simulation-based training, it is the area of life support training. A range of simulators are available that help in basic and advanced cardiovascular life support training. Simple task trainers such as a half body torso are used for demonstrating and performing the skills of assessment of consciousness and breathing where the instructor states whether the patient is responsive and whether patient is apneic or having abnormal breathing, both of which constitute the preliminary steps to identify cardiopulmonary arrest **(Fig. 9)**. The correct location for palpation of a major pulse such as the carotid artery can also be demonstrated, with the instructor needing to vocalize whether it is present or absent (the third cardinal sign for diagnosing cardiopulmonary arrest). Advanced life support trainers are available that can vocalize, breathe, and have a palpable pulse that help in creating a clinical scenario that is even closer to reality. Both these types of mannequins can be used to perform airway opening maneuvers, artificial breathing, and cardiac compressions. These task trainers have clicker devices that provide an audio feedback (in the form of a click) when an adequate depth of cardiac compression has been achieved. Trainers are also available that come with an integral device such as a *skillmeter* that records and provides a report at the end of the session **(Fig. 10)**. The generated report will provide the rate and tidal volume of breaths delivered, as also the rate and depth of cardiac compressions given. Such reports can be used to evaluate oneself during self-evaluation programs. They can also be used as a subjective means for initial certification or subsequent recertification as the case may be.

Performance of the next step of basic life support needs the use of an automated external defibrillator (AED) **(Fig. 9)**. The training unit looks just like the one that is used in clinical practice and has voice prompts that can lead a trainee through the correct steps of defibrillation. It has a built-in timer adjusted for working around 2-minute cycles of cardiopulmonary

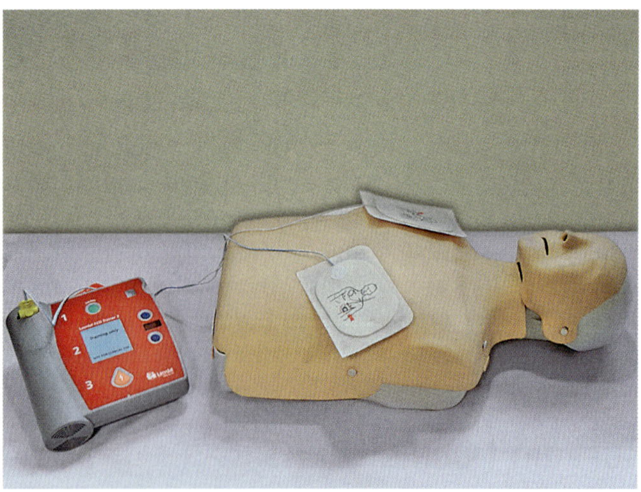

Fig. 9: Adult half torso with automated external defibrillator connected for training in basic life support.

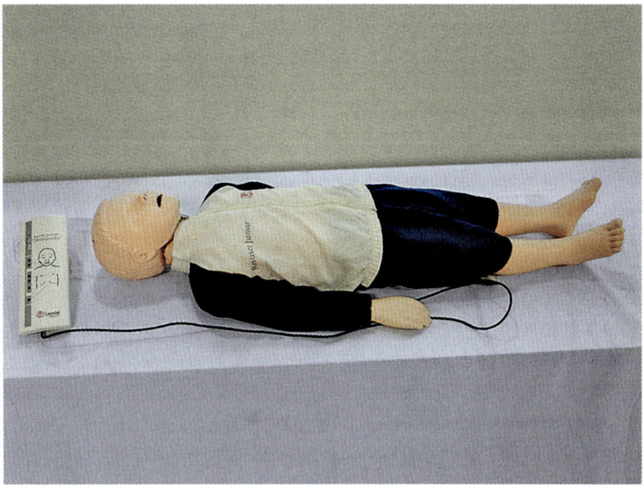

Fig. 10: Full body of older child with skillmeter.

resuscitation. Training AEDs can be programmed to simulate various combinations of outcomes such as how many shocks need to be given before a shockable rhythm converts to normal sinus rhythm, or whether a shockable rhythm deteriorates into a nonshockable one.

Advanced cardiovascular life support techniques require the trainee to be able to recognize the shockable (ventricular fibrillation and pulseless ventricular tachycardia) and nonshockable rhythms (pulseless electrical activity and asystole). Besides the pulseless arrest rhythms that are listed above, the learner should also be able to diagnose several prearrest rhythms. These include bradycardic rhythms such as first-, second-, and third-degree heart block; and tachycardic rhythms such as narrow or wide complex, regular, or irregular tachycardias. A rhythm simulator is a compact device that can be used in conjunction with a defibrillator monitor for demonstrating the multitude of rhythms that one can come across during the course of prearrest and pulseless cardiac arrest **(Fig. 11)**. The type of arrhythmia and the heart rate can be varied by the trainer as required, making the device a very exciting tool to impart training in the area of arrhythmia detection and management.

While the AED allows the trainee to master the steps of defibrillation during a pulseless arrest, a manual defibrillator needs to be used to treat the prearrest rhythms. Defibrillators that are normally in use in the hospital environment are generally brought in at this point of training so that the learner can graduate to performing electrical therapy in the form of cardioversion or defibrillation as is appropriate for the rhythm that is dialed by the instructor. The final arm of treatment of cardiopulmonary arrest (drug therapy) is also added at this stage. This could be in as simple a manner as providing labeled syringes with the trainee announcing what drug is being administered and in what dose so that the trainer can complete the loop by creating the appropriate hemodynamic changes. High-fidelity human

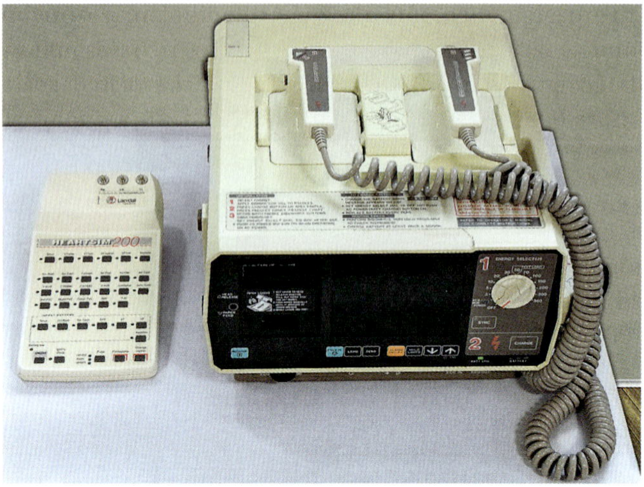

Fig. 11: Rhythm simulator and manual defibrillator.

patient simulators are also available. These have the ability to recognize the drug and dose administered through bar-coded syringes. The injected drug then produces the desired effect through a built-in computerized closed-loop program.

High-fidelity mannequins can also be used to create signs of return of spontaneous circulation (ROSC) with a desired heart rate and rhythm, blood pressure, pulse oximetry, capnography, temperature, pupillary reaction, and altered level of consciousness. Correct interpretation of these parameters helps in imparting to the trainee the steps of postresuscitation care.

SPINAL AND EPIDURAL ANESTHESIA

Mannequins for training in spinal and epidural techniques are available. These consist of a pressurized thecal sac that will allow clear fluid to drip out of the hub of a needle once the tip of the needle enters the subarachnoid space. These mannequins also allow the trainee to appreciate the tissue resistances as the needle passes through the skin, ligaments, and meningeal layers covering the spinal cord. Exposure to these procedures prior to performing them on real patients not only improves dexterity and proficiency but also minimizes failure rates and improves the confidence levels in the trainee before they are placed in the real clinical environment.

SIMULATION OF EMERGENCIES IN ANESTHESIA, TRAUMA, AND EMERGENCY MEDICINE

The highest level of training in anesthesiology (including intensive care and emergency medicine) includes the recognition and logical management of emergencies. To do this in a concise and realistic manner, we need to make use of the highest level of simulators available in the form of computerized

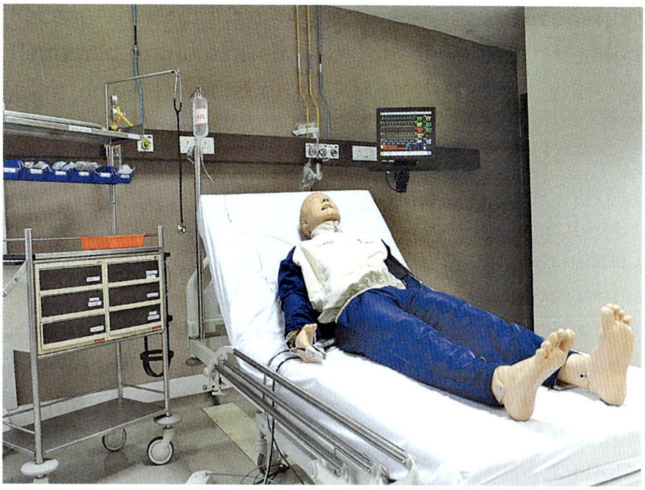

Fig. 12: High-fidelity advanced simulator (Laerdal SimMan™) placed in a simulated intensive care unit environment.

high-fidelity mannequins such as, to quote one, the *Laerdal SimMan*™ **(Fig. 12)**. These advanced simulators are capable of creating as realistic a clinical environment as possible. These mannequins, as mentioned earlier, can create a desired heart rate and rhythm, blood pressure, pulse oximetric traces, capnographic waves and numbers, temperature, pupillary reaction, and altered levels of consciousness.

The simulation instructor can thus create an exercise that normally unfolds in 10–12 minutes. The instructor presents a brief clinical history during the process of prebriefing that gives a group of trainees the necessary information to be able to zero in on the possible clinical emergencies that can present in a similar manner. The team of trainees (usually four to five in number) will then need to examine the patient and elicit the signs and symptoms that would provide a differential diagnosis to a few possible clinical emergencies that could present in a similar manner. The instructor then typically changes the vital signs in a way that would happen in real life such that the team picks up these clues and narrows down their diagnosis. As is true in medicine, diagnosis and management of emergencies should proceed in parallel. The possible scenarios that could unfold will depend on the level of expertise of the team undertaking the simulation exercise. As the correct diagnosis is made and appropriate therapeutic steps are initiated, the patient can be made to improve clinically.

The instructor therefore has the responsibility of varying the clinical parameters as the team progresses in the right direction. However, the instructor can also provide broad hints to a team that is lost in order to bring them back on track. It is always believed that no simulation exercise should end in mortality or significant morbidity as it demoralizes the entire team. A skilled instructor can ensure that the team proceeds toward the correct diagnosis without making it obvious that the team is hopelessly lost. Though one can always bring a dead mannequin back to life, simulation instructors always assist the team to end on a successful note.

Anesthetic emergencies that can be simulated in this manner include conditions as simple and straightforward as anaphylaxis to a drug or a local anesthetic systemic toxicity (LAST) to a rare yet potentially life-threatening condition such as venous air embolism or malignant hyperthermia. Advanced simulation can also be used to simulate the entire spectrum of airway emergencies such as difficult mask ventilation, difficult placement of a supraglottic airway device, difficult laryngoscopy, and difficult intubation. It could also allow a clinical scenario to deteriorate into a *cannot intubate-cannot oxygenate* scenario wherein the team will need to demonstrate their expertise in performing a surgical cricothyrotomy. As mentioned earlier, cardiopulmonary resuscitation is another area that is eminently suited for simulation. Mannequins can be used to impart the entire range of skills from basic life support to advanced cardiovascular life support (including the management of prearrest scenarios and postresuscitation care). As mentioned earlier, the presentation and management of malignant hyperthermia, an infrequent and yet potentially fatal complication of anesthesia, can be ideally learnt in the less stressful environment of a simulation center.

Another area that is eminently suited for simulated learning in the emergency environment is trauma life support. Mannequins can be used to train a team in extrication of a trauma victim from a vehicle at the scene of the accident, transporting a victim with suspected spinal injury using spinal immobilization techniques, decompressing a tension pneumothorax in the field situation, dealing with hemorrhagic shock, securing the airway in a patient with suspected cervical spine injury, and so on. The list is endless, and so are the exciting educational opportunities in medical simulation.

Last but not the least, simulation can be used to impart training in spheres of emergency medicine such as status asthmaticus, myocardial infarction, metabolic emergencies such as diabetic ketoacidosis, electrolyte and acid-base disturbances, status epilepticus and stroke. The list is by no means complete. The sky is the limit when one looks at training opportunities in emergency medicine.

DEBRIEFING

A well thought-out simulation exercise will start with well-defined learning objectives. While a number of intricate and complex scenarios can be created, it is always better to keep the learning points to a minimum of three to four. These could then be clearly demonstrated, making the simulation exercise interesting and less intimidating. Four to five learners typically constitute a team that participates in a scenario. Simulation exercises are best dealt with by a team of at least two instructors, one of whom stays with the team inside the simulation bay while the other is located in the control room so that clinical parameters can be appropriately changed as indicated.

The simulation exercise usually begins with the lead instructor providing a concise history that helps to focus the minds of the team members on the area of simulation being attempted. This step is called a *prebrief*. The lead instructor then performs a handover of the clinical scenario, often allowing the team of trainees to ask a few leading questions in case something is unclear. While the exercise typically starts with certain clinical parameters already dialed in, the trainees should be clearly instructed that they should ask for any information that they believe is crucial to the progress of the clinical scenario. The second simulation instructor usually positions himself/herself inside the simulation bay and makes notes as the scenario unfolds. These notes are immensely useful at the end of the simulation exercise when the team performs a *debrief*.

An audio and visual pickup is not only recorded but can also be transmitted real-time to a room nearby where a bigger group of learners are seated watching the scenario being played out. The lead instructor uses this audiovisual feedback to make changes in the vital signs and any other parameter as deemed necessary (as for instance ROSC, spontaneous breathing or return of varying degrees of consciousness). A typical simulation exercise runs for about 10–12 minutes when the simulation instructors decide to "call it off". This is usually done once most of the learning objectives have been realized. The team of trainees and instructors then assembles in front of the remaining group of learners who have been watching but not actively performing the simulation.

"Debrief" is a term that has been borrowed from a military exercise. It encompasses the process by which a team looks at what happened in order to first identify what the strengths of the exercise were. Though what went right is important to boost the morale of the team, what went wrong is probably more important in order to improve the future performance of a team. The simulation environment lends itself to the possibility of "making nonretractable mistakes that could adversely impact the medical outcome." Such mistakes can be corrected in a manner that does not jeopardize patient's safety had they happened in real-life situations. A typical debrief begins with the team summarizing their impressions of how the scenario unfolded. Self-realization of a mistake is often the most effective means of changing inappropriate medical decisions and actions. The positive reinforcement that such an outcome provides is beyond imagination. The instructors typically allow the team that was actively involved with the simulation exercise to interact freely with the rest of the peer group, providing gentle steering of the discussions in the right direction without dominating the discussions. A period of such peer interactions helps in identifying what went right or wrong during the simulation exercise. One of the simulation instructors then makes a presentation in the form of a learning capsule wherein the important learning objectives are spelt out as take-home messages. The entire process as described beginning with prebrief, actual playing out of the scenario and ending with discussions in the form of peer interaction, and a summary teaching capsule completes the simulation exercise.

SUMMARY

Simulation is a powerful teaching tool that can be used to impart knowledge in various spheres of learning. Anesthesia and emergency medicine are ideally suited for this method of teaching as their practice often involves a series of interlinked steps of diagnosis with appropriate management strategies. The role of simulation in acquiring venous and arterial cannulation skills, airway management skills, central neuraxial skills, and life support skills is unmatched. Simulation-based learning is invaluable in teaching the management of life-threatening clinical situations ranging from management of the anticipated and unanticipated difficult airway to the less common venous air embolism and malignant hyperthermia.

A typical simulation exercise begins with designing a module that has clearly defined learning objectives. It then goes on to the selection of proper mannequins that could impart these learning objectives and also a script that encompasses the relevant actions and verbal clues. Good simulation instructors create an environment that is realistic while at the same time not overwhelming. A well-planned and executed debriefing exercise should form the icing on the cake of learning. It should focus the attention of the learners to the objectives that were being spelt out in a comprehensive manner that leaves both the teacher and the learner satisfied. The capsule that summarizes the entire exercise should be a fitting finale to a well-orchestrated learning exercise. The author sincerely hopes that these various tenets of simulated learning have been clearly enunciated in the preceding discussions.

SUGGESTED READING

1. Gallagher CJ, Issenberg SB. Simulation in Anesthesia. Philadelphia: Elsevier; 2007.
2. Kyle RR, Murray WB. Clinical Simulation: Operations, Engineering and Management. London: Elsevier; 2008.
3. Loyd GE, Lake CL, Greenberg RB. Practical Healthcare Simulations. Philadelphia: Elsevier Mosby; 2004.
4. Rall M, Gaba DM, Dieckmann P, Eich CB. Patient simulation. In: Miller RD (Ed). Miller's Anesthesia. United States: Saunders, Elsevier Inc; 2015. pp. 167-209.e6.
5. Riley RH. Manual of Simulation in Healthcare. Oxford: Oxford University Press; 2008.

Index

Page numbers followed by *b* refer to box, *f* refer to figure, *fc* refer to flowchart, and *t* refer to table.

D

G

H

Q

R